THE CIBA COLLECTION OF MEDICAL ILLUSTRATIONS

VOLUME 3

A Compilation of Paintings on the
Normal and Pathologic Anatomy of the

DIGESTIVE SYSTEM

PART III

LIVER, BILIARY TRACT AND PANCREAS

With a Supplement on
New Aspects of Structure, Metabolism,
Diagnostic and Surgical Procedures
Associated with Certain Liver Diseases

Prepared by

FRANK H. NETTER, M.D.

Edited by

ERNST OPPENHEIMER, M.D.

Commissioned and published by

C I B A

OTHER PUBLISHED VOLUMES OF
THE CIBA COLLECTION OF MEDICAL ILLUSTRATIONS

By

FRANK H. NETTER, M.D.

NERVOUS SYSTEM

REPRODUCTIVE SYSTEM

UPPER DIGESTIVE TRACT

LOWER DIGESTIVE TRACT

ENDOCRINE SYSTEM AND
SELECTED METABOLIC DISEASES

HEART

KIDNEYS, URETERS, AND URINARY BLADDER

(See page 200 for additional information)

FIRST EDITION, 1957
SECOND EDITION (WITH SUPPLEMENT), 1964
SECOND PRINTING OF SECOND EDITION, 1967
THIRD PRINTING OF SECOND EDITION, 1972
FOURTH PRINTING OF SECOND EDITION, 1975
FIFTH PRINTING OF SECOND EDITION, 1979

ISBN 0-914168-05-3
LIBRARY OF CONGRESS CATALOG NO.: 53-2151

PRINTED IN U.S.A.

ORIGINAL PRINTING BY COLORPRESS, NEW YORK, N.Y.
COLOR ENGRAVINGS BY EMBASSY PHOTO ENGRAVING CO., INC., NEW YORK, N.Y.
OFFSET CONVERSION BY R. R. DONNELLEY & SONS COMPANY
FIFTH PRINTING OF SECOND EDITION BY R. R. DONNELLEY & SONS COMPANY

PREFACE TO THE SECOND EDITION

This book, originally printed in 1957, has been so popular that the supply was exhausted three years earlier than expected. The necessity of reprinting Digestive System, Part III, provided the opportunity to make a number of revisions and add a supplementary section on new aspects of structure, metabolism, diagnostic and surgical procedures associated with certain liver diseases. It is regrettable indeed that my predecessor and preceptor, Dr. Ernst Oppenheimer, the first editor of the CIBA COLLECTION, could not collaborate in this revision. He died on February 6, 1962 while working on Volume 4, which portrays the Endocrine System and Selected Metabolic Diseases.

It is a privilege and challenge to serve as editor of this well-known and widely read series, and I trust that our collective efforts, with those of the inimitable artist and physician, Dr. Frank H. Netter, and the various consultants, may result in the production of future volumes that will match the high standards of those now available.

In this revision the anatomical terms were made to conform, in most instances, to the *Nomina Anatomica* of 1961, as revised by the International Anatomical Nomenclature Committee and published by Excerpta Medica Foundation. For his important contribution to this phase of the revision, we are greatly indebted to one of America's leading authorities in this field, Dr. Edward A. Boyden, Emeritus Professor of Anatomy at the University of Minnesota and Research Professor at the University of Washington, Seattle. We express our gratitude for his meticulous assistance, given in such an expeditious, enthusiastic and friendly manner. The extent to which recommended changes in terminology could be incorporated was dictated by expediency; although it was highly desirable to have a revised book as up to date as possible, we wished to keep to a minimum the inevitable increase in cost (see Glossary, page 199).

An additional feature of this new book is the addition of a two-part supplement (see page 167). The first part deals with recent developments in our understanding of the liver's structure and metabolism (normal and disturbed) and with pertinent tests for detecting the latter. This material was prepared by Dr. Frank H. Netter in collaboration with Dr. Hans Popper, the internationally recognized authority on the liver, who served so admirably as chief consultant for the original book and for this revision. The second part includes several plates demonstrating the value of surgical procedures in metastatic disease of the liver. These were prepared by Dr. Netter in collaboration with Dr. George T. Pack. The supplement is available separately to original purchasers who wish to add this new information to their copies of Digestive System, Part III.

It is a pleasure to acknowledge the painstaking editorial assistance of Miss Louise Stemmle, Mrs. Janet A. Yonkman and Mrs. L. A. Oppenheim, and the excellent work of Wallace and Anne Clark as literary consultants. To Mr. A. W. Custer of CIBA and to the staffs of Embassy Photo Engraving Co., Inc., and Colorpress, I express my gratitude for their fine cooperation.

FREDRICK F. YONKMAN, M.D., PH.D.

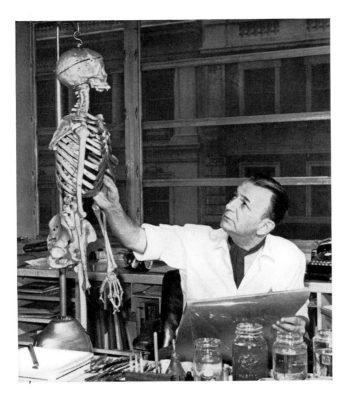

THE ARTIST

Many readers of the CIBA COLLECTION have expressed a desire to know more about Dr. Netter. In response to these requests this summary of Dr. Netter's career has been prepared.

Frank Henry Netter, born in 1906 in Brooklyn, New York, received his M.D. degree from New York University in 1931. To help pay his way through medical school and internship at Bellevue, he worked as a commercial artist and as an illustrator of medical books and articles for his professors and other physicians, perfecting his natural talent by studying at the National Academy of Design and attending courses at the Art Students' League.

In 1933 Dr. Netter entered the private practice of surgery in New York City. But it was the depth of the depression, and the recently married physician continued to accept art assignments to supplement his income. Soon he was spending more and more time at the drawing board and finally, realizing that his career lay in medical illustration, he decided to give up practicing and become a full-time artist.

Soon, Dr. Netter was receiving requests to develop many unusual projects. One of the most arduous of these was building the "transparent woman" for the San Francisco Golden Gate Exposition. This 7-foot-high transparent figure depicted the menstrual process, the development and birth of a baby, and the physical and sexual development of a woman, while a synchronized voice told the story of the female endocrine system. Dr. Netter labored on this project night and day for 7 months. Another interesting assignment involved a series of paintings of incidents in the life of a physician. Among others, the pictures showed a medical student sitting up the night before the osteology examination, studying away to the point of exhaustion; an emergency ward; an ambulance call; a class reunion; and a night call made by a country doctor.

During World War II, Dr. Netter was an officer in the Army, stationed first at the Army Institute of Pathology, later at the Surgeon General's Office, in charge of graphic training aids for the Medical Department. Numerous manuals were produced under his direction, among them first aid for combat troops, roentgenology for technicians, sanitation in the field, and survival in the tropics.

After the war, Dr. Netter began work on several major projects for CIBA Pharmaceutical Company, culminating in THE CIBA COLLECTION OF MEDICAL ILLUSTRATIONS. To date, five volumes have been published and work is in progress on the sixth, dealing with the urinary tract.

Dr. Netter goes about planning and executing his illustrations in a very exacting way. First comes the study, unquestionably the most important and most difficult part of the entire undertaking. No drawing is ever started until Dr. Netter has acquired a complete understanding of the subject matter, either through reading or by consultation with leading authorities in the field. Often he visits hospitals to observe clinical cases, pathologic or surgical specimens, or operative procedures. Sometimes an original dissection is necessary.

When all his questions have been answered and the problem is thoroughly understood, Dr. Netter makes a pencil sketch on a tissue or tracing pad. Always, the subject must be visualized from the standpoint of the physician; is it to be viewed from above or below, from the side, the rear, or the front? What area is to be covered, the entire body or just certain segments? What plane provides the clearest understanding? In some pictures two, three, or four planes of dissection may be necessary.

When the sketch is at last satisfactory, Dr. Netter transfers it to a piece of illustration board for the finished drawing. This is done by blocking the back of the picture with a soft pencil, taping the tissue down on the board with Scotch tape, then going over the lines with a hard pencil. Over the years, our physician-artist has used many media to finish his illustrations, but now he works almost exclusively in transparent water colors mixed with white paint.

In spite of the tremendously productive life Dr. Netter has led, he has been able to enjoy his family, first in a handsome country home in East Norwich, Long Island, and, after the five children had grown up, in a penthouse overlooking the East River in Manhattan.

ALFRED W. CUSTER

CONTRIBUTORS AND CONSULTANTS

The artist, editor and publishers express their appreciation
to the following authorities for their generous collaboration:

OSCAR BODANSKY, M.D.

Chief, Department of Biochemistry and Attending Clinical Biochemist, Memorial Hospital; Head, Research Biochemistry Section, Sloan-Kettering Institute for Cancer Research; Professor of Biochemistry, Sloan-Kettering Division, Cornell University Medical College, New York, N. Y.

EUGENE CLIFFTON, M.D.

Associate Professor of Clinical Surgery, Cornell University Medical College; Attending Staff, New York Hospital, Memorial Hospital, Bellevue Hospital and James Ewing Hospital; Associate, Sloan-Kettering Institute for Cancer Research, New York, N. Y.

DONALD D. KOZOLL, M.D.

Associate Attending Surgeon, Cook County Hospital; Associate Attending Surgeon, Northwestern University Medical School; Research Associate, The Hektoen Institute for Medical Research, Cook County Hospital, Chicago, Ill.; Chief of Surgical Service, St. Francis Hospital, Evanston, Ill.

HANS POPPER, M.D.

Director, Department of Pathology, Cook County Hospital; Scientific Director, The Hektoen Institute for Medical Research; Professor of Pathology, Northwestern University Medical School, Chicago, Ill. (Present Affiliations: Director, Department of Pathology, Mount Sinai Hospital; Professor of Pathology, College of Physicians and Surgeons, Columbia University, New York, N. Y.)

VICTOR M. SBOROV, M.D.

Assistant Clinical Professor of Medicine, University of California Medical School; Consultant, Gastro-enterology, Letterman Army Hospital, San Francisco, Cal. (Formerly, Chief, Department of Hepatic and Metabolic Diseases, Army Medical Service Graduate School, Washington, D. C.)

GEORGE T. PACK, M.D.

Attending Surgeon Emeritus, Memorial Cancer Center; Attending Surgeon, Pack Medical Group, New York, N. Y.

INTRODUCTION

If the number of newly published books on a particular medical topic may be taken as an index of the interest of the profession in such a subject, the diseases of the liver would assuredly belong among those that stand at the top of the list. No less than eight monographs on the liver and/or biliary system have appeared in the last 2 years. This interest was also evidenced in some 7,000 answers CIBA received several years ago to an inquiry as to which subject would be the most desirable for the continuation of the series of medical illustrations, which had been published and distributed over a period of 10 years. At that time the central nervous system held first position, and the anatomy and pathology of the liver was a very close second. Yielding to the wishes of a small majority, Volume 1 of THE CIBA COLLECTION OF MEDICAL ILLUSTRATIONS, *Nervous System,* was published in 1953. With the present book we hope to satisfy the demands for an illustrated description of the anatomy and pathology of the liver and biliary system. In line with the over-all plan of this series of books, according to which a separate volume is devoted to each single system of the human organism (see Preface to Volume 1), the bile-producing and -transporting organs, as well as the pancreas, must be included in Volume 3, designed to cover the digestive system.

To offer the illustrations of the whole digestive system in one single book, as we did with the reproductive system, was considered too impractical. Such an attempt would not only have meant a long wait for a new volume after the appearance of the last one but would also have resulted in a rather voluminous, unwieldy and very expensive tome. The separation of Volume 3 into three parts — each a single book containing from 140 to 160 plates, issued at intervals as short as possible — seemed, therefore, to serve best the needs which this COLLECTION aims to meet. These books concern respectively, the upper digestive tract, the lower digestive tract, and the liver, biliary tract, and pancreas.

The attempt to interpret the anatomic and pathologic features of the liver with pencil and colors and in words, the number of which is restricted to fit into a relatively small space, led to numerous problems for the artist and consultants alike, problems of a kind we had not met in previous volumes. New concepts of the liver structure, new insights into the pathogenesis of hepatic and pancreatic diseases, a new store of knowledge of the functional aspects and their relation to morphologic characteristics and refined discriminations of disease entities necessitated novel forms and approaches to the lucid two-dimensional visual demonstrations, more frequent conferences between the artist and the consultants, more time-consuming studies and more elaborate planning for the presentation of all the important macro- and microscopic, etiologic, functional, etc., facets. Obviously, in spite of the amazing progress medical science has made in this field, numerous problems remain unsolved and not a few differences of opinion await reconciliation by future investigation. In the pictorial part of the present book, controversial issues or claims not definitely established have been circumvented, except in very few instances, in which, however, a question mark indicates a point of view which is not generally accepted. In the text, the problematic aspects or uncertainties of specific allegations are clearly specified as such. Nevertheless, we are aware of the strong possibility that a variety of statements or opinions, though carefully formulated by our consultants, may have to be revised in a relatively short time. Such revisions had to be incorporated in pictures and texts that were prepared during the early period of work on this book (1954). In any event, we have made every possible effort to have this book reflect in all respects the status of the knowledge in this field at the time of going to press (September, 1956).

One of our great problems has been, again as in Volume 2 which deals with the reproductive system, to remain within the limits of the not easily definable "desirable details", with which the scope of this COLLECTION was described in a programmatic fashion at the time the series was launched with Volume 1. Completeness is not our aim, and it seems appropriate to emphasize again that this Part III of Volume 3 (as is the case with the previously published books) does not, and has not been set up to, substitute for a single one of the many available textbooks and monographs on the subject of diseases of the liver, extrahepatic biliary tract and pancreas. As stated before: "The principle that guided each of our consultants, as well as the artist, was to supplement rather than to replace the standard reference works in the physician's library".

With regard to the liver and biliary tract, we have attempted to cover the essential anatomic, functional and pathologic features as completely as possible within the scope indicated above. The same holds true for the pancreas, except for its endocrine aspects, which have been reserved for that volume of this COLLECTION which will illustrate the endocrine system (hypophysis, thyroid, parathyroid, adrenal, thymus and pancreas). A clear-cut separation of the exocrine and endocrine functions of a single gland is, of course, not possible; therefore, some overlapping of features shown in this book and in the future volume will be inevitable. The islet cell tumors, in spite of their obvious involvement with the hormonal situation of the organism, had to be considered together with the pictures on the tumors of the pancreas.

Some readers will observe a few inconsistencies with respect to the terminology for certain anatomic entities. We have adopted wherever possible the terms in common usage, which are in almost every case identical with the descriptive names employed in the standard American textbooks on anatomy. On the other hand, we have also tried to reconcile classical terms with the results of recent investigations and with the new list of *Nomina Anatomica* as revised by the International Nomenclature Committee and accepted by the Sixth International Congress of Anatomists (Paris, July, 1955). The *Nomina Anatomica,* which is supposed the take the place of the first international nomenclature, the famous *Basle Nomina Anatomica* (BNA) of 1895, lists the anatomic terms only in the Latin language. These had to be Anglicized to harmonize with the English names used in this book. While the preparation of this book was in progress, two meetings were held, in which specially appointed committees discussed the nomenclature of liver structures and diseases. We have also accepted terms suggested by these committees whenever they were unanimously recommended by the committee members and when they seemed to clarify the corresponding anatomic, pathologic or pathogenetic situations.

We have adhered to the principle that remarks about therapy remain restricted to a minimum of general directions.

Diagnostic procedures and functional aspects are presented in one special section (XVI). A great number of page references have been entered in the texts to all the plates, and the index has been prepared in such a fashion as to make easy the correlation between the various sections of the book. Italics within the texts that discuss the paintings have been used not exactly to emphasize certain words or terms but to make the reader aware of the fact that he will find such particular items illustrated in the accompanying plate. This technique was innovated in Volume 2, and it seems to have fulfilled the purpose for which it was contrived.

One new feature has been added. Following the suggestion of a few reviewers of Volume 2, we have prepared a record of those books and journal articles that have served as sources for the artist, as references for the editorial work and which the consultants suggested as particularly suitable to support the commentaries and discussions of the most recent developments. Needless to say, this bibliography is not at all complete, because its only aim is to offer a convenience for those interested in checking or following up certain novel or complex points or affairs which, owing to the restricted space available for the text, had to be discussed in a very concise manner. Should the list of special references prove insufficient in any particular case, it will not be difficult to find more bibliographic details in one of the monographs cited under "General References".

No words can express our gratitude to each one of our consultants. The unwavering spirit they exhibited during the many months of work on this book and their unselfish devotion to the task of making this collection of illustrations a didactically valuable contribution have been for us a provocative and at times even reviving stimulus. As indicated above, we faced problems and encountered obstacles, particularly with the series of pictures on the liver, which were not anticipated and were not encountered with the topics in the previous volumes. Dr. Popper's contagious enthusiasm, his indefatigable work power and his stimulating and persuasive personality produced a continuous challenge for us to tackle the difficulties and to surmount the many technical hindrances. Admittedly, when we approached him requesting his co-operation, because of his well-known contributions in the field, we did not realize what we were asking of him, particularly with regard to the time necessary for the many conferences, the assemblage of material, the discussions of the sketches and final paintings and, last but not least, the preparation of the texts. We profited from his knowledge, from his collection of slides and reprints, from his life-long study of the liver and its diseases and from his experience as a teacher and as author of a major monograph, *The Liver; Its Structure and Function,* a book which, fortunately for the present COLLECTION, was just moving toward its final stage when the work on the pictures for this book started. Dr. Popper's remarkable flair for the best didactic arrangement and most instructive demonstration was of indispensable help in presenting the infinite complexities of the structure and pathology of the liver.

In preparing the plates concerned with the structural pattern of the liver (Section XV, Plates 7 to 10), it was our great privilege to have the co-operation of Dr. Hans Elias, whose prudent counseling, skillful suggestions and constructive criticism were of inestimable value. For the solution of a multitude of problems in connection with the effort to demonstrate biochemical features two-dimensionally, we received most effective assistance and guidance from Dr. J. de la Huerga, who graciously and generously gave us not only much of his time but many original ideas and practical answers to some harassing questions. In other parts of the book, we have been supported by the competent advice, discriminating comments and clarifying information received from Dr. J. E. Healey, Jr. (Section XV, Plates 8 and 11),

Dr. J. Higginson (Section XVII, Plate 16) and Dr. A. Grossman (pages 119 and 120). Dr. F. Schaffner showed and maintained a constant and most active interest during all the months we worked on Sections XV, XVI and XVII, liberally giving us his time and experience. Dr. R. M. Terry guided the preparation of Plate 11 in Section XVI. Most sincerely we gratefully acknowledge the help we obtained from all these gentlemen.

For his meticulous attention and expert counsel in the preparation of three decidedly clinical topics concerned with the liver, we render our hearty thanks to Dr. Victor M. Sborov, who also has dedicated many years to the better understanding of hepatic diseases. We regret that our association with him was only relatively short and sincerely hope that future volumes will give us the opportunity to benefit from his sound scientific and practical guidance.

For the presentation of the facial expressions and other features in hepatic coma (Section XVII, Plate 11) we had the good fortune to be able to study leisurely a motion picture made by Dr. W. H. J. Summerskill (Thorndike Memorial Hospital, Harvard University) of patients under the care and observation of Dr. S. Sherlock (Department of Medicine, University of London, England). The film, with Dr. Summerskill's permission, was obligingly placed at our disposal by Dr. L. W. White (Stanford Medical School).

Working on the section on Diseases of the Biliary Tract, we enjoyed the co-operation of Dr. Donald D. Kozoll, a former co-worker of Dr. Popper. Though an exhausting surgical practice laid claim to his time, we found him on all occasions willing to help, to advise us with the selection of topics and to suggest improvements after seeing the preliminary sketches or final pictures.

The pictures on the various aspects of the pancreas (with the exception of Plates 23 and 24 in Section XV) were prepared under the counselorship of Dr. Oscar Bodansky and Dr. Eugene E. Cliffton, both well-known experts in the field. The resumption of former friendly relations with Dr. Bodansky, as a result of our requesting and receiving his co-operation, gave us a personal and heartfelt satisfaction. His experience as a teacher and author in the field of biochemistry, his insistence on simple and instructive presentations, avoiding all speculative concepts, we consider to have been a great advantage for the book. Similarly, we hold in esteem Dr. Cliffton's sincerity in guiding us through the complexities of pancreatic diseases and their anatomic background. The pictures, as they appear in Sections XV and XIX, owe their reliability to his convincing judgment of the things we know and the things of which we are ignorant. Always willing to give his valuable time to this enterprise, he went out of his way in order to provide the necessary material. In his careful selection of the microscopic pictures to be shown, Dr. Cliffton was effectively supported by Dr. J. Ellis. To both gentlemen we extend our sincere thanks.

Without the tireless co-operation of Mrs. L. A. Oppenheim, serving as assistant to the editor and as organizational center between artist, consultants, editor, engraver and printer, the development of Part III of Volume 3 would have taken far longer than it did. The unstinting efforts and gracious devotion to the project of Mrs. Vera Stetson, assistant to Dr. Netter, contributed much to ease and expedite the task. To them and to Mrs. Hans Popper, who voluntarily took over the work of providing us, with the least delay, the 96 typescripts of her husband's descriptive texts, go our special thanks. We acknowledge finally the concurrent efforts of Messrs. A. W. Custer and Felton Davis, Jr., of the CIBA staff, Wallace and Anne Clark of Buttzville, N. J., as literary consultants, and the staffs of Embassy Photo Engraving Co., Inc., and Colorpress.

FRANK H. NETTER, M.D.
E. OPPENHEIMER, M.D.

CONTENTS OF COMPLETE VOLUME 3
DIGESTIVE SYSTEM

CONTENTS

Section XV

NORMAL ANATOMY OF THE LIVER, BILIARY TRACT AND PANCREAS

by

FRANK H. NETTER, M.D.

in collaboration with

EUGENE E. CLIFFTON, M.D.
Plates 25-29

HANS POPPER, M.D.
Plates 1-24

DEVELOPMENT OF LIVER AND ITS VENOUS SYSTEM

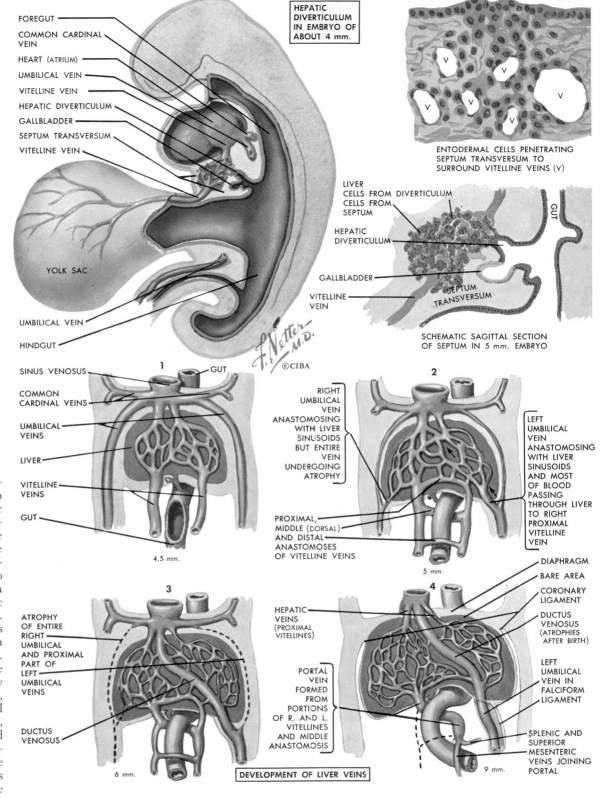

FOREGUT
COMMON CARDINAL VEIN
HEART (ATRIUM)
UMBILICAL VEIN
VITELLINE VEIN
HEPATIC DIVERTICULUM
GALLBLADDER
SEPTUM TRANSVERSUM
VITELLINE VEIN

HEPATIC DIVERTICULUM IN EMBRYO OF ABOUT 4 mm.

ENTODERMAL CELLS PENETRATING SEPTUM TRANSVERSUM TO SURROUND VITELLINE VEINS (V)

LIVER CELLS FROM DIVERTICULUM
CELLS FROM SEPTUM
HEPATIC DIVERTICULUM
GALLBLADDER
VITELLINE VEIN
SEPTUM TRANSVERSUM
GUT

SCHEMATIC SAGITTAL SECTION OF SEPTUM IN 5 mm. EMBRYO

YOLK SAC
UMBILICAL VEIN
HINDGUT

SINUS VENOSUS
COMMON CARDINAL VEINS
UMBILICAL VEINS
LIVER
VITELLINE VEINS
GUT

1   GUT
4.5 mm.

RIGHT UMBILICAL VEIN ANASTOMOSING WITH LIVER SINUSOIDS BUT ENTIRE VEIN UNDERGOING ATROPHY

LEFT UMBILICAL VEIN ANASTOMOSING WITH LIVER SINUSOIDS AND MOST OF BLOOD PASSING THROUGH LIVER TO RIGHT PROXIMAL VITELLINE VEIN

PROXIMAL, MIDDLE (DORSAL) AND DISTAL ANASTOMOSES OF VITELLINE VEINS

2
5 mm.

ATROPHY OF ENTIRE RIGHT UMBILICAL AND PROXIMAL PART OF LEFT UMBILICAL VEINS

DUCTUS VENOSUS

3
6 mm.

HEPATIC VEINS (PROXIMAL VITELLINES)

PORTAL VEIN FORMED FROM PORTIONS OF R. AND L. VITELLINES AND MIDDLE ANASTOMOSIS

DIAPHRAGM
BARE AREA
CORONARY LIGAMENT
DUCTUS VENOSUS (ATROPHIES AFTER BIRTH)
LEFT UMBILICAL VEIN IN FALCIFORM LIGAMENT
SPLENIC AND SUPERIOR MESENTERIC VEINS JOINING PORTAL

4
9 mm.

DEVELOPMENT OF LIVER VEINS

The liver develops from a *diverticulum,* which sprouts in close relation to the *vitelline veins* from the ventral floor of the endodermal foregut at a site corresponding to the future duodenum. The caudal portion of the diverticulum is the origin of the cystic duct and the *gallbladder.* The cephalic portion gives rise to cellular masses (liver cell plates) which extend ventrally into the splanchnic mesoderm of the *septum transversum.* Part of this septum subsequently becomes the diaphragm, while the lower portion serves as the site for the liver formation. A vascular plexus branching out from the *vitelline veins* becomes surrounded by the irregularly arranged endodermal cells, which, apparently as a result of mutual stimulation, differentiate into liver cells, originally in several-cell-thick plates and later in one-cell-thick plates. The endothelial cells of the plexus become the Kupffer cells. The mesenchyma provides also the connective tissue for the capsule and the portal tracts. At 10-mm. embryonal length, bile capillaries, as well as intrahepatic bile ducts and cholangioles (ductules), develop between the liver cell plates. It is still debated whether the epithelium of the bile ductules (cholangioles), and possibly also of the bile ducts, derives from the liver cells or vice versa. The former would explain the formation of ductules from liver cells during regeneration (see page 63). However, on the evidence afforded by electron microscopy, most authorities believe that, in postnatal life, transformations between bile ductular cells and liver cells do not exist. The intrahepatic bile ducts connect subsequently with the extrahepatic bile ducts, which have arisen from the cephalic part of the hepatic diverticulum.

At an early stage the pairs of vitelline veins split into a *plexus within the liver.* Uniting again behind the plexus into pairs, these veins enter into the *sinus venosus* of the heart together with the *umbilical veins* coming from the placenta and with the common *cardinal veins.* Subsequently, the pairs of vitelline veins form more anastomoses, the proximal of them lying within the liver, a middle and distal one extending dorsally and ventrally around the duodenum, so that a vascular ring is formed, part of which obliterates together with the distal portion of the vitelline veins. The remaining venous trunk becomes the *portal vein* which is joined by the *superior mesenteric* and *splenic veins.* The proximal portions of the paired vitelline veins between the plexus and the sinus venosus become the *hepatic veins,* the left of which atrophies, so that the blood of the left half of the liver drains into the right vitelline vein. The

umbilical veins also find contact with the hepatic sinusoidal system, but later the entire right umbilical vein and the part of the left vein proximal to the anastomosis with the hepatic sinusoids atrophy and disappear. For a time the venous blood from the placenta passes through the liver to the right vitelline vein. Eventually, a large venous trunk develops and separates from the hepatic sinusoids to carry as *ductus venosus* pure oxygenated blood directly to the heart. At this stage approximately half of the blood from the umbilical vein goes through the ductus, while the rest passes through the liver.

As the liver protrudes into the abdominal cavity, it remains in contact with the *diaphragm* in the *bare area,* and the attachment to the septum transversum becomes the *coronary ligament.* At the same time the umbilical vein becomes included as ligamentum teres into the *falciform ligament.*

PRENATAL AND POSTNATAL CIRCULATION

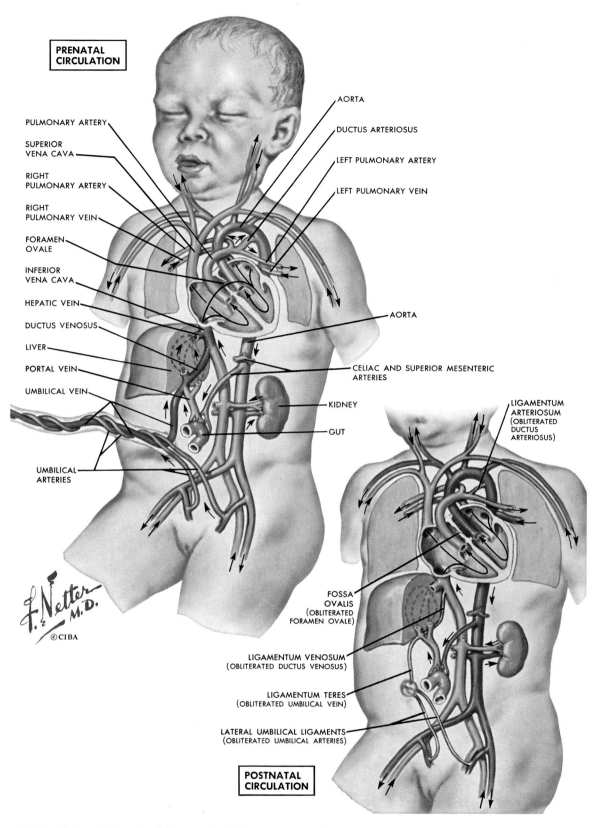

PRENATAL CIRCULATION

PULMONARY ARTERY

SUPERIOR VENA CAVA

RIGHT PULMONARY ARTERY

RIGHT PULMONARY VEIN

FORAMEN OVALE

INFERIOR VENA CAVA

HEPATIC VEIN

DUCTUS VENOSUS

LIVER

PORTAL VEIN

UMBILICAL VEIN

UMBILICAL ARTERIES

AORTA

DUCTUS ARTERIOSUS

LEFT PULMONARY ARTERY

LEFT PULMONARY VEIN

AORTA

CELIAC AND SUPERIOR MESENTERIC ARTERIES

KIDNEY

GUT

LIGAMENTUM ARTERIOSUM (OBLITERATED DUCTUS ARTERIOSUS)

FOSSA OVALIS (OBLITERATED FORAMEN OVALE)

LIGAMENTUM VENOSUM (OBLITERATED DUCTUS VENOSUS)

LIGAMENTUM TERES (OBLITERATED UMBILICAL VEIN)

LATERAL UMBILICAL LIGAMENTS (OBLITERATED UMBILICAL ARTERIES)

POSTNATAL CIRCULATION

In intra-uterine life the fetus receives blood carrying oxygen and nutrients obtained by contact with maternal blood in the placenta (see THE CIBA COLLECTION, Volume 2, page 219) through the *umbilical vein,* except during the very early stages when the yolk sac and vitelline veins still function. While the vitelline veins are transformed (see page 2), the umbilical vein makes contact with the vitelline plexus and anastomoses, so that at one stage (6 mm. fetal length) the entire blood of the umbilical vein passes through the primitive hepatic sinusoids. At the same time, the right umbilical vein branch and the proximal portion of the left undergo atrophy, while subsequently the enlarged distal part of the left umbilical vein courses diagonally through the liver in a channel, the *ductus venosus,* which has formed by rearrangement of early hepatic sinusoids. With the growing of the liver lobes, the ductus venosus comes to lie outside the liver and joins the *inferior vena cava,* in which the small amount of venous blood from the caudal portions of the fetus is mixed with the oxygen-rich blood coming through the ductus venosus. This blood stream, entering the right atrium, hits the interatrial membrane (septum secundum) and is directed through the *foramen ovale* into the *left atrium* and thus keeps the foramen open. In the left atrium the blood mixes with some nonoxygenated blood from the pulmonary veins and passes through the left ventricle into the ascending aorta, whence mixed blood provides the coronary artery, the head, neck and upper extremities. A small amount of blood from the vena cava inferior, together with the inflow from the superior caval vein, is diverted into the *pulmonary artery* supplying the lungs. The greater part of the blood from this artery, however, owing to a higher resistance in the pulmonary vascular tree, is shunted through the *ductus arteriosus* directly into the *aorta descendens,* where it joins

the blood ejected from the left ventricle. This vascular organization is instrumental in providing heart and brain with blood of higher oxygen content than is supplied to other organs less sensitive to hypoxia.

After birth, probably because of a sphincter mechanism at its origin, the ductus venosus closes rapidly. It soon obliterates and is transformed into the *ligamentum venosum,* which connects with the *ligamentum teres* or round ligament, where the obliterated umbilical vein is lodged. The ligamentum teres (see page 5) terminates at the umbilicus, from where also the lateral umbilical ligaments containing the remnants of the *umbilical arteries* spread in the interior abdominal wall to the *internal iliac arteries.* With the closure of the ductus venosus, oxygenated blood no longer reaches the inferior vena cava, and the liver from birth on is provided with oxygen-rich blood only via the hepatic artery. With the first respiration

the resistance in the pulmonary vascular tree diminishes, and this pressure change leads immediately to a shift of the current in the right and left atria, so that no blood passes through the foramen ovale, which, within 1 year, closes in 75 per cent of newborns by fusion of the atrial septa. A *fossa ovalis* indicates in adult life the former site of the foramen. In the remaining 25 per cent of infants, an oblique communication persists between right and left atria, which may be demonstrated anatomically but only in rare cases is patent enough to have functional consequences. The ductus arteriosus closes with breathing, apparently by muscular contraction, and is obliterated gradually by intima proliferation, so that within 3 months after birth only a connective tissue band, the *ligamentum arteriosum,* remains, except in a small percentage of cases wherein a patent ductus arteriosus persists.

Labels on illustration: LATERAL BODY LINE — TRANSPYLORIC LINE — DIAPHRAGM — LIVER COVERED BY DIAPHRAGM, PLEURA AND LUNG (DULLNESS) — LIVER COVERED BY DIAPHRAGM AND PLEURA (FLATNESS) — LIVER COVERED BY DIAPHRAGM (FLATNESS, INTESTINAL RESONANCE) — GALLBLADDER — LIVER — DIAPHRAGM — LIVER COVERED BY DIAPHRAGM, PLEURA AND LUNG (DULLNESS) — LIVER COVERED BY DIAPHRAGM AND PLEURA (FLATNESS) — LIVER COVERED BY DIAPHRAGM, PLEURA AND LUNG (DULLNESS) — LIVER COVERED BY DIAPHRAGM AND PLEURA (FLATNESS) — GALLBLADDER — LIVER EDGE — DIAPHRAGM

F. Netter M.D. ©CIBA

TOPOGRAPHY OF LIVER

The liver (hepar) is located in the upper part of the abdomen, where it occupies the right hypochondriac and the greater part of the epigastric regions. With its left lobe the liver extends, to an individually varying degree, into the left hypochondrium. The liver, the largest organ of the body, weighs from 1400 to 1600 gm. in the adult male and from 1200 to 1400 in the female. In normal, healthy individuals, the *liver margin* extending below the thoracic cage is smooth and offers little resistance to the palpating finger. Downward displacement, enlargement, hardening and formation of nodes or cysts produce impressive palpatory findings. Using percussion, one must consider that the lungs overlay the upper portion of the liver and that the liver, in turn, overlaps the intestines and the stomach.

The *projections of the liver on the body surface* have acquired added significance in the performance of liver biopsy (see page 46). The projections vary, depending upon the position of the individual as well as the body build, especially upon the configuration of the thorax. The liver lies close to the diaphragm, and the upper pole of the right lobe projects as far as the level of the fourth intercostal space or the fifth rib, the highest point being 1 cm. below the nipple near the lateral body line. The upper limit of the left lobe projects to the upper border of the sixth rib. Here, the left tip of the liver is close to the diaphragm.

The *ribs cover* the greater part of the liver's right lobe, while a small part of its anterior surface is in contact with the anterior abdominal wall. In the *erect position* the liver extends downward to the tenth or eleventh rib in the right midaxillary line. Here, the pleura projects downward to the tenth rib, and the lung to the eighth. The inferior margin of the liver crosses the costal arch in the

right lateral body line approximately on the level of the pylorus (*transpyloric line*). In the epigastrium the liver is not covered by the thoracic cage and extends about three fingers below the base of the xyphoid process in the midline. Part of the left lobe is covered again by the rib cage.

Over the upper third of the right half of the liver, percussion gives a *dull zone,* since here diaphragm, pleura and lung overlay the liver. Over the middle portion *flat percussion* is obtained. Over the lowest third of the liver, usually a flat percussion tone is heard, except that sometimes *intestinal resonance* is produced by gas-filled intestinal loops. The border between dullness and flatness moves on respiration and is altered by enlargement or displacement of the liver, and also by conditions within the thoracic cage which change the percussion qualities of the thoracic organs.

In the *horizontal position* the projection of the liver moves a little upward, and the area of flatness appears slightly enlarged. The portion of the flat sound, best percussed in the horizontal position, permits information about the size of the organ.

The projections of the liver are altered in some diseases of the liver, such as tumor infiltration, cirrhosis or syphilitic hepar lobatum, and are changed by displacements of the organ or more often by thoracic conditions pushing the liver downward. Subphrenic abscesses, depending upon location and size, also displace the liver downward. Ascites, excessive dilation of the colon or abdominal tumors may push the liver upward, and retroperitoneal tumors may move it forward. Kyphoscoliosis or a barrel shape of the chest alters the position of the liver. Sometimes the liver is abnormally movable (hepatoptosis), causing peculiar palpatory findings.

RIGHT TRIANGULAR LIGAMENT
DIAPHRAGM (PULLED UP)
CORONARY LIGAMENT
LEFT TRIANGULAR LIGAMENT
APPENDIX FIBROSA
LEFT LOBE
RIGHT LOBE
ANTERIOR ASPECT
FALCIFORM LIGAMENT
INFERIOR MARGIN
LIGAMENTUM TERES (TO UMBILICUS)
COSTAL IMPRESSION
GALLBLADDER

LEFT TRIANGULAR LIGAMENT
INFERIOR VENA CAVA
CORONARY LIGAMENT
SUPRARENAL IMPRESSION
RIGHT TRIANGULAR LIGAMENT
LEFT HEPATIC VEIN
BARE AREA
APPENDIX FIBROSA
ESOPHAGEAL IMPRESSION
CAUDATE LOBE
GASTRIC IMPRESSION
FISSURE FOR LIGAMENTUM VENOSUM
PAPILLARY PROCESS
CAUDATE PROCESS
PORTAL VEIN
HEPATIC ARTERY
COMMON BILE DUCT
COMMON HEPATIC DUCT
FISSURE FOR LIGAMENTUM TERES
PORTA HEPATIS
QUADRATE LOBE
FALCIFORM LIGAMENT
LIGAMENTUM TERES
CYSTIC DUCT
DUODENAL IMPRESSION
GALLBLADDER
RENAL IMPRESSION
COLIC IMPRESSION
VISCERAL SURFACE
LEFT TRIANGULAR LIGAMENT

LEFT TRIANGULAR LIGAMENT
FALCIFORM LIGAMENT
CORONARY LIGAMENT
RIGHT TRIANGULAR LIGAMENT
BARE AREA
FISSURE FOR LIGAMENTUM VENOSUM
SULCUS FOR INFERIOR VENA CAVA
POSTERIOR ASPECT

INF. VENA CAVA
UPPER RECESS
BARE AREA
ADRENAL GLAND
LESSER SAC
STOMACH
KIDNEY
EPIPLOIC FORAMEN (WINSLOW)
COLON
LIVER BED

f. Netter M.D.
©CIBA

SURFACES AND BED OF LIVER

The liver is a large, wedge-shaped organ molded to the underside of the diaphragm and resting upon the upper abdominal viscera. Its *diaphragmatic surface* is divided into a *pars superior* (which includes the *cardiac impression*), a *pars anterior* (which extends beyond the diaphragm onto the anterior abdominal wall), a *pars dextra* and a *pars posterior* (attached to the diaphragm by the coronary ligament). The border between the *anterior aspect* and *visceral surface* is the *inferior margin*. Its consistency, sharpness of edge, smoothness of surface and movement upon respiration provide clinical information. On laparotomy the inferior margin and the anterior aspect are first exposed. Otherwise, the hepatic surfaces are not separated by distinct margins.

The liver is covered by peritoneum, except for the gallbladder bed, the porta, adjacent parts surrounding the inferior vena cava, and a space to the right of the vena cava inferior called *"bare area"*, which is in contact with the right *suprarenal gland* (*suprarenal impression*) and the right kidney (*renal impression*). The peritoneal duplications, which extend from the anterior abdominal wall and from the diaphragm to the organ, form the ligaments of the liver, which, formerly, were thought to maintain the liver in its position but probably add little to its fixation. It is now held that the liver is kept in place by intra-abdominal pressure. The diaphragmatic peritoneal duplication is the *coronary ligament,* the upper layer of which is exposed if the liver is pulled away from the diaphragm. The right free lateral margin of the coronary ligament forms the *right triangular ligament,* whereas the *left triangular ligament* surrounds and merges with the left tip of the liver, the *appendix fibrosa hepatis.* Over the right lobe the space between the upper and lower layers of the coronary ligament is filled with areolar connective tissue. Below the insertion of

the lower layer of the right coronary ligament, the hepatorenal space extends behind the liver.

From the middle portion of the coronary ligament originates another peritoneal duplication, the *falciform ligament,* which extends from the liver to the anterior abdominal wall between the diaphragm and the umbilicus. Its insertion on the liver divides the organ into a *right* and *left lobe.* As the falciform ligament crosses the inferior margin of the liver it releases the *ligamentum teres* (the obliterated left umbilical vein) which then enters a fissure on the visceral surface of the liver. Inferiorly, this *fissure of the ligamentum teres* separates the *quadrate lobe* from the left lobe of the liver. Beyond the *porta hepatis* it is continued superiorly as the *fissure of the ligamentum venosum* (the obliterated *ductus venosus* of the fetus). The two fissures may be regarded as the left limb of an H-shaped pattern characteristic of the vis-

ceral surface of the liver. The right limb is formed by the *gallbladder fossa* and the *sulcus of the vena cava inferior.* The horizontal limb is marked by the *porta hepatis,* which contains the *common hepatic duct, hepatic artery, portal vein,* lymphatics and nerves. The *quadrate lobe,* between the gallbladder and the fissure for the umbilical vein, is in contact with the pylorus and the first portion of the duodenum (*duodenal impression*). Above the porta hepatis lies the *caudate lobe* between the fissure for the ligamentum venosum and the vena cava inferior, its caudal projection being the *papillary process.* The visceral surface of the liver reveals further impressions of the organs with which it is in contact: the *impressions for the colon and the right kidney,* and on the left lobe the *impressions for the esophagus and the stomach.* The superior surface is related to the diaphragm and forms the domes of the liver.

LIGAMENTUM TERES
QUADRATE LOBE
GALLBLADDER
EPIPLOIC FORAMEN (WINSLOW)
RIGHT LOBE
LEFT LOBE
CAUDATE LOBE SEEN THROUGH LESSER OMENTUM
WINDOW CUT IN LESSER OMENTUM
HEPATIC ARTERY
COMMON BILE DUCT
PORTAL VEIN
LESSER OMENTUM
KIDNEY (UNDER PERITONEUM)
STOMACH
COLON
COLON
GREATER OMENTUM

LESSER OMENTUM, VARIATIONS IN FORM OF LIVER

VARIATIONS IN FORM OF LIVER

VERY SMALL LEFT LOBE; COSTAL DEPRESSIONS

COMPLETE ATROPHY OF LEFT LOBE (LEFT PORTAL VEIN COMPRESSION)

TRANSVERSE "SADDLELIKE" LIVER; RELATIVELY LARGE LEFT LOBE

"TONGUELIKE" PROCESS OF RIGHT LOBE

VERY DEEP RENAL IMPRESSION AND "CORSET CONSTRICTION"

"DIAPHRAGMATIC" GROOVES

If the *inferior margin* of the liver is lifted, the *lesser omentum* is exposed. It represents a peritoneal fold, which extends from the first portion of the duodenum and the lesser curvature of the stomach and the diaphragm to the liver, where it is inserted in the fissure of the ligamentum venosum and continues to the porta hepatis. Here, the layers are separated to accommodate the structures running to and from the liver. On the free right edge of the lesser omentum is the thick hepatoduodenal ligament. It is the anterior boundary of the *epiploic foramen (of Winslow)*, which is the entrance to the lesser abdominal cavity (*omental bursa*). The posterior wall of this cavity is formed by the *vena cava inferior* and the *caudate lobe* of the liver (see page 5). Near the right margin of the lesser omentum is found the *common bile duct* dividing into the cystic and common hepatic ducts. To its left lies the *hepatic artery* and behind both, the *portal vein*. The nerves (see page 21) and the lymph vessels (see page 20) of the liver accompany these structures. The porta hepatis is limited inferiorly by the *quadrate* and superiorly by the caudate lobes (see page 5). On the right side of the porta, the right and left hepatic ducts branch from the main hepatic duct and enter the liver. To the left of them, the hepatic artery (see page 14) enters the liver behind the ductal branches. The forking portal vein enters posteriorly to the ductal and arterial ramifications.

The shape of the liver varies. Its great regenerative ability, as well as the plasticity of the liver tissue, permits a wide variety of forms, which depend in part upon pressure exerted by neighboring organs and in part upon disease processes or vascular alteration. A *greatly reduced left lobe* is compensated by enlargement of the right lobe, which reveals very conspicuous and deep costal impressions. Occasionally, the *left lobe* is completely *atrophic,* with a wrinkled and thickened capsule and, microscopically, an impressive approximation of the portal triads (see page 11), with hardly any lobular parenchyma between them. In the majority of such cases, vascular aberrations have been demonstrated, such as partial obstruction of the lumen of the left branch of the portal vein by a dilated left hepatic duct or obstruction of the bile ducts. Therefore, this lesion has been considered the effect of a local nutritional deficiency, especially since the nutritional condition of the left lobe is poor to begin with (see page 18). In other instances, associated with a transverse position of the organ, the left lobe is unduly large. Formerly, disfiguration of the liver frequently resulted from laced corsets or from tight belts or straps. Such physical forces may flatten and elongate the liver from above downward, with reduction of the superior diaphragmatic surface and sometimes with peculiar *tonguelike extension of the right lobe*. In other instances the *"corset liver"* is displaced, and the *renal impression* is exaggerated. Clinical symptoms (dyspepsia, cholelithiasis, chlorosis) were ascribed to the "corset liver", but it is questionable whether the "corset liver" actually leads to clinical manifestations other than peculiar findings on palpation. Indentations on the liver are normally produced by the ribs, by diaphragmatic insertions and by the costal arch. In kyphoscoliosis the rib insertions may become very prominent. Parallel sagittal furrows on the hepatic convexity have been designated as *"diaphragmatic"* grooves. Functionally, none of the described variations are today considered significant.

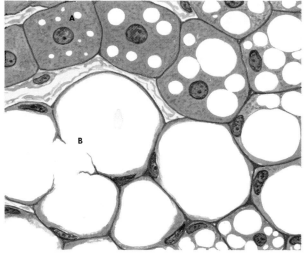

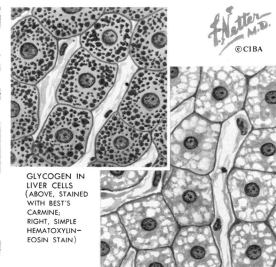

©CIBA

CELLULAR ELEMENTS OF LIVER

The cytoplasm of the liver cells normally contains various defined particles which can be visualized by histochemical methods. Neutral fat is found in the form of droplets, which are stainable in frozen sections by fat stains but appear as vacuoles after dissolution of fat with the routine use of organic solvents in histologic techniques. The *fat droplets* or *vacuoles* in normal liver cells do not exceed 4 microns in diameter. They usually line up on the free margin of the cells, like pearls on a string. Enlargement of the fat droplets (fatty metamorphosis) is the result of an imbalance between the transport of fat to the liver from either the intestine or the peripheral tissue, or of its formation or catabolism within the liver (see pages 36 and 37). The imbalance in fat metabolism may be focal, then mainly resulting from disturbances of the blood flow and local anoxia, or may be diffuse (fatty liver, see pages 78 and 79). The fat droplets become gradually larger until the liver cell cytoplasm is studded with droplets of different size, the nucleus, however, still remaining in the center. Subsequently, the droplets merge, and one large drop pushes the nucleus to the side. Eventually, large drops of neighboring liver cells coalesce to form *fatty cysts,* in which the fat is actually extracellular and the remnants of several cells line the cyst (Hartroft).

Glycogen, if previously precipitated by alcohol fixation, appears as fine red particles in the cytoplasm after staining with Best's carmine or periodic acid and Schiff's reagent. In routinely fixed and stained sections or biopsy specimens of normal liver, the dissolved glycogen produces a fine, granulated and vacuolated appearance of the cytoplasm. In severe disease of any kind, particularly in the agonal period, the glycogen content becomes markedly reduced, so that, as a rule, in autopsy specimens little glycogen is found. The glycogen content of the liver cells is an index of its functional status.

The cytoplasm of the normal cell contains many fine basophilic granules which, in *methyl green-pyronine stain,* appear distinctly red, as does the nucleolus. This reaction is caused by pentose nucleic acids in contrast to the desoxypentose nucleic acids in the nuclear chromatin, which stain green. The specificity of the reactions requires further confirmation. The cytoplasmic pentose nucleic acids have been tentatively asso-

LIVER CELLS WITH VARIOUS DEGREES OF FAT ACCUMULATION RANGING FROM FINE DROPLETS (A) TO LARGE FATTY CYSTS (B)

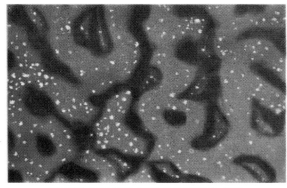

GLYCOGEN IN LIVER CELLS (ABOVE, STAINED WITH BEST'S CARMINE; RIGHT, SIMPLE HEMATOXYLIN-EOSIN STAIN)

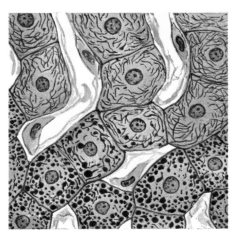

LIVER CELLS WITH METHYL GREEN–PYRONINE STAIN (METHYL GREEN STAINS CHROMATIN; PYRONINE STAINS CYTOPLASMIC INCLUSIONS AND NUCLEOLUS)

VITAMIN A IN LIVER CELLS AND KUPFFER CELLS MADE VISIBLE BY FLUORESCENCE

VARIFORM MITOCHONDRIA IN LIVER CELLS REFLECTING DIFFERENCES IN FUNCTIONAL ACTIVITY (JANUS GREEN STAIN)

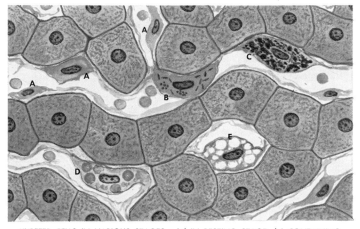

KUPFFER CELLS IN VARIOUS STAGES — (A) IN RESTING STAGE; (B) CONTAINING BACTERIA; (C) CONTAINING PIGMENT; (D) CONTAINING RED BLOOD CELLS; (E) CONTAINING FAT DROPLETS

ciated with protein formation, and attention has been drawn to a parallelism between cytoplasmic basophilia of the liver cells and their capacity to form proteins (see page 39).

Under the fluorescence microscope in frozen section, a rapidly fading yellow-green fluorescence of the cytoplasm of liver and Kupffer cells is caused by *vitamin A,* mainly in fat droplets. This fluorescence decreases in malnutrition and increases upon the administration of large amounts of vitamin A. In liver damage the distribution of the fluorescence, never quite regular, becomes patchy and more irregular.

The *mitochondria,* stainable, for instance, supravitally with Janus green, are globular elements in the center and rod-shaped in the periphery of the lobule. They contain, as in all cells of the body, phospholipids and a great number of enzyme systems.

The *Kupffer cells* assume in the normal liver a great variety of shapes as an expression of different activity stages, primarily phagocytosis. Some of them are flat, similar to endothelial cells in other organs. Others have a large cytoplasm which contains various inclusions, not necessarily an expression of disease. Some of these inclusions are *bacteria,* other *pigments, red cells* or *fat droplets.* In various abnormal conditions, the phagocytosis is exaggerated. Vital microscopic studies have demonstrated that a resting endothelial-like Kupffer cell can very rapidly change into the large phagocytic type.

Electron microscopy (see page 170) and histochemistry (see page 174) have given new meaning to many structures formerly observed only by conventional microscopy. Moreover, numerous previously known features become understandable when they are interpreted in the light of knowledge of their shape, which is made possible by higher magnification.

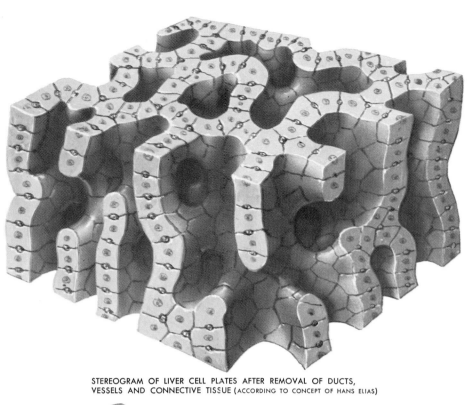

STEREOGRAM OF LIVER CELL PLATES AFTER REMOVAL OF DUCTS,
VESSELS AND CONNECTIVE TISSUE (ACCORDING TO CONCEPT OF HANS ELIAS)

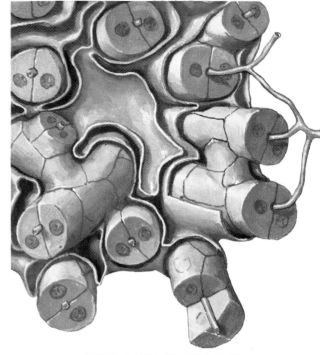

FORMER CONCEPT OF LIVER STRUCTURE
AS COMPOSED OF CELL CORDS

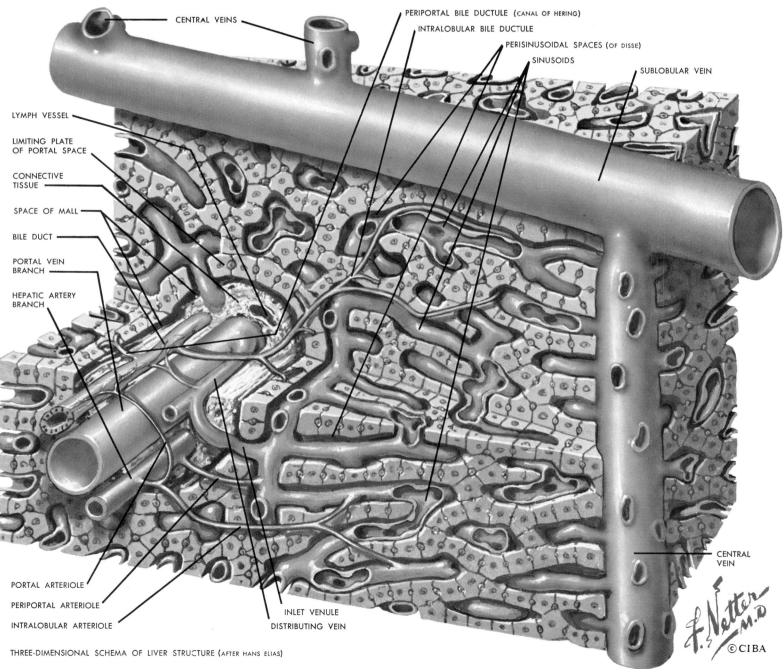

CENTRAL VEINS

PERIPORTAL BILE DUCTULE (CANAL OF HERING)

INTRALOBULAR BILE DUCTULE

PERISINUSOIDAL SPACES (OF DISSE)

SINUSOIDS

SUBLOBULAR VEIN

LYMPH VESSEL

LIMITING PLATE
OF PORTAL SPACE

CONNECTIVE
TISSUE

SPACE OF MALL

BILE DUCT

PORTAL VEIN
BRANCH

HEPATIC ARTERY
BRANCH

CENTRAL
VEIN

PORTAL ARTERIOLE

PERIPORTAL ARTERIOLE

INTRALOBULAR ARTERIOLE

INLET VENULE

DISTRIBUTING VEIN

THREE-DIMENSIONAL SCHEMA OF LIVER STRUCTURE (AFTER HANS ELIAS)

INTRAHEPATIC STRUCTURES

Liver Cell Arrangement

Until about 10 years ago the standard description of the pattern of liver cell arrangement, as presented in all textbooks, was considered securely settled. The *liver cells* were supposed to *form cords* composed of opposing cells which were thought to be arranged on either equal or alternate levels. The cords were believed to extend in an irregular and frequently crooked and angular fashion from the periphery of the lobule (marked by the final termination of the portal vein) toward the central vein. The existence of many communications between the various cords as well as their corresponding central bile capillaries had to be assumed. These cords were considered to be surrounded by the blood sinusoids, which thus were visualized as forming a large pool around the liver cell cords. Few investigators dissented from the "cord theory", but it is noteworthy that Hering, for instance, almost 100 years ago described the rabbit liver as a continuous cellular mass traversed by blood capillaries. A few years ago Elias challenged the cord theory as a result of his attempt to draw, in three-dimensional fashion, the structure of the liver, especially as it would appear to a microorganism inhabiting the liver. He was unable to conceive a pattern which would agree with the standard description of the liver and at the same time conform to its appearance in histologic slides and, especially, to three-dimensional reconstructions made from serial sections. He realized that if the cord theory were correct the histologic sections, representing a cross section through the liver, should exhibit, mainly, isolated groups of two cells with a central bile capillary between them. Where the cords were cut obliquely, short rows of cells up to three and four in number should be seen. Actual observation, however, generally revealed long rows of cells almost always in single file, with an occasional multicellular group. The appreciation of these pictures, well known to any anatomist or pathologist, prompted Elias to statistical geometrical analysis, as well as to reconstructions of liver tissue. As a result of his studies, he proposed the "plate theory" of the liver to replace the cord structure. This theory, to a great extent in agreement with the old concept of Hering, is also well reconciled

with the histologic picture and with various older reconstruction models, such as the classical model of Braus in which the presence of both plates and cords is demonstrated.

The plate concept assumes that the mature *liver* is *composed of plates,* as a rule one cell thick, which are only in part straight but otherwise curved in all directions. An irregular wallwork comes into existence because of the many holes of various sizes in the plates and because of their fusing together at different angles. Where one or several plates meet each other, the cut surface seen in the histologic sections reveals an aggregation of several cells, whereas otherwise the liver cells appear usually as long rows of cells in single file, with the nucleus being in the center of the plate and a relatively great part of its border a free surface. As Elias has also shown, the size and the shape of the individual liver cell vary greatly, depending upon the cell's position in the plate. Cells near a hole in the plate are usually small, whereas cells at the corners, where several cells meet, are large. He even proposes that the frequently encountered presence of two or more nuclei in the normal liver cell depends upon the location of the cell and the thus determined size. Two-cell-thick plates are hardly ever found in the normal mature human liver. They are the rule in lower vertebrates and also in the embryologic stage of the human liver, when gradual maturation from several-cell-thick plates to the one-cell-thick plate takes place (see page 2). Similarly, in adult regeneration (see page 63) or tumor development (see page 113), two-and-more-cell-thick plates are found. The two-cell-thick plate is far less efficient than the one-cell-thick plate, because in the former the free surface in contact with the blood stream is much smaller, probably only one eleventh of its entire surface, whereas in the one-cell-thick plate one fifth of the total surface is free. Moreover, the one-cell-thick plate responds to stretching or other mechanical stresses with far less distortion than does the two-cell-thick plate and is, therefore, considerably more stable.

The liver is thus conceived to consist not of a communicating system of cords surrounded by the sinusoids but rather of an irregular, almost spongelike wallwork or cellular mass tunneled by a communicating system of cavities, to which the term lacunae has been applied. The diameter of these lacunae in man is usually considerably wider than the diameter of a single liver cell, and only occasionally is it found narrow and cylindrical, as seen in rodents and the horse. The lacunae contain the blood capillaries of the liver, the sinusoids, which have a basement membrane. Their endothelial lining is formed by the Kupffer cells. The sinusoids differ from capillaries elsewhere in the body by the specific functions of the Kupffer cells which may increase in size (see page 7), as well as owing to the greater permeability of their membrane for macromolecular substances, especially proteins. This faculty permits a better exchange of large-sized compounds between liver cell and sinusoid. The exchange of nutrients and waste products of large or small size takes place through a very narrow tissue space separating the sinusoidal wall from the liver cell plates. This interstice, known as Disse's space (see also page 20), has been wrongly assumed to act as a lymphatic space. It is probably correct that the tissue fluid in this

space may be drained by the lymphatic vessels, especially when the blood capillaries or the liver cells are unable to absorb excessive amounts of fluid accumulating in it, which happens in hepatic edema caused, *e.g.,* by abnormal permeability of the sinusoidal wall. The tissue spaces in the human liver, examined after death, may thus appear unduly wide because of the edema developing in the agonal period (see pages 20 and 63). In vivo, therefore, under normal circumstances this space, traversed by a few reticular fibers, is hardly existent, and, therefore, the lacunae between the liver cell plates are almost entirely filled out by the blood in the sinusoids. The arrangement of the cells in the liver cell plates is fairly fixed; however, the shape and direction of the plates are highly variable and depend, *e.g.,* on the blood stream which creates the lobular arrangement (see Plate 8, page 10).

The mass of epithelial cells is traversed by two mesenchymal tracts arranged around the vessels and bile ducts of the liver; one is the portal tract and around it the cellular mass assumes a characteristic arrangement. A *limiting plate envelops the portal tract* along its entire circumference and is perforated only where *bile ductules* enter the portal tract and where blood vessels enter the parenchyma. This plate is actually continuous throughout the liver. It is separated from the connective tissue of the portal tract by a very narrow tissue space, the *space of Mall* (see also page 20). From the limiting plate the other plates seem to originate at almost a right angle. The cells of the limiting plate differ cytologically from the cells of the other plates by being flatter, by being markedly basophilic because of the presence of pentose nucleic acids (see page 7) and by being relatively poor in glycogen. Moreover, these cells are more prone to regeneration, not only because of their cytologic characteristics but also because of their close relation to the portal vein, since portal vein blood, so important in stimulating regeneration, reaches them in highest concentration. Actually, nodular regeneration (see pages 63, 66 and 67) has a tendency to develop especially from the vicinity of the portal tract, and some evidence also exists that primary hepatic cancer (see page 112) seems to start in this location. If in the course of inflammatory and degenerative processes around the portal tracts the limiting plate is destroyed, healing is completed when a new limiting plate is formed. Around the other mesenchymal tract, the *central canal,* the liver cell plates end abruptly (frequently perpendicularly). An enveloping plate is encountered only around larger hepatic veins.

Connective Tissue, Vascular and Ductal Relations (Plate 8, page 10)

The liver is covered by thick collagenous fibers and membranes, intermixed with elastic elements which form the *perivascular fibrous capsule* (Glisson's: see Plate 8, page 10). In the deeper layers it carries a lymphatic network, a few blood vessels and nerves. Though representing vestigial structures, some aberrant bile ducts (see page 22) also found in the capsule are of clinical interest because of their becoming markedly dilated in extrahepatic biliary obstruction, so as to cause
(Continued on page 10)

(Continued from page 9)

biliary peritonitis by their spontaneous rupture or as a result of liver biopsy. Over the normally smooth capsular convexity, fibrin may be deposited when plasma proteins ooze from the liver, *e.g.*, in passive congestion, and the surface may become uneven when such exudates become organized and form adhesions or firm white ridges, sometimes to the extent that a white platelike icing over the liver can be seen ("Zuckergussleber" or chronic perihepatitis). At the porta hepatis (and also in the neighborhood of the inferior vena cava), Glisson's capsule thickens and extends along the branches of the *portal vein, hepatic artery* and *bile duct*. Bundles of collagenous fibers accompany the vessels and ducts continuously to their terminal ramifications where, markedly reduced in size and number, they emerge with the adventitia of veins and arteries forming the interlobular spaces or *portal tracts* or *triads*. In these the branches of the portal vein terminate, while the smallest arterioles and ductules, and probably also lymphatics (see page 20), still frequently covered with a thin sheet of connective tissue, extend into the lobular parenchyma. Similarly, connective tissue strands escort in an attenuating fashion the hepatic veins* from their entry into the vena cava inferior via *sublobular veins* to their origins, the *central veins*. The covering, however, is much thinner than that of the structures of the portal triads, which explains the easy yielding of the hepatic vein system to compression (see page 69). The ramifications of the hepatic vein and of the portal vein cross each other in an interdigitated fashion and, under normal circumstances, never touch each other; nowhere do they run parallel. The distance between the ramifications of both systems is said to be equal throughout the liver, to guarantee equal blood flow, but moderate variations (about ½ mm.) of the distance are found.

Liver Lobules (Plate 8)

Between the ramifications of portal triads and hepatic vein tributaries, the hepatic parenchyma, arranged as described above (cell plates) (see Plate 9, page 11), is surrounded by a fine framework of argentaffin reticulum fibers, which, in turn, are anchored at the portal triads and the hepatic vein branches and appear to have an arrangement concentric toward the central vein. This characteristic pattern has led to the description of the classical *liver lobule* which is said to be arranged *around the central vein*. The portal triads mark the peripheral meeting place of several lobules. Otherwise, the periphery of the human liver lobule is not sharply defined. Under abnormal cir-

*In the upper schematic picture of Plate 8, which makes no effort to represent the exact pattern of the vascular arrangement (see page 13), only one hepatic vein has been drawn. Usually, three hepatic veins converge but enter the inferior caval vein separately.

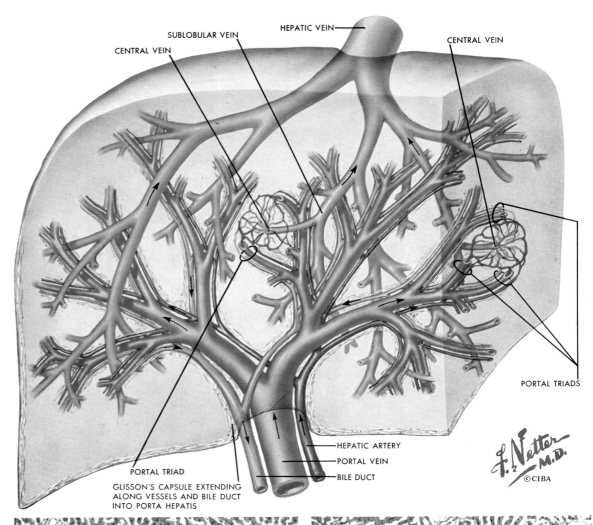

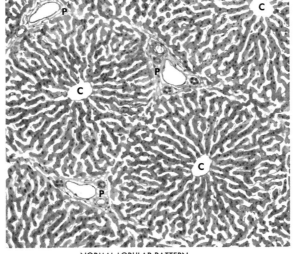

NORMAL LOBULAR PATTERN
P—PORTAL TRIAD; **C**—CENTRAL VEIN

REVERSAL OF LOBULAR PATTERN DUE
TO ELEVATED PRESSURE IN HEPATIC VEIN

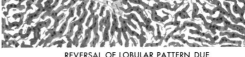

Upper picture after John E. Healey, Jr.

cumstances, however, as, *e.g.*, in perilobular fibrosis, a sharper lobular delineation may be found in man. The lack of demarcation led some observers to assume a portal unit, in the center of which the draining bile ducts of the portal tracts were thought to be located — a concept which emphasizes the glandular function of the liver. According to modern concepts (Elias), the direction of the liver cell plates depends upon the blood flow and the blood-pressure gradient from the portal vein and hepatic artery branches to the hepatic vein tributaries. In the embryo no lobular architecture is recognized in the absence of a significant gradient. It develops after birth, when the liver cell plates become convergent. Alteration of the normal blood-pressure gradient, for instance by stasis in passive congestion, alters the positions of the liver cell plates which then appear almost to converge toward the portal triad, producing the pic-

ture of a *reversal of the lobular architecture* in subacute passive congestion. The liver lobules, thus, are not fixed structures but depend upon the blood flow and the vascular ramifications.

Intrahepatic Biliary System
(Plate 9, page 11)

The biliary passages start with the fine bile capillaries or canaliculi between the hepatic cells (see Plate 9). It has been claimed that their finest ramifications extend into the cytoplasm of the parenchymal cells, but the evidence for this assumption is dubious. The bile canaliculi can best be demonstrated by injections of dyes excreted into the bile. The use of fluorescent dyes has greatly enhanced the visualization of the bile capillaries, which fluoresce bright yellow-

(Continued on page 11)

(*Continued from page 10*)

green under ultraviolet light shortly after injection of fluorescein, in vital microscopy or in tissue sections. In such preparations diverticuli, sometimes of vacuolated appearance, have been observed frequently, but it is now realized that they represent artefacts brought about by anoxia or other alterations of the animals observed under such conditions. It is, therefore, now assumed that the *bile canaliculi* have a fairly straight lining with only small extensions between neighboring liver cells, a theory that agrees with the picture seen in tissue sections if the bile capillaries are stained with proper techniques, such as with mordant hematoxylin. In jaundice the bile canaliculi become dilated and filled with bile, sometimes precipitating to bile casts or plugs which probably contain a core of precipitated protein. Under these circumstances the arrangement of the bile canaliculi is readily visualized without special stains. Although in liver tissue preparations, made by teasing, the bile capillaries readily separate from the liver cells, they actually represent merely an enforcement of the membrane of the liver cell. With injuries to the liver cells, therefore, the continuity of the bile capillary wall is also destroyed, which explains the backflow of bile from the bile capillaries into the tissue spaces in jaundice caused by hepatocellular damage (see page 48).

The bile capillaries form a chickenwirelike, intercommunicating network within the center of the liver cell plates. They are surrounded by the liver cells and appear to lie within grooves in them, though they actually constitute a part of them. Nowhere in the normal liver are the bile capillaries close to the tissue space; as a rule, they are separated from it by half the diameter of a liver cell. Even if, *e.g.*, in severe cholestasis, the bile capillaries and their intercellular extensions are dilated, they hardly ever reach the tissue spaces to permit regurgitation of bile. The network of bile canaliculi is drained by the smallest *intralobular bile ducts,* the *cholangioles* or *ductules.* They are mostly found in the periportal zone of the parenchyma, where they are also designated as *canals of Hering.* Far less frequent are ductules connecting with bile capillaries deep within the lobule. They form communicating loops, which eventually either unite with the periportal cholangioles or independently perforate the *limiting plate.* The intralobular cholangioles are surrounded by a connective tissue sheet which also envelops the arterioles and possibly very small lymphatic vessels. The epithelial cells of the cholangioles are cuboidal, the nucleus is central and the cytoplasm is less basophilic than that of the liver cells, but the lumen is usually so narrow that it may be difficult to separate them from two-cell-thick liver cell plates. The separation can be made much more easily when the basement membrane is made visible by connective

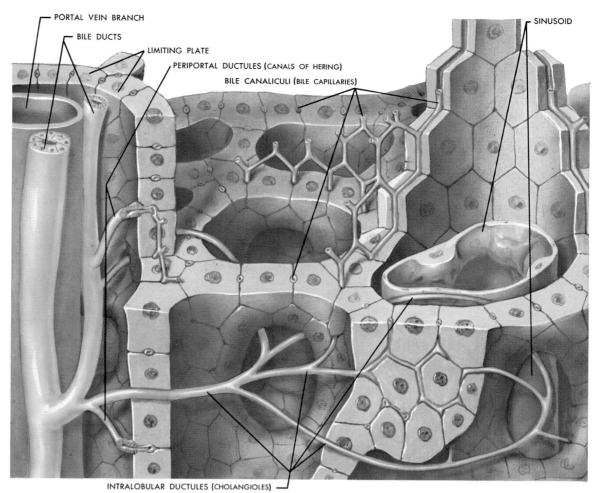

PORTAL VEIN BRANCH
BILE DUCTS
LIMITING PLATE
PERIPORTAL DUCTULES (CANALS OF HERING)
BILE CANALICULI (BILE CAPILLARIES)
SINUSOID
INTRALOBULAR DUCTULES (CHOLANGIOLES)

THREE-DIMENSIONAL SCHEMA OF INTRAHEPATIC BILIARY SYSTEM (AFTER HANS ELIAS)

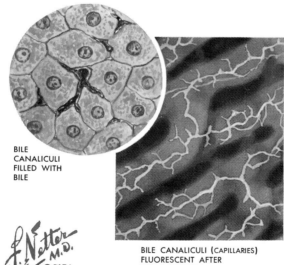

BILE CANALICULI FILLED WITH BILE

BILE CANALICULI (CAPILLARIES) FLUORESCENT AFTER DYE INJECTION

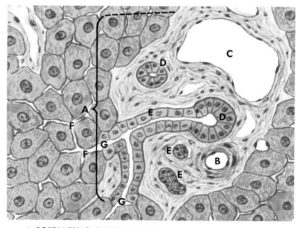

A–PORTAL TRIAD; B–HEPATIC ARTERY BRANCH; C–PORTAL VEIN BRANCH; D–BILE DUCTS; E–BILE DUCTULES; F–BILE CANALICULI (CAPILLARIES); G–JUNCTION OF CANALICULI WITH DUCTULES

tissue stains. In the portal tracts the cholangioles communicate with the smallest interlobular bile ducts, while their epithelial cells become cylindrical, with basal nuclei. As the ducts become wider, owing to the confluence of the smaller ones, and while they approximate the hilus, their epithelium becomes high columnar and, occasionally, mucus-producing. Mucus is also added to the duct's content by small adnexal secretory glands.

Intrahepatic Vascular System
(Plate 10, page 12)

After the *portal vein* has forked into main branches and has divided consecutively into smaller branches, eventually small portal tracts are reached in which a central *distributing vein,* less than 0.3 mm. in diameter, discharges short *inlet venules* at right angles.

Finally, the smallest portal vein divides into two terminal twigs entering the parenchyma. The inlet venules extend through the *limiting plate* into the *peripheral sinusoids* within the liver lobules, supplying the bulk of the portal vein blood to the parenchyma. From the sinusoids running peripherally along the limiting plate, the blood flows through *radially arranged sinusoids* to the *central vein.* Contractibility of the sinusoids probably forces some of the blood to take a longer route and thus provides equal contact of all points of the liver cell plates with blood. Portal vein branches with a diameter of above 0.3 mm. fail to discharge inlet venules directly into the sinusoidal system and have been called *conducting veins* (Elias). These veins lie in the larger portal tracts and are accompanied by parallel-running, small distributing veins which carry blood sometimes in

(*Continued on page 12*)

(Continued from page 11)

the same and sometimes in the opposite direction to the current in the larger conducting vein. The simultaneous presence of both distributing and conducting veins in the larger portal tracts guarantees the direct supply of portal vein blood to the parenchyma around the larger portal tracts. The arborization of the portal vein varies in different species, a fact which has significance in the development of fibrosis and cirrhosis. In the rat, *e.g.*, distributing veins are not found so regularly in the vicinity of conducting veins, and the parenchyma around the middle-sized portal tract receives its portal blood supply not from the portal tract itself but rather from a distant smaller one.*

The blood supply and drainage of the structures in the portal tract, especially of the bile ducts, differ from those of the hepatic parenchyma in that the portal vein branches act as blood-draining rather than -supplying vessels. Small venules collecting blood from the capillary plexus in the portal tracts, and especially around the bile ducts, transport it into the lobular parenchyma by uniting with inlet venules acting as "internal roots" of the portal vein. Malignant hepatic tumors frequently have a blood supply more similar to that of the structures of the portal tract rather than to those of the parenchyma, and the efferent portal vein branches corresponding to the "internal roots" may become large trunks — facts which might suggest that these tumors derive from structures in or near the portal tracts.

The *hepatic artery* ramifies parallel with the portal vein branches. *Arterioles* are released into the lobular parenchyma and terminate at different levels of the lobule, thus providing fresh arterial blood to all of its parts. The bulk seems to be released, however, in the periportal area by short arterioles. The arterial branches in the portal tracts also supply the peribiliary plexus, whence the blood is drained to the "internal roots" of the portal vein. This blood supply over the capillary plexus in the portal tracts has been wrongly interpreted as direct arterioportal anastomoses, which do not exist under normal circumstances, although they are an important feature in cirrhosis (see page 69).

The draining hepatic vein starts with the *central vein* into which the sinusoids enter freely in the absence of a limiting plate. The central veins unite to sublobular veins, which, in turn, form larger intrahepatic veins and finally join the inferior vena cava. In contrast to some animals such as the rat, no sinusoids

*In a functional sense the parenchyma around the middle-sized and larger portal tracts in rats is "nonportal", as Hartroft pointed out, and has the tendency to exhibit similar pathologic changes, as does the centrolobular area. If fibrosis follows fatty metamorphosis in rats on experimental diets, fibrous septa connect portal with central canals and thus produce cirrhosis by fatty metamorphosis alone, a process different from that in human beings (see pages 66 and 67).

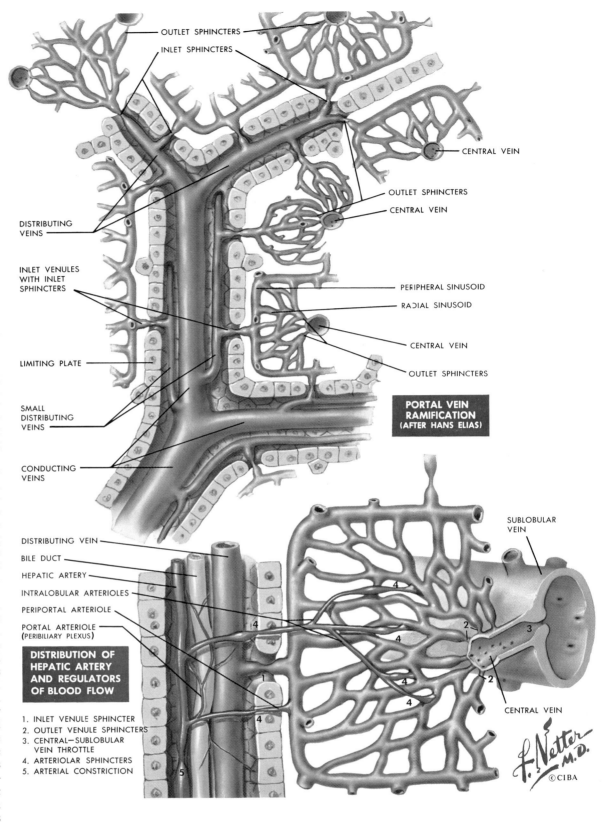

PORTAL VEIN RAMIFICATION (AFTER HANS ELIAS)

OUTLET SPHINCTERS
INLET SPHINCTERS
CENTRAL VEIN
OUTLET SPHINCTERS
CENTRAL VEIN
PERIPHERAL SINUSOID
RADIAL SINUSOID
CENTRAL VEIN
OUTLET SPHINCTERS
DISTRIBUTING VEINS
INLET VENULES WITH INLET SPHINCTERS
LIMITING PLATE
SMALL DISTRIBUTING VEINS
CONDUCTING VEINS

DISTRIBUTING VEIN
BILE DUCT
HEPATIC ARTERY
INTRALOBULAR ARTERIOLES
PERIPORTAL ARTERIOLE
PORTAL ARTERIOLE (PERIBILIARY PLEXUS)

DISTRIBUTION OF HEPATIC ARTERY AND REGULATORS OF BLOOD FLOW

1. INLET VENULE SPHINCTER
2. OUTLET VENULE SPHINCTERS
3. CENTRAL—SUBLOBULAR VEIN THROTTLE
4. ARTERIOLAR SPHINCTERS
5. ARTERIAL CONSTRICTION

SUBLOBULAR VEIN
CENTRAL VEIN

enter sublobular and larger hepatic vein tributaries in the human. That situation represents a potential difficulty for the drainage of the hepatic parenchyma and might explain the relatively great tendency to centrolobular congestion and necrosis in the human. Comparatively small veins frequently enter larger hepatic vein tributaries at right angles, a design which provides a possibility for a reduced drainage by contraction of the larger vessel. Such a *throttle* mechanism, in the absence of true muscular sphincters, is morphologically recognized by a dilatation of the smaller vessel just before it pierces the wall of the larger one. This drainage regulation corresponds to the far more efficient throttle mechanisms in animals such as the dog. In them, formidable spiral muscles in the hepatic vein branches act as a veritable sphincter regulating blood drainage from the liver.

Less obvious mechanisms regulating the blood flow

in the liver are found throughout the entire intrahepatic vasculature. Knisley has demonstrated *inlet sphincters* on the *venules* supplying the portal sinusoids and also *outlet sphincters* where the sinusoids join the central veins. The arteries are known to be subjected to regulation of their blood flow, and Elias has emphasized the variation in the arterial blood supply to different levels of the lobule by alternating contractions of periportal and intralobular arterioles. Vital microscopic observations (Wakin-Mann) have indicated such an intralobular arterial blood supply and also the great variations of blood flow throughout the liver in different parts of the lobule. These sphincter mechanisms, which regulate blood supply and drainage from different parts of the liver and vary the time a given unit of blood is in contact with a given part of the liver cell plate, represent a most efficient device for the regulation of liver functions.

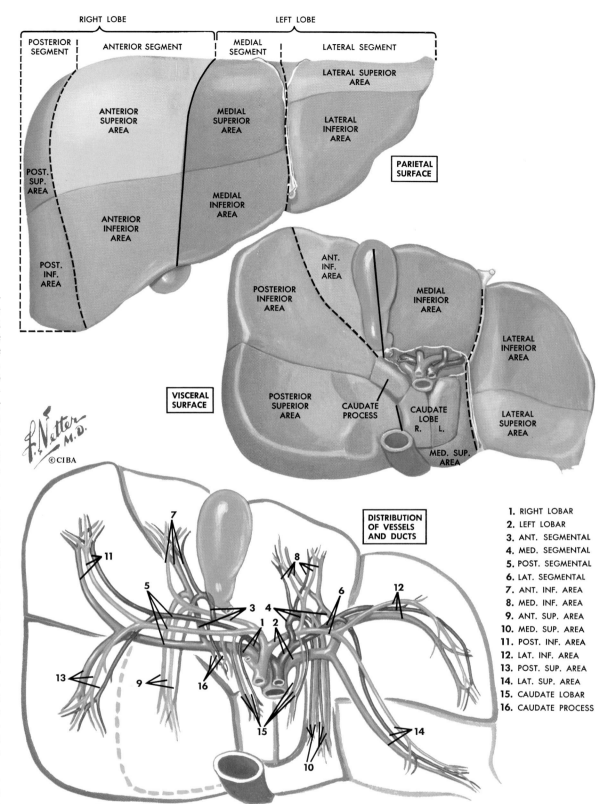

VESSEL AND DUCT DISTRIBUTION, LIVER SEGMENTS

The intrahepatic distribution of vessels and bile ducts was successfully studied on casts prepared by injecting a chemically impregnable plastic into the vascular and biliary conduits before removing the tissue by corrosive agents. The knowledge thus obtained proved to be a valuable asset for the cholangiographic demonstration of the vascular apparatus in vivo but was also of more than theoretical interest in view of the recognition of segmental divisions, similar to those in the lungs, which opened up the possibility of partial hepatectomy or the excision of single metastatic nodules. Although the human liver, in contrast to the liver of some animals, fails to display surface lobulation, the parallel course of the branches of the hepatic artery, portal vein and bile ducts and the appearance of clefts in these preparations of vessels and ducts pointed to a distinct lobular composition. A major lobar fissure extends obliquely downward from the fossa for the inferior vena cava (see page 5) to the gallbladder fossa, which does not coincide with the surface separation between the right and left lobes running along the insertion of the falciform ligament and the fossa for the ductus venosus. Through this fissure extends one of the main trunks of the hepatic vein, the tributaries of which never follow the distribution of the other vessels but cross the portal vein branches in an interdigitated fashion.

Each lobe is partitioned by a segmental division and is drained by a lobar bile duct of the first order. The right division extends obliquely from the junction of the anterior and posterior surfaces downward toward the lower border of the liver and continues on the inferior surface toward the porta, dividing the *right lobe* into an *anterior* and a *posterior segment,* each of which is drained by a bile duct of the second order. The left segmental cleft runs on the anterior surface along the attachments of the falciform ligament and on the visceral surface through the fissure of the ligamentum teres and ligamentum venosum. This fissure divides the *left lobe* into a *medial* and a *lateral segment,* but in a significant number of cases it is crossed by bile ducts and vessels. The lateral segment corresponds to the classical descriptions of the left lobe, whereas the aspect of the

medial segment on the visceral liver surface corresponds to the quadrate lobe. The four bile ducts of the second order fork into those of the third order, which drain either the superior or the inferior area of the corresponding segments. Thus, the bile ducts and the accompanying vessels can be designated according to the lobes, segments and areas to which they belong. The anatomically distinct *caudate lobe* has a vascular arrangement which divides it into a *left portion* drained by the left and a *right portion* drained by the right lobar duct. The *caudate process,* connecting the caudate lobe with the right lobe of the liver, has a separate net of vessels, which, in the majority of cases, communicates with branches of the right lobar duct. Neither the caudate lobe nor other parts of the liver provide an effective communication between the right and left lobar duct systems. Intrahepatic anastomoses between intraparenchymal branches of the arteries also have not been found, but in one fourth of the cases interconnections between the right and left systems exist through small extrahepatic or subcapsular anastomosing vessels.

The distribution of draining bile ducts and afferent blood vessels, as described and pictorialized in a schematic fashion, is valid in the majority of instances, but individual variations are met in abundance. They concern, especially, the lateral superior vessels and ducts for the appendix fibrosa. Rudimentary bile ducts are frequent in this region. The incidence of segmental bile duct variation is greater on the right, whereas that of segmental arteries is greater on the left side. Furthermore, the observations of several investigating groups are, in some respects, still at variance. The above description, as well as the illustration, follows Healey's account, which is based on the most extensive material.

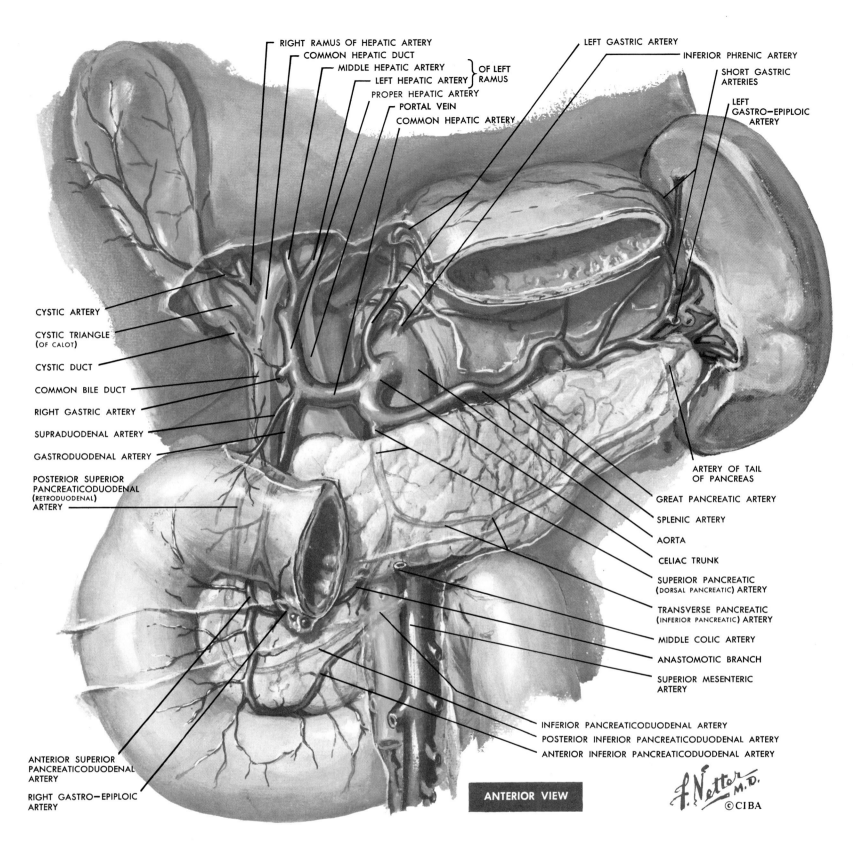

RIGHT RAMUS OF HEPATIC ARTERY
COMMON HEPATIC DUCT
MIDDLE HEPATIC ARTERY } OF LEFT
LEFT HEPATIC ARTERY } RAMUS
PROPER HEPATIC ARTERY
PORTAL VEIN
COMMON HEPATIC ARTERY

LEFT GASTRIC ARTERY
INFERIOR PHRENIC ARTERY
SHORT GASTRIC ARTERIES
LEFT GASTRO—EPIPLOIC ARTERY

CYSTIC ARTERY
CYSTIC TRIANGLE (OF CALOT)
CYSTIC DUCT
COMMON BILE DUCT
RIGHT GASTRIC ARTERY
SUPRADUODENAL ARTERY
GASTRODUODENAL ARTERY
POSTERIOR SUPERIOR PANCREATICODUODENAL (RETRODUODENAL) ARTERY

ANTERIOR SUPERIOR PANCREATICODUODENAL ARTERY
RIGHT GASTRO—EPIPLOIC ARTERY

ARTERY OF TAIL OF PANCREAS
GREAT PANCREATIC ARTERY
SPLENIC ARTERY
AORTA
CELIAC TRUNK
SUPERIOR PANCREATIC (DORSAL PANCREATIC) ARTERY
TRANSVERSE PANCREATIC (INFERIOR PANCREATIC) ARTERY
MIDDLE COLIC ARTERY
ANASTOMOTIC BRANCH
SUPERIOR MESENTERIC ARTERY
INFERIOR PANCREATICODUODENAL ARTERY
POSTERIOR INFERIOR PANCREATICODUODENAL ARTERY
ANTERIOR INFERIOR PANCREATICODUODENAL ARTERY

ANTERIOR VIEW

f. Netter M.D.
©CIBA

SECTION XV—PLATES 12 AND 13

ARTERIAL BLOOD SUPPLY OF LIVER, BILIARY SYSTEM AND PANCREAS

Recent studies, especially the painstaking dissections of Michels, have disclosed considerable variations (see page 16) in the arterial supply of the liver, biliary system and pancreas. According to the conventional description, which was found in only 55 per cent of examined specimens, the *celiac trunk* is a very short, thick artery originating from the aorta just below the aortic hiatus

in the diaphragm. It extends horizontally and forward above the pancreas, and splits into the *left gastric,* the *common hepatic* and *splenic* arteries. An *inferior phrenic artery,* usually starting from the aorta, or a dorsal pancreatic artery, otherwise departing from the splenic artery, the hepatic artery or the aorta, may exceptionally derive from the celiac trunk. The *left gastric artery,* the smallest of the three celiac branches, starting at the cardia, extends along the lesser curvature of the stomach to anastomose with the *right gastric artery.*

The *splenic artery,* largest of the three celiac branches (in the adult), takes a somewhat tortuous course to the left, along and behind the upper border of the pancreas. At a variable distance from the spleen, it breaks up into a number of terminal branches which enter the hilus of the

spleen. The *left gastro-epiploic artery* and the *short gastric arteries* usually take origin from one of these terminal branches.

The *common hepatic artery,* intermediate in size, passes forward and to the right to enter the right margin of the lesser omentum (see page 6), in which it ascends, lying to the left of the common bile duct and anterior to the portal vein. As the *common hepatic artery* turns upward, it gives origin first to the *gastroduodenal artery* (see below), then usually to the *supraduodenal* and, finally, to the *right gastric artery.* The *supraduodenal artery,* which may also originate from the *right hepatic* or *retroduodenal artery,* descends to supply the anterior, superior and posterior surfaces of the first inch of the duodenum. The *right gastric artery* passes to the left along the

(*Continued on page 15*)

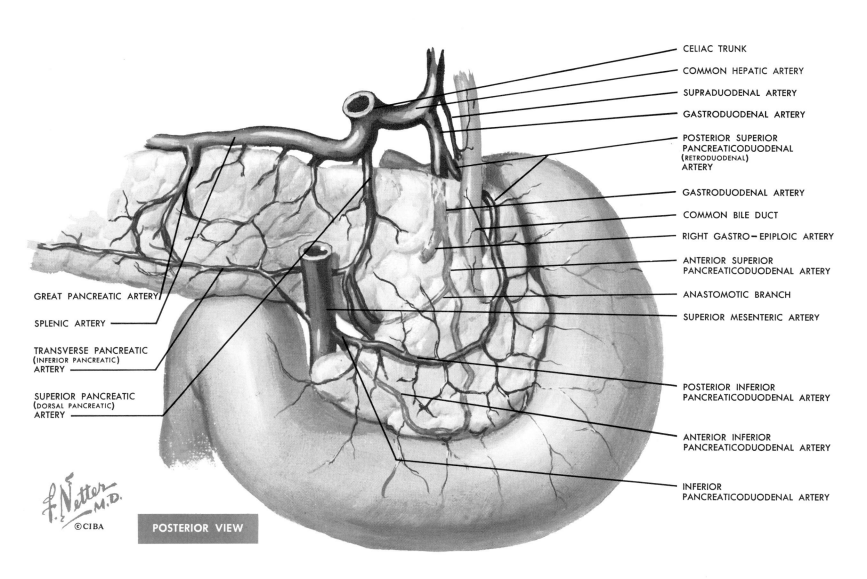

CELIAC TRUNK

COMMON HEPATIC ARTERY

SUPRADUODENAL ARTERY

GASTRODUODENAL ARTERY

POSTERIOR SUPERIOR
PANCREATICODUODENAL
(RETRODUODENAL)
ARTERY

GASTRODUODENAL ARTERY

COMMON BILE DUCT

RIGHT GASTRO−EPIPLOIC ARTERY

ANTERIOR SUPERIOR
PANCREATICODUODENAL ARTERY

ANASTOMOTIC BRANCH

SUPERIOR MESENTERIC ARTERY

POSTERIOR INFERIOR
PANCREATICODUODENAL ARTERY

ANTERIOR INFERIOR
PANCREATICODUODENAL ARTERY

INFERIOR
PANCREATICODUODENAL ARTERY

GREAT PANCREATIC ARTERY

SPLENIC ARTERY

TRANSVERSE PANCREATIC
(INFERIOR PANCREATIC)
ARTERY

SUPERIOR PANCREATIC
(DORSAL PANCREATIC)
ARTERY

POSTERIOR VIEW

©CIBA

(Continued from page 14)

lesser curvature of the stomach to anastomose with the *left gastric*. The continuation of the common hepatic artery beyond the origins of these vessels is known as the *hepatic artery proper* (arteria hepatica propria). It ascends and divides into several branches, most commonly into a *right ramus* and a *left ramus*. The *middle* hepatic artery usually arises from the left ramus. The right hepatic artery generally passes behind the common hepatic duct to enter the *cystic triangle* (*of Calot*), formed by the cystic duct, the hepatic duct and, cephalad, by the liver. In a minority of cases, however, the right hepatic artery crosses in front of the bile duct (see page 16). All terminal branches of the hepatic artery enter the liver at the porta hepatis. The *cystic artery* and its many variations are described on page 17.

The arterial supply to the *pancreas, common bile duct* and adjacent portions of the duodenum comes, in general, from branches of the gastroduodenal, the superior mesenteric and the splenic arteries. The *gastroduodenal artery*, after its origin from the common hepatic, passes downward to course behind the first portion of the duodenum and in front of the head of the pancreas. Before or immediately after passing behind the duodenum, it gives origin to the *posterior superior pancreaticoduodenal artery* (the *retroduodenal artery* of Michels). Its origin is often hidden by dense fibrous tissue, and, passing to the right and downward over the common bile duct, it gives off a branch comprising the principal blood supply of that duct. The retroduodenal artery continues downward behind the head of the pancreas and between the duodenum and common bile duct, finally turning to the left to

unite with the *posterior branch* of the *inferior pancreaticoduodenal artery*, also known as *posterior inferior pancreaticoduodenal artery*.

At the lower border of the pylorus, the *gastroduodenal artery* divides into a larger *right gastro-epiploic artery* and a *smaller anterior superior pancreaticoduodenal artery*. The right gastro-epiploic enters the greater omentum to follow the greater curvature of the stomach. The anterior superior pancreaticoduodenal artery continues downward on the anterior surface of the head of the pancreas as far as its lower border, where it turns upward to unite with the anterior branch of the inferior pancreaticoduodenal artery, also known as the *anterior inferior pancreaticoduodenal artery*. In approximately 40 per cent of the cases, no common inferior pancreaticoduodenal artery exists, and the anterior and posterior vessels originate separately from the superior mesenteric artery.

The head of the pancreas and the second and third portions of the duodenum are thus supplied by two arcades — an anterior and a posterior arch. The posterior arch is formed by the posterior superior pancreaticoduodenal (retroduodenal) artery uniting with the posterior inferior pancreaticoduodenal artery. The anterior arch is formed by the gastroduodenal and anterior superior pancreaticoduodenal arteries uniting with the anterior inferior pancreaticoduodenal artery. The posterior span is situated at a somewhat higher level than the anterior. Both give off branches which anastomose with each other through and around the pancreas, supplying that organ as well as the duodenum.

The body and tail of the pancreas are supplied chiefly by branches from the splenic artery (*rami

pancreatici*). Some of these are small twigs given off by the splenic artery, as it courses along the upper border of the pancreas. Three of them, however, are usually larger than the others and have achieved the distinction of individual names. Of these the *dorsal pancreatic artery*, also known as the *superior pancreatic artery*, while usually originating from the beginning of the splenic artery, may also arise from the hepatic artery, celiac trunk or from the *aorta*. It runs downward behind and in the substance of the pancreas, dividing into left and right branches. The left branch generally comprises the *transverse pancreatic artery*. The right branches constitute an anastomotic vessel to the anterior pancreatic arch and also a branch to the *uncinate process*. The *great pancreatic artery* originates from the splenic further to the left and passes downward, dividing into branches which anastomose with the transverse or inferior pancreatic artery. The artery for the tail of the pancreas (*arteria cauda pancreatis*) originates from the splenic artery, or from its terminal branches at the tail of the pancreas, and divides into branches which anastomose with the terminal twigs of the transverse pancreatic artery. The transverse pancreatic artery, usually the left branch of the dorsal pancreatic, courses behind the body and tail of the pancreas close to its lower border. It may originate from or communicate with the superior mesenteric artery.

The other branches of the splenic artery are variable terminal branches to the spleen, the left gastro-epiploic artery, short gastric arteries to the fundus of the stomach and, usually also, branches which anastomose with the left inferior phrenic artery.

15

HEPATIC ARTERY VARIATIONS

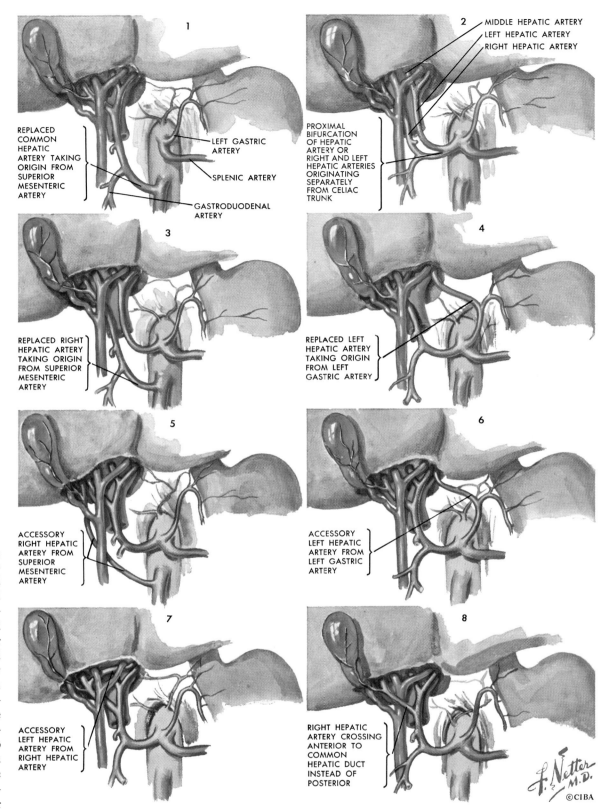

1 — REPLACED COMMON HEPATIC ARTERY TAKING ORIGIN FROM SUPERIOR MESENTERIC ARTERY / LEFT GASTRIC ARTERY / SPLENIC ARTERY / GASTRODUODENAL ARTERY

2 — MIDDLE HEPATIC ARTERY / LEFT HEPATIC ARTERY / RIGHT HEPATIC ARTERY / PROXIMAL BIFURCATION OF HEPATIC ARTERY OR RIGHT AND LEFT HEPATIC ARTERIES ORIGINATING SEPARATELY FROM CELIAC TRUNK

3 — REPLACED RIGHT HEPATIC ARTERY TAKING ORIGIN FROM SUPERIOR MESENTERIC ARTERY

4 — REPLACED LEFT HEPATIC ARTERY TAKING ORIGIN FROM LEFT GASTRIC ARTERY

5 — ACCESSORY RIGHT HEPATIC ARTERY FROM SUPERIOR MESENTERIC ARTERY

6 — ACCESSORY LEFT HEPATIC ARTERY FROM LEFT GASTRIC ARTERY

7 — ACCESSORY LEFT HEPATIC ARTERY FROM RIGHT HEPATIC ARTERY

8 — RIGHT HEPATIC ARTERY CROSSING ANTERIOR TO COMMON HEPATIC DUCT INSTEAD OF POSTERIOR

In over 40 per cent of dissections, *variations in the origin and course of the hepatic artery* or its branches were found (Michels). They concern with equal incidence the right and left hepatic arteries and are of more than passing surgical significance, mostly because of the liver necrosis which follows their unintended ligation. A "replaced" hepatic artery originates from a source different from that in the standard description and substitutes for the typical vessel (see page 14). An accessory artery is a vessel additional to those originating according to standard descriptions. An example of a replacement is the *origin of the common hepatic artery from the superior mesenteric artery* (1). It passes through or behind the head of the pancreas, and its ligation during a pancreaticoduodenal resection deprives the liver of its arterial blood supply. Under these circumstances, only the left gastric and splenic arteries arise from the celiac trunk. Sometimes, *right or left hepatic arteries originate independently from the celiac trunk or fork off from a very short common hepatic artery* (2). Under these conditions the *gastroduodenal artery* originates from the right hepatic artery. Very frequently, the *right hepatic artery,* giving off the gastroduodenal artery, takes off *from the superior mesenteric artery,* while the left hepatic artery, in turn giving off the middle hepatic artery, derives from the celiac

trunk (3). Ligation of the replaced right hepatic artery, especially where it crosses the junction of the cystic and the common ducts, for instance during cholecystectomy, deprives the right lobe of the liver of its blood supply. In contrast, ligation of an *accessory right hepatic artery, coming from the superior mesenteric* (5), is far less significant, since another right hepatic artery runs its typical course. Under these circumstances two right hepatic arteries may be found in Calot's triangle. A replaced right hepatic is far more frequent than an accessory. An aberrant *left hepatic artery,* originating *from the left gastric artery,* is, in half of the cases, replaced (4) and, in the other half, accessory (6). If it is replaced, only the right hepatic artery comes from the celiac trunk, while in the presence of an accessory vessel the common and proper

hepatic arteries take their usual course. Ligation of a replaced left hepatic artery, for instance during gastrectomy, endangers the blood supply to the left lobe of the liver.

An *accessory left hepatic artery* may also come *from the right hepatic artery* (7). In about 12 per cent of the cases the *right hepatic artery,* originating at its typical site of departure, *crosses in front of the common hepatic duct instead of behind it* (8), a variation worthy of being remembered in the exploration of the duct. The described variations are also significant in the formation of collaterals after obstruction or ligation of an artery (see page 107). Other variations not described here are less frequent, but their potential existence should not be ignored when operating in this field.

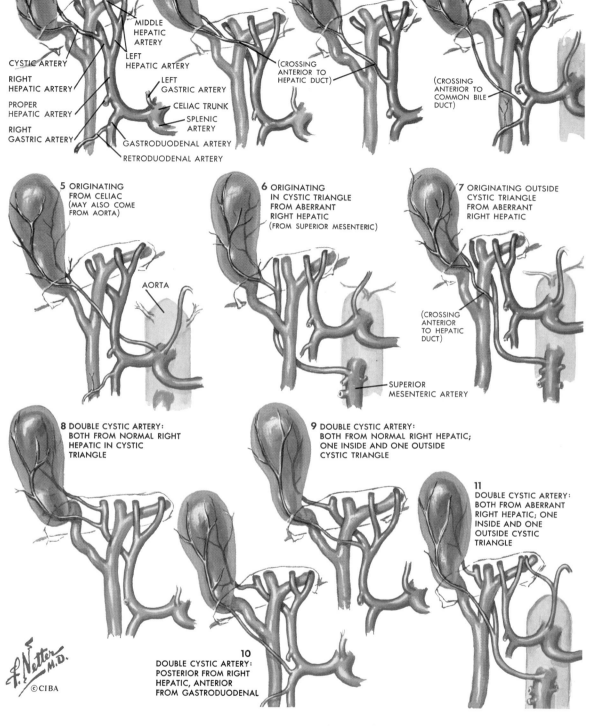

1 ORIGINATING FROM NORMAL RIGHT HEPATIC, <u>OUTSIDE</u> CYSTIC TRIANGLE

2 ORIGINATING FROM MIDDLE HEPATIC (MAY ALSO COME FROM LEFT HEPATIC)

3 ORIGINATING FROM PROPER HEPATIC

4 ORIGINATING FROM GASTRODUODENAL

MIDDLE HEPATIC ARTERY

LEFT HEPATIC ARTERY

CYSTIC ARTERY

RIGHT HEPATIC ARTERY

LEFT GASTRIC ARTERY

PROPER HEPATIC ARTERY

CELIAC TRUNK

SPLENIC ARTERY

RIGHT GASTRIC ARTERY

GASTRODUODENAL ARTERY

RETRODUODENAL ARTERY

(CROSSING ANTERIOR TO HEPATIC DUCT)

(CROSSING ANTERIOR TO COMMON BILE DUCT)

5 ORIGINATING FROM CELIAC (MAY ALSO COME FROM AORTA)

6 ORIGINATING IN CYSTIC TRIANGLE FROM ABERRANT RIGHT HEPATIC (FROM SUPERIOR MESENTERIC)

7 ORIGINATING OUTSIDE CYSTIC TRIANGLE FROM ABERRANT RIGHT HEPATIC

AORTA

(CROSSING ANTERIOR TO HEPATIC DUCT)

SUPERIOR MESENTERIC ARTERY

8 DOUBLE CYSTIC ARTERY: BOTH FROM NORMAL RIGHT HEPATIC IN CYSTIC TRIANGLE

9 DOUBLE CYSTIC ARTERY: BOTH FROM NORMAL RIGHT HEPATIC; ONE INSIDE AND ONE OUTSIDE CYSTIC TRIANGLE

11 DOUBLE CYSTIC ARTERY: BOTH FROM ABERRANT RIGHT HEPATIC; ONE INSIDE AND ONE OUTSIDE CYSTIC TRIANGLE

10 DOUBLE CYSTIC ARTERY: POSTERIOR FROM RIGHT HEPATIC, ANTERIOR FROM GASTRODUODENAL

CYSTIC ARTERY AND ITS VARIATIONS

The cystic artery, according to textbook descriptions, originates from the right hepatic artery within the cystic triangle of Calot, to the right of the common hepatic duct (see page 14). Variations, of great significance in cholecystectomy, are frequent and are best recognized by careful dissection of the structures in the cystic triangle. Typically, the artery divides into an anterior branch, going to the free peritoneal surface of the gallbladder, and a posterior branch to the nonperitoneal surface and the gallbladder bed. Both branches communicate with each other by means of numerous twigs. In about 20 per cent of the cases, the cystic artery does not originate in the triangle but *arises from the right hepatic artery* (1) *outside the triangle, from the middle* (2) *or left hepatic artery* or even less frequently, *from the proper hepatic artery* (3) before it forks into its branches. In all these instances it crosses the anterior and sometimes the posterior aspect of the common hepatic duct. Rare replacements include an *origin from the gastroduodenal artery* (4), and even *from the celiac trunk* (5), or independently *from the aorta*. In these instances the cystic artery originates caudally from the cystic duct and crosses the common duct. The cystic artery may also derive *from an aberrant right hepatic artery* coming from the superior mesen-

teric artery, the origin being either within the cystic triangle (6) or outside of it (7). In the latter instance it again crosses in front of the common hepatic duct.

Double cystic arteries are also frequent variations, occurring in approximately 25 per cent of the cases. Under these circumstances both the superficial or anterior branch and the deep posterior may arise *within the triangle* from the right hepatic artery (8). The origin of the posterior as a rule is much higher in the triangle, whereas the anterior branch may swing caudally around the proximal part of the cystic duct. Less frequently does one or both of the cystic arteries originate *outside the triangle*, in which case the most frequent pattern is an origin of the anterior cystic artery outside the triangle from the right hepatic artery with crossing in front of the bile duct, while the poste-

rior branch to the deeper structures of the gallbladder originates high within the triangle (9). Rare is an origin of the anterior cystic artery from the gastroduodenal artery (10). For the surgeon it is well to remember that an important vessel may have a caudad origin and accompany the cystic duct, in case the entire cystic artery or its superficial branch starts from the gastroduodenal artery or other intestinal arteries. Double cystic arteries may also arise within or without the triangle *from an aberrant right hepatic artery* (11). The number of possible variations is great, and their incidence is not negligible. It should be emphasized that an artery resembling the cystic artery in its course and paralleling the cystic duct is not necessarily the cystic artery but may be a branch of the hepatic artery.

PORTAL VEIN TRIBUTARIES, PORTACAVAL ANASTOMOSES

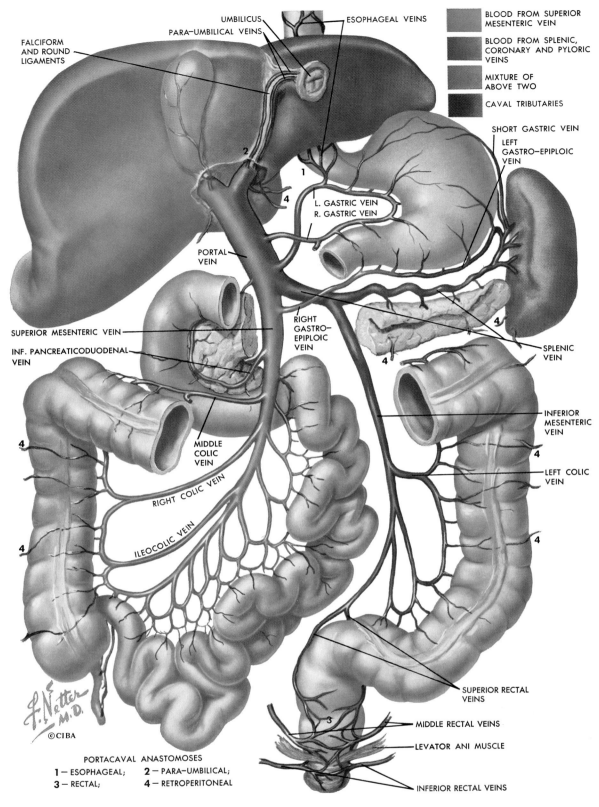

FALCIFORM AND ROUND LIGAMENTS

UMBILICUS
PARA-UMBILICAL VEINS

ESOPHAGEAL VEINS

BLOOD FROM SUPERIOR MESENTERIC VEIN

BLOOD FROM SPLENIC, CORONARY AND PYLORIC VEINS

MIXTURE OF ABOVE TWO

CAVAL TRIBUTARIES

SHORT GASTRIC VEIN

LEFT GASTRO-EPIPLOIC VEIN

L. GASTRIC VEIN
R. GASTRIC VEIN

PORTAL VEIN

SUPERIOR MESENTERIC VEIN

INF. PANCREATICODUODENAL VEIN

RIGHT GASTRO-EPIPLOIC VEIN

SPLENIC VEIN

MIDDLE COLIC VEIN

RIGHT COLIC VEIN

ILEOCOLIC VEIN

INFERIOR MESENTERIC VEIN

LEFT COLIC VEIN

SUPERIOR RECTAL VEINS

MIDDLE RECTAL VEINS

LEVATOR ANI MUSCLE

INFERIOR RECTAL VEINS

PORTACAVAL ANASTOMOSES
1 — ESOPHAGEAL; 2 — PARA-UMBILICAL;
3 — RECTAL; 4 — RETROPERITONEAL

The portal vein forms behind the head of the pancreas at the height of the second lumbar vertebra by confluence of the superior mesenteric and splenic veins. It runs behind the first portion of the duodenum and then in the right border of the lesser omentum to the porta hepatis, where it splits into its hepatic branches. The portal vein receives the *left gastric (coronary) vein* which communicates with the esophageal venous plexus. The latter, in turn, connects with the *short gastric veins,* the azygos and hemi-azygos veins in the lower and middle parts and with various branches of the superior vena cava, such as the innominate and inferior thyroid veins in the upper part of the esophageal region. The portal vein further accepts the *right gastric (pyloric) vein* which with the *left gastric (coronary) vein* forms a loop. The left main branch of the portal vein admits the *para-umbilical veins* and, occasionally, a persisting umbilical vein.

The *superior mesenteric vein,* one of the constituents of the vena portae, originates at the root of the mesentery, mainly from the *middle colic, right colic* and *ileocolic veins,* receiving in addition many small veins. It runs in front of the third portion of the duodenum and the uncinate process of the pancreas and receives the *inferior pancreaticoduodenal vein.* The *right gastro-epiploic vein* coming from the right aspects of the greater curvature of the stomach enters the superior mesenteric vein.

The *splenic vein* usually receives the *inferior mesenteric vein* behind the body of the pancreas (see also page 28). The inferior mesenteric vein starts with the *superior rectal veins* and continues in the posterior abdominal wall, receiving many tributaries, especially the *left colic vein.* The splenic vein begins at the hilus of the spleen and admits the *left gastro-epiploic vein,* short gastric veins (both communicating with esophageal veins) and pancreatic veins which anastomose with retroperitoneal veins, thus with the caval system.

The shortness of the main stem of the portal vein prevents under certain cir-

cumstances mixing of the blood coming from its constituents, so that the right extremity of the liver may receive chiefly blood coming from the superior mesenteric vein. The left lobe may receive blood from the left gastric (coronary), inferior mesenteric and splenic veins, whereas the left part of the right lobe, including the caudate and quadrate lobes, receives mixed blood. These streamlines, demonstrated in experimental animals, are not seen during portal venography and are not certain to occur in the human being. Their existence has been assumed, however, to explain the localization of tumor metastases and abscesses and also the predominance of massive necrosis in acute fatal viral hepatitis in the left lobe, which supposedly does not receive nutrient-rich protective blood from the small intestine.

The portacaval anastomoses have great clinical significance. They dilate when the blood flow in the

portal vein and through the liver is restrained; they relieve portal hypertension (see pages 71, 73 and 74) and may be lifesaving in acute portal hypertension but, as in chronic obstruction, may shunt blood from the liver, depriving the organism of the liver's vital functions and, therewith, they contribute to hepatic insufficiency. Dilatation of the rectal veins results in hemorrhoidal piles, with the danger of hemorrhage, thrombosis and inflammation. The varicosities of the esophageal veins (and less so of the cardiac veins of the stomach) may lead to esophageal hemorrhage, the most dangerous complication of portal hypertension (see page 72). The various *retroperitoneal varicose portacaval anastomoses* have less clinical significance. The *para-umbilical anastomoses* lead to a marked dilatation of the veins in the anterior abdominal wall. If these veins converge toward the umbilicus, they form what is called "caput medusae".

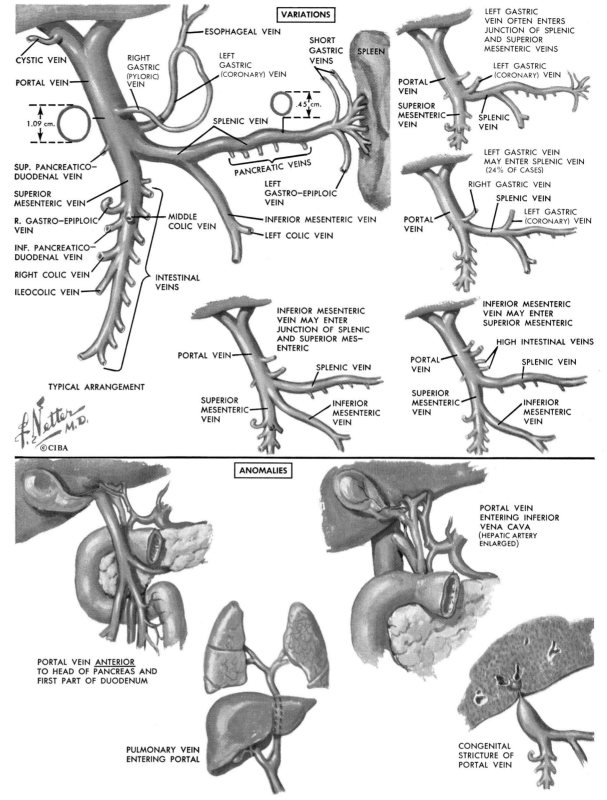

VARIATIONS

CYSTIC VEIN
PORTAL VEIN
RIGHT GASTRIC (PYLORIC) VEIN
ESOPHAGEAL VEIN
LEFT GASTRIC (CORONARY) VEIN
SHORT GASTRIC VEINS
SPLEEN
1.09 cm.
.45 cm.
SPLENIC VEIN
SUP. PANCREATICO-DUODENAL VEIN
PANCREATIC VEINS
SUPERIOR MESENTERIC VEIN
R. GASTRO-EPIPLOIC VEIN
INF. PANCREATICO-DUODENAL VEIN
RIGHT COLIC VEIN
ILEOCOLIC VEIN
MIDDLE COLIC VEIN
LEFT GASTRO-EPIPLOIC VEIN
INFERIOR MESENTERIC VEIN
LEFT COLIC VEIN
INTESTINAL VEINS
TYPICAL ARRANGEMENT

LEFT GASTRIC VEIN OFTEN ENTERS JUNCTION OF SPLENIC AND SUPERIOR MESENTERIC VEINS
PORTAL VEIN
SUPERIOR MESENTERIC VEIN
LEFT GASTRIC (CORONARY) VEIN
SPLENIC VEIN

LEFT GASTRIC VEIN MAY ENTER SPLENIC VEIN (24% OF CASES)
RIGHT GASTRIC VEIN
SPLENIC VEIN
PORTAL VEIN
LEFT GASTRIC (CORONARY) VEIN

INFERIOR MESENTERIC VEIN MAY ENTER JUNCTION OF SPLENIC AND SUPERIOR MESENTERIC
PORTAL VEIN
SPLENIC VEIN
SUPERIOR MESENTERIC VEIN
INFERIOR MESENTERIC VEIN

INFERIOR MESENTERIC VEIN MAY ENTER SUPERIOR MESENTERIC
HIGH INTESTINAL VEINS
PORTAL VEIN
SPLENIC VEIN
SUPERIOR MESENTERIC VEIN
INFERIOR MESENTERIC VEIN

F. Netter M.D.
©CIBA

ANOMALIES

PORTAL VEIN ANTERIOR TO HEAD OF PANCREAS AND FIRST PART OF DUODENUM

PULMONARY VEIN ENTERING PORTAL

PORTAL VEIN ENTERING INFERIOR VENA CAVA (HEPATIC ARTERY ENLARGED)

CONGENITAL STRICTURE OF PORTAL VEIN

PORTAL VEIN
Variations and Anomalies

The anatomy of the portal vein system is said to reveal less major anatomic variations than the hepatic arterial system. Nevertheless, the newly developed shunt operations for portal hypertension (see page 73) have created considerable interest in the anatomy of the portal vein, and dissections of several groups in a great number of individuals have indicated frequent minor variations of surgical importance. The length of the portal vein varies between 5.5 and 8 cm., with an average of approximately 6.5 cm., the mean diameter being normally 1.09 cm. In cirrhosis, however, the diameter is considerably wider. It is of practical importance that in only slightly over 10 per cent of the studied cases no vessel enters the main stem of the portal vein, but that in the vast majority several veins are admitted which may be torn during the dissection for portacaval anastomoses. Dangerous hemorrhage may result, and their ligation may interfere with the size of the portal vein and the performance of the anastomosis. In more than two thirds of the cases the *left gastric vein,* which is of major significance as portal drainage from esophageal varices, enters into the left aspect of the portal vein. Otherwise it enters at the junction of the *splenic and superior mesenteric veins,* while in almost one fourth of the cases it *joins the splenic vein.* Under all these circumstances the *pyloric vein* may enter into the portal vein stem. On its right aspect the portal vein may admit the *superior pancreaticoduodenal vein,* and close to the liver the *cystic vein,* which frequently joins the right branch of the portal vein. The usual anatomic

description of the formation of the portal vein is found only in about half of the cases. In the remainder the *inferior mesenteric vein* enters the junction of splenic and superior mesenteric veins or joins the *superior mesenteric vein.*

The size of the splenic vein, of major importance in splenorenal shunt, is said to average less than ½ cm. between the splenic hilus and the junction with the inferior mesenteric vein. As a rule the splenic vein is widened to a lesser degree in portal hypertension than is the portal vein. Since the splenic vein is more or less embedded into the cephalic portion of the pancreas, the many pancreatic venous tributaries are so short that they may be easily torn during shunt operation, and their ligation again creates technical problems.

Of the rare congenital anomalies of the portal vein, the one of surgical significance concerns an abnormal *position anterior to the head of the pancreas and the duodenum.* Another rare but physiologically interesting anomaly is the *entrance of the portal vein into the inferior vena cava.* It would indicate that the morphologically normal-appearing liver can function without portal vein blood. With this anomaly the hepatic artery is considerably enlarged. A great rarity is an entrance of the *pulmonary vein into the portal vein,* probably the consequence of some disturbance in the development of the venous systems at an early fetal stage (see page 2). Again, extremely rare are *congenital strictures* of the portal vein at the porta hepatis, producing severe portal hypertension which may not be relieved by surgical anastomoses.

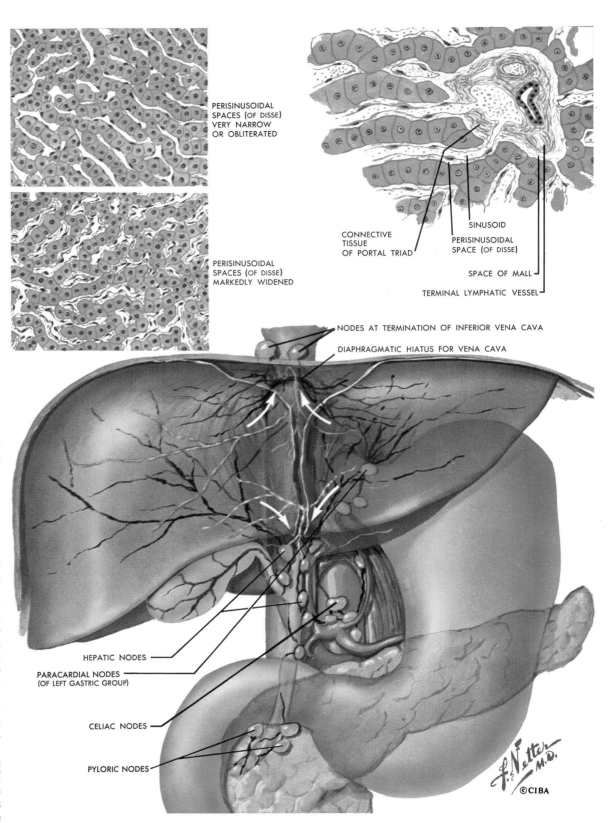

PERISINUSOIDAL SPACES (OF DISSE) VERY NARROW OR OBLITERATED

PERISINUSOIDAL SPACES (OF DISSE) MARKEDLY WIDENED

CONNECTIVE TISSUE OF PORTAL TRIAD

SINUSOID

PERISINUSOIDAL SPACE (OF DISSE)

SPACE OF MALL

TERMINAL LYMPHATIC VESSEL

NODES AT TERMINATION OF INFERIOR VENA CAVA

DIAPHRAGMATIC HIATUS FOR VENA CAVA

HEPATIC NODES

PARACARDIAL NODES (OF LEFT GASTRIC GROUP)

CELIAC NODES

PYLORIC NODES

LYMPHATIC DRAINAGE OF LIVER AND BILE TRACT

The tissue spaces in the hepatic parenchyma, the *perisinusoidal spaces of Disse,* separate the sinusoidal wall from the liver cell plates. The spaces are traversed by fine arcuate reticular fibers, extending from the basement membrane of the capillaries to the liver cell plates, which themselves do not rest on a basement membrane. Through these spaces the exchange of fluid, and especially solids from the liver cells to the sinusoidal lumen and vice versa, takes place. Under normal circumstances the perisinusoidal spaces are almost completely obliterated, and the arcuate reticular fibers can hardly be separated from the sinusoidal basement membranes. However, in the agonal period, and especially in passive congestion, in anoxia or in various toxic conditions, hepatic edema sets in, with widening of the sinusoidal spaces, which are filled by a protein-rich fluid. This widening may develop very rapidly, probably as a result of an abnormally increased permeability for serum protein brought about, for instance, by hypoxia. Therefore, in autopsy specimens of even normal livers, as a rule, the perisinusoidal spaces are expanded, whereas in biopsy specimens they are usually invisible. In toxic conditions or congestion, this widening may be markedly exaggerated. The perisinusoidal spaces communicate with a tissue space on the periphery of the portal tracts, the *space of Mall.* The fluid in the spaces of Disse and Mall is not lymph, but it is drained into the lymphatic vessels, which probably terminate in the portal tracts. In the human, in contrast to some animals, especially such as the dog, few lymphatics are present in the central canals around the tributaries of the hepatic vein. It is possible, but still not established, that in addition very small lymphatic vessels accompany the arterioles within the lobular parenchyma. Glisson's capsule contains a subperitoneal dense network of lymphatics which communicates with both a lymphatic network in the gallbladder bed and with the intraparenchymal lymph vessels. These widespread intercommunications make the hepatic lymphatic system a functional unit.

The lymphatic drainage of the liver follows several main routes, at least judging from studies in the dog. The bulk of the hepatic lymph collects in lymph vessels around the intrahepatic branches of the portal vein. The accompanying bile ducts contain a dense lymphatic network, extending sometimes beneath the epithelium. At the porta hepatis several lymphatic vessels are found, which reach the *hepatic lymph nodes* around the common duct and the main stem of the portal vein. The lymphatic vessels continue to a chain of *celiac nodes* around the celiac trunk and the vena cava inferior. From there, lymphatic vessels proceed to the cisterna chyli, while a few extend directly from the porta hepatis to the thoracic duct. Another quantitatively less significant route follows within the hepatic parenchyma from the central vein to the larger tributaries of the hepatic veins and, after assembling around the intrahepatic portion of the vena cava inferior, the lymphatics pass through the *diaphragmatic*

hiatus for the vena cava into the thoracic cage. There, they either reach *nodes at the termination of the vena cava inferior* or enter directly the thoracic duct.

The lymphatic network in Glisson's capsule or in the immediate subcapsular zone is also drained into lymphatic channels, passing through the diaphragmatic hiatus along the vena cava inferior directly to the thoracic duct. In addition, a few vessels from the left side of the posterior surface drain to the *paracardial group of the left gastric nodes* and some from the right side of the posterior surface drain directly to the celiac nodes. The lymph vessels from the gallbladder and from most of the extrahepatic bile ducts drain to the hepatic nodes, but a few vessels from the common bile duct also run to the *pyloric nodes.* Anastomoses of the hepatic lymphatics with duodenal and pancreatic lymphatics are noted only in the presence of adhesions.

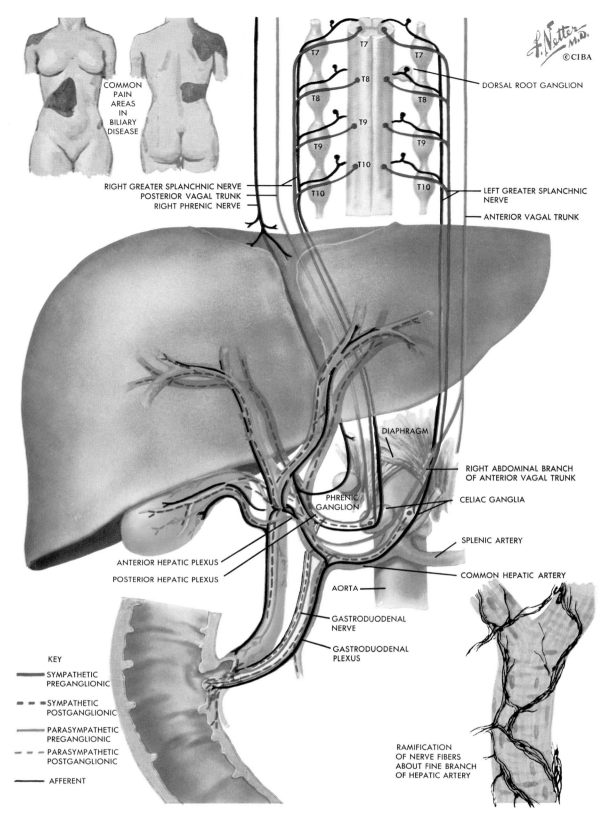

COMMON PAIN AREAS IN BILIARY DISEASE

T7 T7 T7
T8 T8 T8
T9 T9 T9
T10 T10 T10

DORSAL ROOT GANGLION

RIGHT GREATER SPLANCHNIC NERVE
POSTERIOR VAGAL TRUNK
RIGHT PHRENIC NERVE

LEFT GREATER SPLANCHNIC NERVE

ANTERIOR VAGAL TRUNK

DIAPHRAGM

PHRENIC GANGLION

RIGHT ABDOMINAL BRANCH OF ANTERIOR VAGAL TRUNK

CELIAC GANGLIA

SPLENIC ARTERY

COMMON HEPATIC ARTERY

ANTERIOR HEPATIC PLEXUS

POSTERIOR HEPATIC PLEXUS

AORTA

GASTRODUODENAL NERVE

GASTRODUODENAL PLEXUS

KEY
— SYMPATHETIC PREGANGLIONIC
- - - SYMPATHETIC POSTGANGLIONIC
— PARASYMPATHETIC PREGANGLIONIC
- - - PARASYMPATHETIC POSTGANGLIONIC
— AFFERENT

RAMIFICATION OF NERVE FIBERS ABOUT FINE BRANCH OF HEPATIC ARTERY

INNERVATION OF LIVER AND BILE TRACT

The liver, gallbladder and biliary tract receive their nerve supply from the sympathetic and parasympathetic systems and from the right phrenic nerve. The *sympathetic innervation* comes chiefly from the seventh to the tenth spinal segments, passes through the corresponding *sympathetic ganglia* and reaches the celiac ganglia by way of the splanchnic nerves. Most of the sympathetic postganglionic fibers originate probably in the *celiac ganglia;* some of them may start in one of the small ganglia present at the porta hepatis. The *parasympathetic innervation* is provided by both vagal trunks, the posterior of which traverses, with some branches, the right portion of the celiac plexus. The anterior vagal trunk with its right abdominal branch takes its course through the hepatogastric ligament.

At the porta hepatis, the nerves form the anterior and posterior hepatic plexuses, of which the former lies near the hepatic artery. It is composed mostly of fibers from the left portion of the celiac plexus and from the right abdominal branch of the anterior vagal trunk. The posterior plexus, behind the portal veins and the bile ducts, receives fibers from the right celiac ganglion and the posterior vagal trunk. Within the liver the nerves follow the branches of the blood vessels and bile ducts. The distribution within the liver is still argued. The portal tracts contain small nonmyelinated fibers, sometimes intermixed with larger myelinated fibers. In the wall of the bile ducts a nerve fiber network extends close to the epithelium. Fine fibers have been demonstrated in the interlobular tissue spaces, but it remains undecided whether they reach the liver cells themselves. Apparently the *branches of the common hepatic artery* are supplied entirely by sympathetic fibers, while the musculature of the bile ducts is innervated by both autonomic nerves. The *extrahepatic bile ducts* and the *gallbladder* receive branches from the anterior and posterior hepatic plexuses. An irregular intercommunicating plexus is seen in the lower layer of the mucosa, the muscularis and the adventitia.

The afferent nerve supply from the liver and extrahepatic biliary system is believed to pass via sympathetic afferent fibers through both splanchnic nerves, and often also by way of the right phrenic nerve. When the latter enters the liver, sometimes joined by sympathetic fibers, branches are distributed to the coronary and falciform ligaments and to the capsule of the liver. The innervation of the intrahepatic blood vessels is analogous to that of other blood vessels. Whereas the afferent innervation of the liver itself is poorly understood, it is well established that the splanchnic nerves inhibit gallbladder contraction, while the stimulating impulses arrive through the vagus fibers. Some contradictory experimental evidence points to the possibility that both sympathetic and parasympathetic nerves contain stimulating as well as inhibitory fibers (see page 52). The *choledochoduodenal junction* is innervated by fibers coursing along the gastroduodenal artery (gastroduodenal plexus) and also by the independent gastroduodenal nerve derived from both the hepatic plexuses and the right vagus.

Pain elicited in the liver is usually of the dull type, associated with diffuse tenderness over the liver and pain in the right shoulder. A *beltlike area* of *skin hypersensitivity,* limited corresponding to the ninth thoracic and first lumbar vertebrae, is found on the right side of the body. Acute enlargement of the liver is frequently painful (stretching of the capsule and traction on the hepatic ligaments). This and the *shoulder pain on the right side* reflect innervation by the phrenic nerve. Biliary tract pains are either circumscribed tenderness in the gallbladder region or colicky pain. Pain radiates to the back just below the tip of the right scapula, to the right shoulder, to the substernal area and sometimes also to the anterior left chest. Involvement of the subserosa produces sharply defined knifelike pain associated with hyperesthesia of the skin.

R. AND L. HEPATIC DUCTS
R. AND L. HEPATIC ARTERIES
COMMON HEPATIC DUCT
CYSTIC DUCT
PROPER HEPATIC ARTERY
COMMON BILE DUCT
R. GASTRIC ARTERY
GASTRODUODENAL ARTERY
CYSTIC ARTERY
LIVER
GALL-BLADDER
DUODENUM
STOMACH
COLON
PANCREAS
NECK OF GALLBLADDER
HARTMANN'S POUCH (INFUNDIBULUM)
CORPUS (BODY) OF GALL-BLADDER
FUNDUS OF GALL-BLADDER
CUT EDGE OF ANTERIOR LAYER OF LESSER OMENTUM

CYSTIC DUCT (PARS GLABRA)
CYSTIC DUCT (PARS SPIRALIS)
RIGHT HEPATIC DUCT
LEFT HEPATIC DUCT
COMMON HEPATIC DUCT
GLAND ORIFICES
SUPRA-DUODENAL
RETRO-DUODENAL
INFRA-DUODENAL
INTRA-DUODENAL
COMMON BILE DUCT
PANCREATIC DUCT
MAJOR PAPILLA (OF VATER)

GALLBLADDER AND BILE DUCTS
Anatomy and Histology

MUCOSAL FOLD
EPITHELIUM
EPITHELIAL POCKET
TUNICA PROPRIA
MUSCLE
ADVENTITIA

GALLBLADDER—MICROSCOPIC SECTION
(HEPATIC SIDE)

EPITHELIUM
FIBRO-ELASTIC TISSUE WITH SCANT MUSCLE FIBERS
GLANDS AND DUCTS
ADVENTITIA

COMMON BILE DUCT—MICROSCOPIC SECTION

LIVER
PERITONEAL REFLECTION
ADVENTITIA
MUSCLE
EPITHELIUM
1 ABERRANT BILE DUCT (LUSCHKA)
2 INFLAMMATORY PSEUDODIVERTICULUM (ROKITANSKY-ASCHOFF)
3 NECK GLANDS

TYPES OF DUCTS IN GALLBLADDER WALL
(SCHEMATIC)

GALLBLADDER MUSCLE (SCHEMATIC)

BLUE: DIAGONAL FIBERS
RED: LONGITUDINAL FIBERS BRANCHING OFF TO DEEPER LEVEL

The pear-shaped *gallbladder* (vesica fellea) is attached to the inferior surface of the right and quadrate lobes of the liver (see also pages 5 and 6). Areolar tissue, in which blood vessels, lymphatics and nerves run, fills the gallbladder bed — an impression in the liver. Otherwise, the gallbladder is covered by peritoneum, the reflection of which continues into the hepatic serosal surface. Usually about 10 cm. long and 3 to 5 cm. in diameter, the gallbladder projects with its *fundus* beyond the anterior liver margin. This is the part which is palpable in vivo and cholecystographically visible as "Phrygian cap" when a kinking or folding of the fundus prevails. The *corpus* (body) is in contact with the second portion of the duodenum and the colon. The *infundibulum,* or Hartmann's pouch, located at the free edge of the lesser omentum bulges forward toward the *cystic duct,* hiding it from surgical exposure but serving as a landmark for its identification. The part between the body of the gallbladder and the cystic duct is called the *neck.*

The gallbladder consists of (1) a *mucous layer* thrown in *folds* and lined by tall columnar surface *epithelium;* (2) a *muscular layer;* (3) a subserous layer; and (4) a serosal layer, mentioned above. The irregular folds, easily seen in contracted state, disappear on extreme distention. The *tunica propria* is richly vascularized and contains lymphocytes. The organ possesses no muscular fibers in the mucosa and no submucosal layer. The fibers of the *gallbladder muscle* below the mucosa are discontinuous, separated by connective tissue and course longitudinally in the inner and diagonally in the outer layer. The latter surround the organ in a spiral fashion.

Mucous glands are found only in the neck. *Pocketlike invaginations* of the surface epithelium occur normally and con-

tribute to the formation of folds. As a result of inflammation, they may extend as *pseudodiverticula* (Rokitansky-Aschoff) into and through the muscular layer. Aberrant vestigial *bile ducts* (Luschka) of the liver, not connected with the gallbladder lumen, may enter the adventitial layer and may serve as a path for infections from the liver to the gallbladder bed.

The *cystic duct,* a few centimeters long, is tortuous (*pars spiralis*) in its first portion and "smooth" (*pars glabra*) in its short end-piece. In the former the *spiral fold* (*of Heister*) is produced by mucosal duplications which regulate filling and emptying of the gallbladder according to the pressure in the biliary system. The *right* and *left hepatic ducts* emerging from the liver unite to become the 2 to 3 cm. long *common hepatic duct,* which, in turn, combines with the cystic duct to form the *common bile duct,* also known as ductus choledochus. The latter, 10 to 15 cm. long, descends

in the free margin of the lesser omentum (see page 6) and continues behind the pars superior of the duodenum and through the pancreas in a downward and slightly rightward direction to enter the descending part of the duodenum at the *major papilla* (*of Vater*). The common bile duct, thus, may be divided into *supraduodenal, retroduodenal, infraduodenal* and *intraduodenal portions.*

The extrahepatic bile ducts are lined by high *columnar epithelium* which is thrown sometimes into irregular folds. The *subepithelial connective tissue* is rich in elastic fibers but contains few and irregularly arranged muscle fibers. Mucus-producing *glands* in the deep layers are connected with the lumen by long *ducts.* Their white viscous secretion, together with that of the neck glands, amounts to about 20 ml. per day. It accounts for the mucous material admixed to the bile.

VARIATIONS OF EXTRAHEPATIC BILE DUCTS, ACCESSORY HEPATIC DUCTS

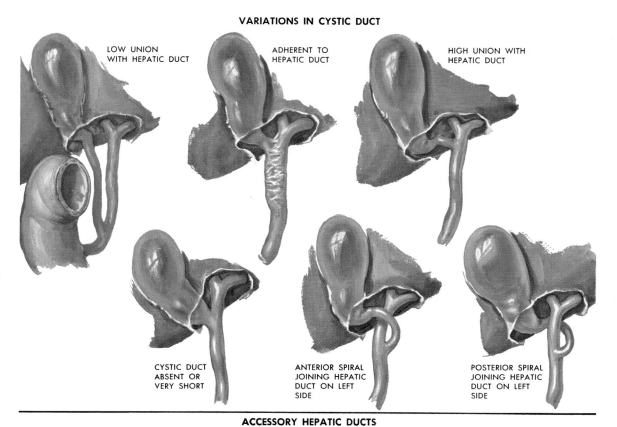

VARIATIONS IN CYSTIC DUCT

LOW UNION WITH HEPATIC DUCT

ADHERENT TO HEPATIC DUCT

HIGH UNION WITH HEPATIC DUCT

CYSTIC DUCT ABSENT OR VERY SHORT

ANTERIOR SPIRAL JOINING HEPATIC DUCT ON LEFT SIDE

POSTERIOR SPIRAL JOINING HEPATIC DUCT ON LEFT SIDE

ACCESSORY HEPATIC DUCTS

JOINING COMMON HEPATIC DUCT

JOINING CYSTIC DUCT

JOINING COMMON BILE DUCT

JOINING GALLBLADDER

TWO ACCESSORY DUCTS

While operating on the biliary system, it is of utmost importance to identify carefully each single structure, because anatomical variations in this field are common and because a series of dreaded consequences may ensue if such variations are overlooked. The course of the cystic duct is liable to vary fairly frequently and may escape ligation, with resultant postoperative bile leakage. The common bile and, even more so, the hepatic ducts are exposed during surgery to unintended injuries, which may mean complete separation of the ducts or strictures (see page 133) at a later date.

The variable site of the union of hepatic and cystic ducts determines the length of the common bile duct, which varies accordingly anywhere between a point close to the duodenum to almost the porta hepatis (see pages 6 and 14). If *this union lies low, i.e.,* far away from the porta hepatis and near the duodenum, the supraduodenal portion of the common bile duct is very short or may be completely absent, while correspondingly the cystic and common hepatic ducts run parallel for a considerable length, inviting difficulties during cholecystectomy. This situation is compounded if the two ducts are encircled by a *common sheath* of dense connective tissue; a stone in the cystic duct may lead not only to compression of the hepatic duct but also to added difficulties at surgery. The *cystic duct* may be duplicated or may be very *short* or *absent,* and then the gallbladder appears to empty directly into

the hepatic duct. As a rule the cystic duct joins the right aspect of the hepatic duct, but sometimes its opening may be found on its anterior aspect and, in rare instances, also on the left aspect of the duct. The *cystic duct* in such a situation crosses in a *spiral fashion* either the *anterior* or the *posterior aspect* of the *common hepatic duct,* again creating problems at surgical dissection.

Accessory hepatic ducts have been found in one fifth of all instances dissected. It has been pointed out (Michels) that they are not actually accessory but rather aberrant, because the drainage of bile from a circumscribed portion of the liver depends upon them. They are readily injured at cholecystectomy, for instance, if they traverse the cystic triangle of Calot. In half of the cases in which an *accessory duct* is found, it *joins* the *common hepatic duct* somewhere along its course. Far less frequently, the *accessory*

duct joins the right branch of the hepatic duct or the *common bile duct.* In the latter instance, it may cross the cystic duct. Sometimes the *cystic duct* may *join the accessory hepatic duct,* and both together combine with the common hepatic duct to form the common bile duct. Most accessory ducts are on the right side. Those on the left side enter the common bile duct. This may be associated with the presence of a right accessory duct joining the hepatic duct. An *accessory hepatic duct* may run through the gallbladder bed and may sometimes even *enter the gallbladder* itself. This duct is readily torn during cholecystectomy, and, if not recognized or if it is mistaken for fibrous strands, postoperative leakage into the gallbladder bed will occur. The relation of accessory vessels to the arteries also poses surgical predicaments, particularly with respect to a high cystic artery which may cross the low hepatic duct, and vice versa.

CHOLEDOCHODUODENAL JUNCTION

The *interior of the second portion of the duodenum* harbors the *major papilla* of Vater as a rule, on the medial aspect, between the *circular folds of the intestine (valvulae conniventes)*. This papilla (1) with the longitudinal fold (3) constitute the *choledochoduodenal junction*, an oblique passageway through the duodenal wall traversed by the common bile duct (*ductus choledochus*) and the main *pancreatic duct* of Wirsung. These ducts may open separately or through the medium of a common chamber, the *hepatopancreatic ampulla* of Vater (Boyden). A *minor papilla* is often seen about 2 cm. above the papilla of Vater, where the accessory pancreatic duct of Santorini empties into the duodenum. This duct communicates usually with the main pancreatic duct within the head of the pancreas (see pages 26 and 27).

The *union between the common bile duct and the main pancreatic duct* varies individually. Most frequently, both ducts join within the wall of the duodenum and have a short common terminal portion. In other instances each duct has its own opening either at the papilla or, occasionally, at some distance — as much as 2 cm. apart. The third possibility is the union of both ducts before entering the duodenum, thus forming a long common terminal portion which transverses the duodenal wall. A slightly elevated longitudinal fold in the duodenum is a projection of the *ampulla of Vater*, which is a dilated part of the common terminal portion of both ducts. It is this common portion which may permit reflux of pancreatic juice into the biliary system or of bile into the pancreas. The potential reflux has been used to explain the etiology of cholecystitis or acute and chronic pancreatic necrosis, respectively. Such etiologic associations, however, have been questioned and are now considered to occur only rarely, despite the incidence of a sufficiently long common channel (29 to 64 per cent of cases studied by several investigators) which would favor a postulated reflux. Obstruction of the papillary orifice by a biliary calculus or a muscular spasm, naturally, is apt to facilitate reflux, except when the common portion is extremely short. Actually, bile flow from the common bile duct into the pancreatic duct has been found in only 16 per cent of individuals studied roentgenologically. Pancreatic enzymes have been demonstrated in gallbladder bile.

As the result of Boyden's painstaking studies of the papillary and ampullary structures, including the muscular arrangement designated as the sphincter

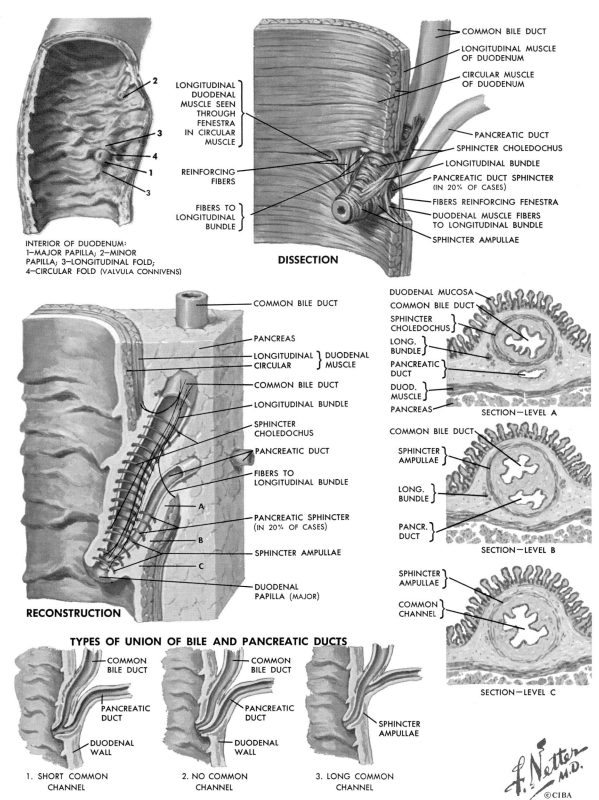

INTERIOR OF DUODENUM:
1–MAJOR PAPILLA; 2–MINOR PAPILLA; 3–LONGITUDINAL FOLD; 4–CIRCULAR FOLD (VALVULA CONNIVENS)

DISSECTION

Labels: COMMON BILE DUCT; LONGITUDINAL MUSCLE OF DUODENUM; CIRCULAR MUSCLE OF DUODENUM; PANCREATIC DUCT; SPHINCTER CHOLEDOCHUS; LONGITUDINAL BUNDLE; PANCREATIC DUCT SPHINCTER (IN 20% OF CASES); FIBERS REINFORCING FENESTRA; DUODENAL MUSCLE FIBERS TO LONGITUDINAL BUNDLE; SPHINCTER AMPULLAE; LONGITUDINAL DUODENAL MUSCLE SEEN THROUGH FENESTRA IN CIRCULAR MUSCLE; REINFORCING FIBERS; FIBERS TO LONGITUDINAL BUNDLE

RECONSTRUCTION

Labels: COMMON BILE DUCT; PANCREAS; LONGITUDINAL / CIRCULAR } DUODENAL MUSCLE; COMMON BILE DUCT; LONGITUDINAL BUNDLE; SPHINCTER CHOLEDOCHUS; PANCREATIC DUCT; FIBERS TO LONGITUDINAL BUNDLE; PANCREATIC SPHINCTER (IN 20% OF CASES); SPHINCTER AMPULLAE; DUODENAL PAPILLA (MAJOR); A; B; C

SECTION—LEVEL A
Labels: DUODENAL MUCOSA; COMMON BILE DUCT; SPHINCTER CHOLEDOCHUS; LONG. BUNDLE; PANCREATIC DUCT; DUOD. MUSCLE; PANCREAS

SECTION—LEVEL B
Labels: COMMON BILE DUCT; SPHINCTER AMPULLAE; LONG. BUNDLE; PANCR. DUCT

SECTION—LEVEL C
Labels: SPHINCTER AMPULLAE; COMMON CHANNEL

TYPES OF UNION OF BILE AND PANCREATIC DUCTS

1. SHORT COMMON CHANNEL — COMMON BILE DUCT; PANCREATIC DUCT; DUODENAL WALL

2. NO COMMON CHANNEL — COMMON BILE DUCT; PANCREATIC DUCT; DUODENAL WALL

3. LONG COMMON CHANNEL — SPHINCTER AMPULLAE

of Oddi, it is now recognized that the common bile and pancreatic ducts with their sphincters pass through the duodenal wall in the form of an eye-shaped window, the size of which determines the influence of duodenal tonus and peristalsis upon bile flow as well as the passing of gallstones. Though the architecture of the sphincter muscles depends upon the various types of union discussed above, the prototype of this complex sphincter arrangement consists of the following parts:

1. The *sphincter choledochus* surrounds the common bile duct from its entrance into the duodenal wall to its junction with the pancreatic duct; it regulates the bile flow and, retrogressively, the filling of the gallbladder (see page 52).

2. The *pancreatic sphincter*, present only in a variable number of instances, surrounds the intraduodenal portion of the pancreatic duct.

3. The *sphincter ampullae*, variably developed, is an annular muscle extending from the junction of the ducts to the tip of the papilla; it is the muscle of the common channel and is responsible for the potential reflux mentioned before.

4. *Longitudinal muscle bundles*, extending from the entrance of the ducts into the duodenal wall to the tip of the papilla, connect the ducts with each other as well as with the duodenal muscles; their activity retracts or erects the papilla.

5. *Reinforcing fibers*, extending from the duodenal muscles to the longitudinal fibers, enforce the duodenal window and prevent its dilatation.

The choledochoduodenal junction (in the cat) is supplied by fibers which course as a gastroduodenal plexus along the gastroduodenal artery and also by way of an independent gastroduodenal nerve derived from both hepatic plexuses and the right vagus nerve.

DEVELOPMENT OF PANCREAS

LIVER
FOREGUT
DORSAL PANCREAS
STOMACH

HEPATIC DIVERTICULUM
HEPATIC DUCT
COMMON BILE DUCT
GALLBLADDER
HEPATICO-PANCREATIC DUCT
VENTRAL PANCREAS

YOLK SAC (CUT AWAY)

HINDGUT

1. BUD FORMATION

COMMON HEPATIC DUCT
PORTAL VEIN
GALL-BLADDER
COMMON BILE DUCT
VENTRAL PANCREAS
DORSAL PANCREAS
SUPERIOR MESENTERIC VEIN

2. BEGINNING ROTATION OF COMMON DUCT AND OF VENTRAL PANCREAS

DORSAL PANCREAS
VENTRAL PANCREAS

3. ROTATION COMPLETED BUT FUSION HAS NOT YET TAKEN PLACE

ACCESSORY PANCREATIC DUCT (SANTORINI'S)
PANCREATIC DUCT (WIRSUNG'S)

4. FUSION OF VENTRAL AND DORSAL PANCREAS AND UNION OF DUCTS

FORMATION OF ACINI AND ISLETS FROM DUCTS. A—ACINI; I—ISLETS IN VARIOUS STAGES OF DEVELOPMENT

RELATIONSHIP OF INTERCALATED DUCT AND CENTRO-ACINAR CELLS TO ACINI

The pancreas arises in 3- to 4-mm.-long embryos from two diverticula of the foregut in a region which later becomes the duodenum. A larger bud develops dorsal and proximal just above the level of the hepatic diverticulum (see page 2). Growing fairly rapidly and extending into the dorsal mesentery of the duodenum near the developing omental bursa, the *dorsal pancreas bud* passes in front of the developing portal vein. The *ventral and distal bud* is smaller and consists initially of paired anlagen of which the left regresses. It originates in close approximation to (or directly from) the *gallbladder* part of the *hepatic diverticulum,* between the latter and the yolk sac. Because of the more rapid growth of the duodenum, the ventral bud, together with the developing *common bile duct,* rotates backward behind the duodenum. When the *rotation* is completed, the original ventral bud comes to lie close to and below and somewhat behind the dorsal pancreas, and eventually its tip lies behind the *superior mesenteric vein* and the root of the portal vein. It also grows into the mesoduodenum, and both *pancreas anlagen fuse.* As the pancreas becomes flattened and attached to the posterior abdominal wall, the right leaflet of the mesoduodenum is absorbed, so that the pancreas is covered only by the left leaflet and appears to lie retroperitoneally.

From the larger dorsal bud originates the cephalic part of the head as well as the body and tail, whereas the caudal part of the head and the uncinate process derive from the smaller ventral bud. Ducts develop in both buds but anastomose when the buds interlock. The secretion of body and tail is subsequently shunted into the duct of the smaller ventral pancreas, which thus becomes the *pancreatic duct (of Wirsung).* Only the upper portion of the head is finally drained by the original duct of the dorsal pancreas, the *accessory pancreatic duct (of Santorini).* A common terminal ampulla of the pancreatic and common bile ducts exists in the adult if the embryonic hepatopancreatic duct persists (see pages 2 and 24).

In early embryonal stages the pancreas consists of tubules from which laterally, as well as at their blind ends, vesicles, the future *acini,* arise. These are first solid but soon develop a central cavity. The budding vesicles, while subsequently partially or completely subdividing, become lined by a single layer of conical epithelium which retains the ability of division. Some acinar cells in the incompletely subdivided vesicles may fail to develop into secreting elements and retain a ductal character, to *connect the acini with the intercalated ducts.* At many places of the same embryonal ductal system which gives rise to the acini and ducts, some cells are pushed out from the tubules. These cells divide and grow into cell masses, which become the *pancreatic islands.* According to available evidence, the acini cannot be transferred into islands; however, the ducts retain the ability to form islands if excessive regeneration takes place during extra-uterine life.

PANCREAS
Anatomy and Histology

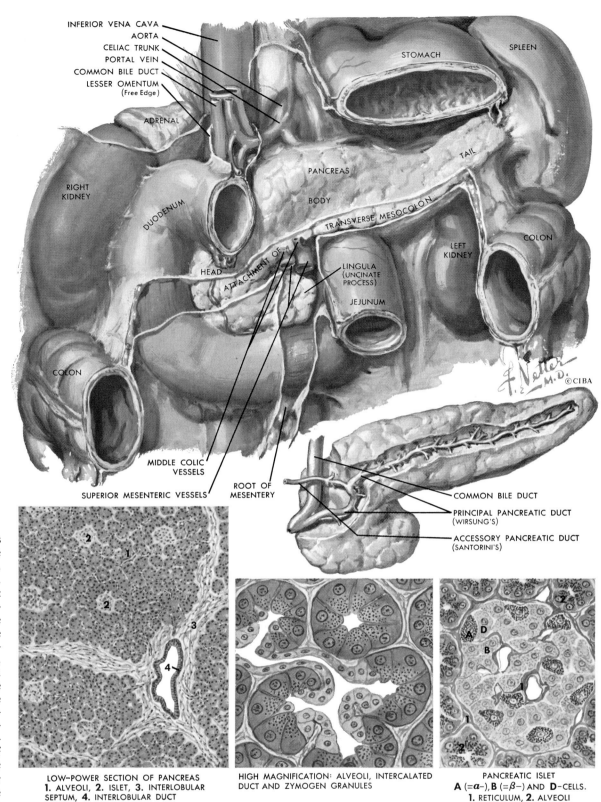

LOW-POWER SECTION OF PANCREAS
1. ALVEOLI, 2. ISLET, 3. INTERLOBULAR SEPTUM, 4. INTERLOBULAR DUCT

HIGH MAGNIFICATION: ALVEOLI, INTERCALATED DUCT AND ZYMOGEN GRANULES

PANCREATIC ISLET
A (=α-), B (=β-) AND D-CELLS.
1. RETICULUM, 2. ALVEOLI

The pancreas, 4 to 6 in. long, extends transversely across the abdomen from the concavity of the duodenum to the spleen. Its color is yellow with a reddish hue. Located deep in the epigastrium and left hypochondrium behind the lesser omental sac, approximately on the level of the first and second lumbar vertebrae, the pancreas escapes direct physical examination. The right extremity of the pancreas, the *head*, is globular in shape with an inferior extension, the *lingula* (uncinate process), projecting like a hook to the left and crossed anteriorly by the *superior mesenteric vessels*. The head, covered anteriorly by the pylorus and transverse colon, fits snugly into the loop of the duodenum, so that the *common bile duct* passes either through a groove or through the substance of the gland. The posterior surface of the head touches the *inferior vena cava*, left renal vein and *aorta*. The head narrows into the body from caudad right to cephalad left behind the pylorus and in front of the origin of the *portal vein*. The prismatic body then bulges upward as the *tuber omentale* in its right half to reach almost the level of the *celiac trunk*. The splenic artery extends along its upper edge. Its anterior surface, covered by serosa, is separated by the omental bursa from the posterior wall of the *stomach*. The inferior surface, below the attachment of the *transverse mesocolon*, is related to the duodenojejunal junction and to the splenic flexure of the colon. The posterior surface is in contact with the aorta, the splenic vein and the *left kidney*, where the body tapers off into a short *tail*.

The *pancreatic duct (of Wirsung)* starts in the tail by confluence of several small ducts and extends into the head, where it turns downward and backward to approximate the infraduodenal portion of the *common bile duct*. It terminates at the papilla in the duodenum (see pages 24 and 27). This principal duct drains the greater part of the gland. As a rule, only a small upper anterior part of the head uses the *accessory pancreatic duct (of Santorini)* which enters the duodenum at a small accessory papilla.

The glandular *alveoli*, bound together by tracts of connective tissue forming the interlobular septa, are composed of high cuboidal or conical cells arranged in single layers around a basement membrane. The nuclei are surrounded by basophilic cytoplasm, whereas the cytoplasm near the lumen varies in appearance, depending on secretory activity. During the resting stage the acinar lumen is small, and the cytoplasm of the secretory cells is filled with refractile *zymogen granules*. They disappear during secretion, and the lumen widens to contain secretory material. Frequently, flat cells without zymogen granules extend as centro-acinar cells into the alveolar lumen. The *interlobular ducts*, surrounded by dense collagenous tissue, are lined by columnar epithelium which becomes cuboidal when the ducts terminate with the *intercalated ducts*.

The *islands (of Langerhans)*, scattered all over the gland, consist of cells structurally and tinctorially different from the exocrine parenchyma. The most frequent cell is the β-cell, which in routine stains has faintly recognizable granules, probably presenting the precursor of insulin. The α-cells have distinct acidophilic granules readily impregnated with silver and represent possibly the precursor of glucagon. The sparse D-cells are free of granules.

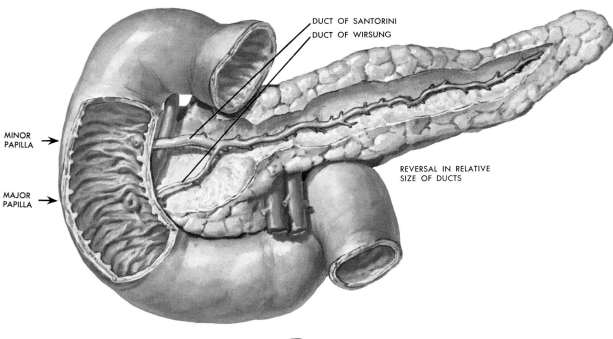

DUCT OF SANTORINI
DUCT OF WIRSUNG

MINOR PAPILLA →

MAJOR PAPILLA →

REVERSAL IN RELATIVE SIZE OF DUCTS

PANCREATIC DUCTS AND VARIATIONS

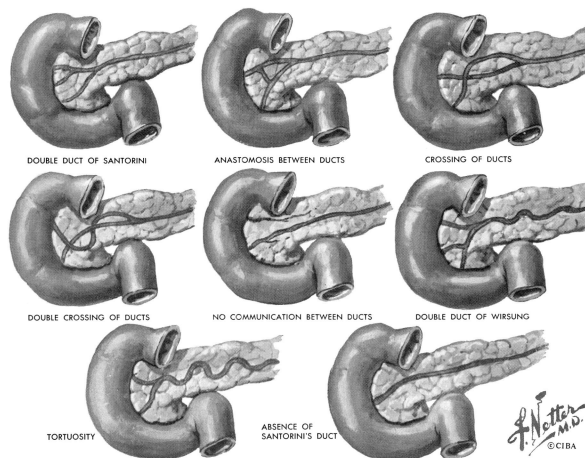

DOUBLE DUCT OF SANTORINI   ANASTOMOSIS BETWEEN DUCTS   CROSSING OF DUCTS

DOUBLE CROSSING OF DUCTS   NO COMMUNICATION BETWEEN DUCTS   DOUBLE DUCT OF WIRSUNG

TORTUOSITY   ABSENCE OF SANTORINI'S DUCT

The arrangement of the pancreatic ducts within the gland varies considerably and even more so in their relationships with the terminal common bile duct (see also pages 22 and 24). The main pancreatic duct (duct of Wirsung) arises from the liver primordium as the ventral anlage of the pancreas (see page 25), and the accessory pancreatic duct (duct of Santorini) originates as the dorsal anlage from the foregut itself. During the developmental period the dorsal pancreas makes up the major part of the body and the tail, so that the accessory duct courses through the major extent of the gland. At the time of fusion, the duct of Wirsung of the ventral anlage joins the duct of the dorsal anlage and becomes the main pancreatic duct. Occasionally, the *relative size* of the two *ducts* is *reversed,* so that the duct of Santorini remains the main duct. The accessory duct ordinarily inserts into the duodenum proximally, on a separate papilla (minor, see page 24). The main pancreatic duct enters the duodenum on the papilla of Vater either through a separate orifice or through a common channel, the ampulla of Vater. The ampulla varies in width from 1.5 to 4.5 mm. and in length from 1 to 14 mm., according to the individual distance from its opening in the duodenum to the start of the septum, which divides the common bile duct and the pancreatic duct. With a short ampulla the contracting sphincter of Oddi closes both ducts together, so that reflux cannot occur. With a longer ampulla, a common channel is present above the sphincter, so that reflux of bile into the pancreas or pancreatic juice into the biliary system can occur. This common channel with reflux remains one of the favored, though not generally accepted, etiologic explanations for acute pancreatitis and chronic or recurrent pancreatitis.

Within the gland itself the main pancreatic duct begins in the tail. It is centrally located as it courses to the right through the body and neck, being joined by tributaries which usually enter at right angles, alternating from opposite sides. In the head the main duct usually turns caudally and dorsally and comes in close proximity to the common bile duct or joins it as it courses through the substance of the pancreas. The main duct commonly drains the tail and body, as well as the caudal and dorsal portions of the head. In rare instances the main duct may collect only from these portions of the head.

The accessory duct usually communicates with the main duct, although occasionally they may have *no communication.* Several of the more common *variations in the course of the ducts* within the gland are illustrated. Their significance is not well documented, but it is conceivable that they may explain the marked variability in results with the numerous surgical procedures for pancreatitis (see page 144). A large accessory duct continuous or *anastomosing* with the main pancreatic duct could well relieve the pressure and damage from reflux produced as a result of a common ampulla of the biliary and pancreatic ducts, whereas completely separate ducts or narrow connections would have an opposite effect and could produce serious damage.

The smaller ductules ramify to connect with the lobules of the gland and in the alveoli, which are tubular, convoluted and almost filled with secreting cells.

PERITONEAL RELATIONS OF PANCREAS

During embryonal development (see also page 25) the anlagen of the body of the pancreas grow into the mesoduodenum and the dorsal mesogastrium. After the rotation of the stomach and intestine has taken place, the pancreas with its posterior peritoneal layer comes in contact with the parietal peritoneum over the posterior abdominal wall; both peritoneal layers fuse and obliterate, so that the pancreas becomes a retroperitoneal organ. The tail of the pancreas reaches the spleen and kidney and becomes fixed in the lienorenal ligament. After its rotation the transverse mesocolon becomes fused to the posterior layer of the greater omentum and so it appears to originate from the inferior border of the body and tail of the pancreas.

The dorsal surface of the tail reclines upon the *left kidney* and renal vessels at the level of the twelfth thoracic and first lumbar vertebrae. The hilus of the *spleen* usually lies behind the tip of the tail. When the pancreas enlarges in its superior inferior diameter, it passes to the right and caudally, crossing the *aorta* and spine at the level of the first lumbar vertebra, overlapping the dorsal twelfth and lumbar second vertebrae. The *body* is anterior to the superior *mesenteric vessels,* which occasionally pass through the posterior portion of the gland, and the tip of the *uncinate process* lies behind these vessels on the aorta and *vena cava* at the level of the second lumbar vertebra. The splenic vein passes behind the central portion of the gland, where it joins the superior mesenteric vein to form the portal vein (see page 18), which then extends cephalad and to the right behind the superior portion of the gland. It may actually pass through the gland substance. The *head* lies to the right of the spine on the inferior vena cava, and still more to the right it comes in contact with the right renal vein. The *common bile duct* passes caudally and to the right behind the upper portion of the head of the pancreas and then enters the substance of the gland, to reach the posteromedial border of the duodenum in company with the main pancreatic duct, with which it enters the duodenum on the *major papilla* (*of Vater*) (see pages 24, 26 and 27).

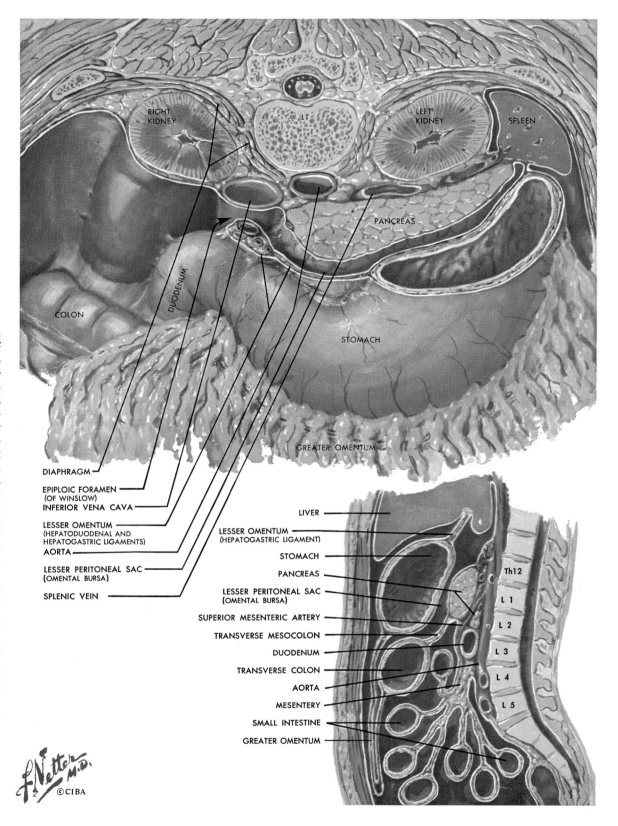

DIAPHRAGM

EPIPLOIC FORAMEN (OF WINSLOW)
INFERIOR VENA CAVA

LESSER OMENTUM (HEPATODUODENAL AND HEPATOGASTRIC LIGAMENTS)
AORTA

LESSER PERITONEAL SAC (OMENTAL BURSA)

SPLENIC VEIN

RIGHT KIDNEY · L1 · LEFT KIDNEY · SPLEEN · PANCREAS · DUODENUM · COLON · STOMACH · GREATER OMENTUM

LIVER
LESSER OMENTUM (HEPATOGASTRIC LIGAMENT)
STOMACH
PANCREAS
LESSER PERITONEAL SAC (OMENTAL BURSA)
SUPERIOR MESENTERIC ARTERY
TRANSVERSE MESOCOLON
DUODENUM
TRANSVERSE COLON
AORTA
MESENTERY
SMALL INTESTINE
GREATER OMENTUM
Th12 · L1 · L2 · L3 · L4 · L5

The anterior surface of the pancreas and the superior edge of the tail and body are normally covered by the posterior peritoneum of the omental bursa, or *lesser peritoneal sac.* This sac is frequently partially or completely obliterated by adhesions. The stomach, *hepatogastric* mesentery and gastrocolic omentum come to be in more or less close contact with the anterior surface. With severe gastroptosis almost the entire gland may be covered only by the hepatogastric mesentery or the edge of the liver. The attachment of the mesentery of the transverse colon lies along the inferior margin of the gland except over the head, where it passes across the midportion of the head from left to right (see page 26). The pylorus and first portion of the *duodenum* lie anterior to the superior edge of the head of the pancreas, and the head is surrounded by the loop of the duodenum, with the third portion of the duodenum lying behind the inferior edge of the uncinate process. The pancreas tends to overlap the duodenum in the second part, especially posteriorly, and this may reach any stage to complete encirclement, as in annular pancreas (see page 141).

The inferior portion of the head, and sometimes the *body,* may lie in the posterior wall of the greater peritoneal cavity, covered only by peritoneum and in contact with the redundant transverse colon or loops of small bowel.

The major difficulties of exposure and removal of the pancreas (see page 29) lie in this close approximation of the vessels (see pages 14 and 15) with their accompanying lymphatics, and particularly the superior mesenteric vessels and portal vein which are frequently invaded by tumor, or lie within the substance of the gland, making removal impossible without damage to the vessels.

SURGICAL APPROACHES TO PANCREAS

The posterior position of the pancreas, completely covered by the stomach, colon and gastrocolic ligament (see page 28), and its close proximity to important vessels (see pages 14 and 15) make difficult the adequate exposure of this organ.

The *anterior surface* of the head, body and tail is best exposed through the gastrocolic omentum. The gastro-epiploic vessels (see pages 14 and 15) may be spared, and the middle colic vessels must be gently dissected off the pancreas. The transverse mesocolon is in contact with the anterior surface of the head and passes along the inferior border of the gland, so in order to get adequate exposure of the head it may be necessary to mobilize the hepatic flexure and the right half of the transverse mesocolon.

The *tail of the gland* lies in the phrenicolienal ligament in the hilus of the spleen. All its surfaces — anterior, posterior, superior and inferior — may be explored by mobilizing the tail together with the spleen and splenic vessels. The splenic artery courses along the superior surface of the gland but is very tortuous and may overlap the gland and send short branches to the body and the tail (see pages 14 and 15). Entrance may be made through the hepatogastric ligament (see pages 6 and 28) for limited exposure of the superior surface of the gland and especially for exposure of many false cysts (see page 145), which frequently lie in the lesser sac, presenting above the lesser curvature of the stomach.

The uncinate process of the head can be visualized and explored but poorly, since it is superposed by the superior mesenteric artery and veins at the point of origin of the middle colic and inferior pancreaticoduodenal vessels. Though the superior mesenteric vessels may be freed and retracted to the right, it remains still difficult to palpate this portion of the gland.

Exposure of the posterior surface of the head of the pancreas and the extra- and intrapancreatic portions of the lower common bile duct is frequently most desirable to clarify early the causes of jaundice or of an ampullary obstruction. Through a generous upper abdominal incision, the common duct and gallbladder are examined for distention due to obstruction. The peritoneum is incised around the loop of the duodenum, the

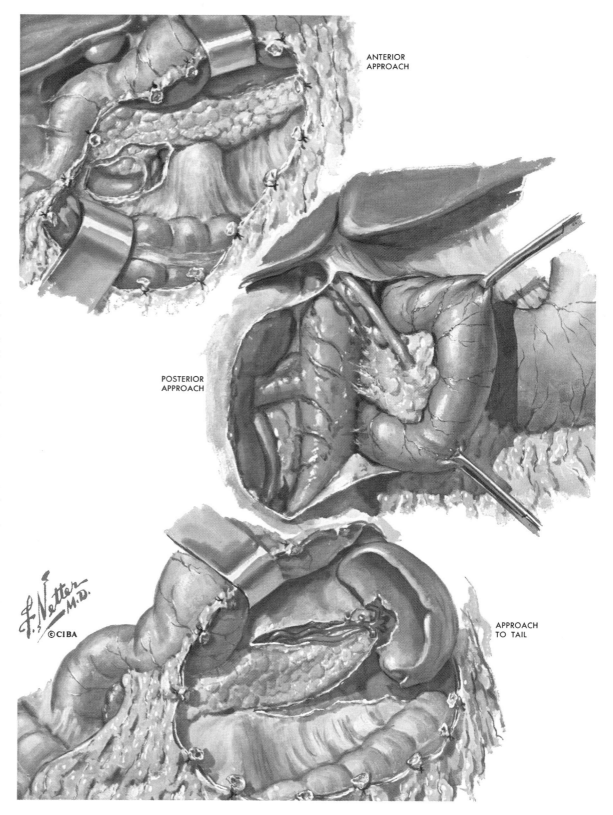

ANTERIOR APPROACH

POSTERIOR APPROACH

APPROACH TO TAIL

plane posterior to the duodenum and pancreas is entered and the organs are lifted upward and to the left. The limitation of this exposure, once again, is the superior mesenteric vessels and their branches, especially the inferior pancreaticoduodenal vessels (see page 15), which hold the gland in place against the posterior wall by either actually passing through its substance or over the uncinate process and the duodenum. The common bile duct may be palpated throughout its entire course, and the lymph nodes around the duct may be visualized and examined. By careful dissection close to the duodenal wall, the pancreatic duct may also be visualized. Dilatation of the pancreatic duct can usually be seen or palpated through the gland substance.

The posterior surface of the head may be explored further by dividing the right gastric and gastroduodenal arteries at their origin from the hepatic, mobilizing the common duct further and visualizing the superior surface of the portal vein. A finger can then be passed downward between the head of the pancreas and the portal vein to appear below the body of the pancreas over the superior mesenteric vessels.

Biopsy of the gland during operation must be approached with caution, especially on the posterior surface of the head. An opening into a large duct can result in prolonged drainage from a pancreatic fistula, which is extremely irritating to the tissues and skin and very debilitating because of loss of electrolytes in the pancreatic secretions. Biopsy may fail to capture tumor tissue even though a tumor is present, and this may lead to false diagnosis and treatment. Chronic pancreatitis distal to the tumor, or overlying it, may be difficult, if not impossible, to distinguish grossly from the tumor and may thus be biopsied erroneously.

LYMPHATIC DRAINAGE OF PANCREAS

The lymphatics of the pancreas arise as fine perilobular capillaries, combining to form larger vessels, in the interlobular spaces and extending along the blood vessels to the surface of the gland. Where the pancreas is closely attached to other organs, such as the duodenum, direct lymphatic connections exist. Although the lymphatic vessels are believed to have valves directing the flow in the proper direction, this mechanism could easily be broken, causing a flow from pancreas to duodenum and vice versa. This situation may explain, in part, the frequent involvement of both organs by carcinoma, arising primarily in one or the other, but it also has been considered that infection might spread from acute duodenitis and cause pancreatitis.

On the anterior surface of the tail and body, the lymphatic trunks emerge from the gland and pass largely to the superior edge and to the tail, to collect in lymph nodes and lymphatic channels along the splenic artery and vein. These trunks and nodes drain primarily into the *celiac nodes* and lymphatics, which have direct connection with the left *gastric nodes* and the chain of *hepatic nodes*. Secondary connections with the mediastinal and cervical nodes explain the appearance of cancer metastases in the supraclavicular nodes (Virchow's node). The lymphatics of the tail are intimately associated with the splenic and the *pancreaticolienal nodes* at the hilus of the spleen and around the splenic vessels, respectively.

The anterior surface of the right half of the body and head drains into two systems. The first of these, the *pancreaticolienal* nodes and the *pyloric* nodes, constitute the upper draining system. These are spaced along the superior pancreaticoduodenal vessels, are connected with celiac and hepatic nodes, and have a direct continuity with the gastric lymphatics along the right gastric vessels. The second system is constituted by the so-called retropancreatic nodes which collect trunks from the anterior, posterior and inferior surfaces of the head and the uncinate process. They follow the

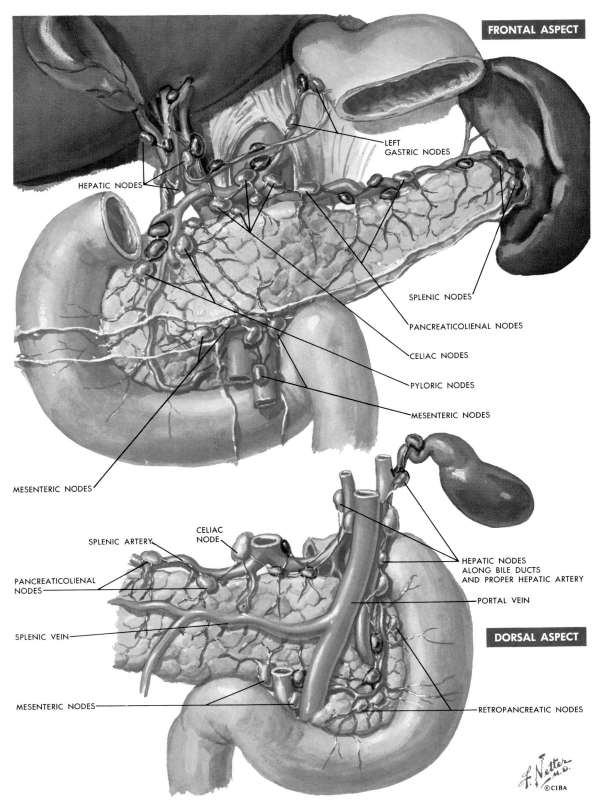

FRONTAL ASPECT

LEFT GASTRIC NODES

HEPATIC NODES

SPLENIC NODES

PANCREATICOLIENAL NODES

CELIAC NODES

PYLORIC NODES

MESENTERIC NODES

MESENTERIC NODES

SPLENIC ARTERY

CELIAC NODE

PANCREATICOLIENAL NODES

SPLENIC VEIN

MESENTERIC NODES

HEPATIC NODES ALONG BILE DUCTS AND PROPER HEPATIC ARTERY

PORTAL VEIN

DORSAL ASPECT

RETROPANCREATIC NODES

posterior superior pancreaticoduodenal vessels to the hepatic and celiac nodes and the posterior inferior pancreaticoduodenal vessels to the *mesenteric nodes,* thence to the peri-aortic chain. *Mesenteric* nodes lying in the root of the transverse mesocolon also drain adjacent portions of the pancreas.

The posterior surface of the head of the gland actually drains directly into all these nodes except the pancreaticolienal nodes. Anastomoses with the duodenal lymphatics are frequent. The primary drainage from the posterior surface is cephalad along the common bile duct to drain into the lymphatics along the bile ducts and thus to the hepatic nodes (see page 20). Since the posterior surface of the pancreas is in direct contact with the areolar tissue of the posterior abdominal wall without peritoneal covering, direct lymphatic connections exist with the posterior abdominal wall and other retroperitoneal structures, includ-

ing the perineural lymphatics. It is this profuse intermingling of the pancreatic lymphatics with lymphatic channels of other organs and the retroperitoneal tissues, with the lack of restraining peritoneal or fascial covering, which explains the rapid spread of carcinoma or infections within the pancreas to other structures, making diagnosis and treatment in many cases so difficult. These lymphatic relations are also of importance in determining the extent of surgery in carcinoma, particularly of the stomach. The duodenal lymphatics and those of the head of the pancreas, particularly of the upper system, are intimately related. As a matter of fact, some of the duodenal lymphatic channels pass through the pancreas and cannot be distinguished from the lymph vessels of the pancreas itself. This contingence has been supposed to represent a possible route for the spreading of infections leading to pancreatitis.

INNERVATION OF PANCREAS

As are the liver (see page 21) and other intra-abdominal organs, the pancreas is innervated by the sympathetic and parasympathetic systems. The sympathetic nerves reach the pancreas through the greater and lesser splanchnic trunks arising from the fifth to the ninth, sometimes to the tenth or eleventh, thoracic ganglia. It is generally agreed that the major sympathetic innervation is through the greater splanchnic nerve. The parasympathetic fibers reach the gland through the vagi. All the nerves of the pancreas, both afferent and efferent, pass through the *celiac plexus*, and complete excision of the celiac plexus thoroughly denervates the gland. The sympathetic preganglionic fibers terminate in the *celiac* or *superior mesenteric ganglia*, whereas the parasympathetics terminate in intrinsic pancreatic ganglia. From the celiac and superior mesenteric ganglia, the nerve fibers proceed along the vessels to the pancreas. The major number accompany the pancreatico-duodenal vessels. Some fibers accompany the splenic vessels, but most of those escorting the splenic vessels terminate in the spleen. The sympathetic (splanchnic) fibers are distributed only, or at least primarily, to the blood vessels of the pancreas, though this concept is still controversial. The parasympathetic fibers (vagi) accompany the vessels as far as the arterioles and then disperse between the pancreatic lobules and around the acini, ultimately finding their *endings* on individual cells (see *schema of intrinsic nerve supply*). These nerves serve both the external secreting acini and the islet cells, and it is stated that the same single fibers may innervate both types of cell. The smooth muscle of the duct is innervated by parasympathetic fibers.

Afferent pain fibers from the pancreas are believed to traverse both the sympathetic and vagus pathways passing through the celiac ganglia but are apparently limited to the greater splanchnic nerves. The level of the *common areas of pancreatic pain* (epigastric, left upper quadrant and back) and the relief of pain by splanchnicectomy are in keeping with this opinion.

A definite knowledge of the results of nerve stimulation on pancreatic secretion is somewhat obscured by the hormonal effects of secretin deriving from the duodenal mucosa (see page 55). The understanding of the influence of nerve stimulation is, furthermore, complicated by the simultaneous action of the nerves on the pancreatic vessels, ducts and secretory cells. The innervation of the vascular apparatus and its surgical interruption may be of some importance for the origin of pain in acute pancreatitis and its relief, respectively.

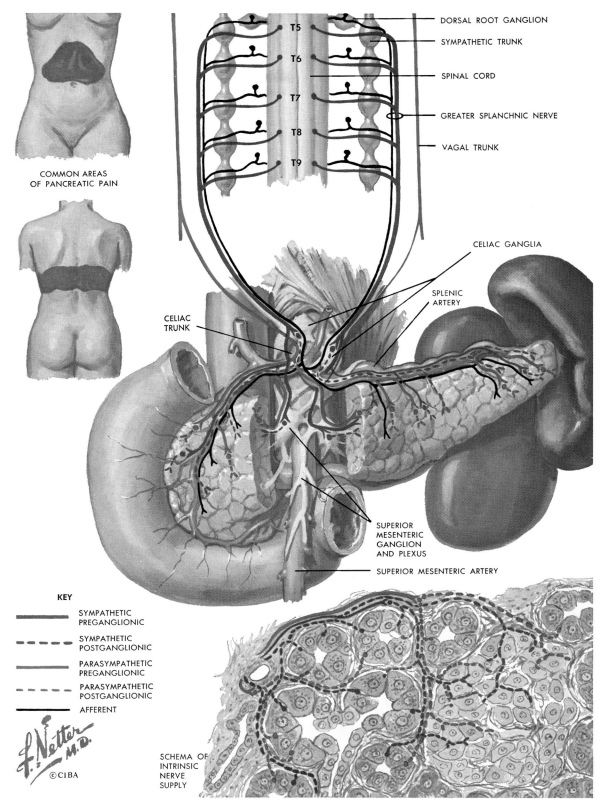

COMMON AREAS OF PANCREATIC PAIN

DORSAL ROOT GANGLION

SYMPATHETIC TRUNK

SPINAL CORD

GREATER SPLANCHNIC NERVE

VAGAL TRUNK

T5

T6

T7

T8

T9

CELIAC GANGLIA

SPLENIC ARTERY

CELIAC TRUNK

SUPERIOR MESENTERIC GANGLION AND PLEXUS

SUPERIOR MESENTERIC ARTERY

KEY

SYMPATHETIC PREGANGLIONIC

SYMPATHETIC POSTGANGLIONIC

PARASYMPATHETIC PREGANGLIONIC

PARASYMPATHETIC POSTGANGLIONIC

AFFERENT

SCHEMA OF INTRINSIC NERVE SUPPLY

Stimulation of the vagus nerves increases the enzyme content of the pancreatic secretions. A similar but slight effect attributed to sympathetic stimulation is probably to be explained by the interference of vascular responses. Vagotomy and atropine both markedly reduce the secretion of enzymes in the pancreatic juice, whereas pilocarpine significantly increases such secretion. Stimulation of the ducts should also be considered in studies of this kind, since constriction of the ducts resulting from splanchnic stimulation slows passage of the pancreatic juice. In general, it can be said that splanchnicectomy will frequently give relief of pain for varying periods of time and anesthetic block of the splanchnic or celiac plexus frequently results in relief of the severe pain of acute pancreatitis. Left splanchnicectomy is most commonly used for relief of pancreatic pain and is frequently successful, but in some cases a right splanchnicectomy becomes necessary later, and, therefore, some surgeons do both at the original operation. Vagotomy, if effective, acts in two ways: first, by decreasing acid secretion in the stomach and so decreasing secretin formation and, second, by directly decreasing the stimulation of pancreatic secretion. To prevent recurrent attacks of pancreatitis, neither splanchnicectomy nor vagotomy nor both has been successful in most cases. With progressive pancreatic disease, the process extends beyond the gland substance and, eventually, involves the peripheral nerves in the area, particularly in the posterior abdominal wall. This results in persistent or recurrent pain, which is completely unaffected by attacks on the sympathetic or parasympathetic nerves. With carcinoma of the pancreas, the perineural lymphatics are frequently involved, leading not only to spread of the tumor by this path but to intractable pain.

Section XVI

PHYSIOLOGY AND PATHOPHYSIOLOGY OF THE LIVER, BILIARY TRACT AND PANCREAS, INCLUDING HEPATIC AND PANCREATIC TESTS

by

FRANK H. NETTER, M.D.

in collaboration with

OSCAR BODANSKY, M.D.
Plates 20-23

HANS POPPER, M.D.
Plates 1-19

LIVER FUNCTIONS

The liver, ranking first in size as a parenchymal organ, takes also first position in number, variety and complexity of functional accomplishments. Only the most essential features of the liver's physiology and those which are of principal interest for the practice of medicine are illustrated and discussed in the following pages of this section. In the accompanying plate an attempt has been made to present a classifying and summarizing survey.

Holding a strategic position between the intestinal and general circulation and harboring, according to its dimensions, a large amount of blood and extracellular fluid, the liver exercises a major influence upon the volume of circulating blood and its constituents. The liver *acts as a sponge* or "flood chamber", which can be filled or congested (see page 106) as, *e.g.,* in failure of the right heart, or which may be emptied, causing an overload of the pulmonary circulation. The *"filter action"* of the liver also results from its peculiar anatomic location, since all nutrients, and also injurious materials absorbed by the intestines, are brought to the organ via the portal system. The effect of the liver on *water and electrolyte balance,* though it is regulated mainly by the kidneys, lungs, adrenals and the hypophysis, should not be underestimated, not only because of the large parenchymal mass of the organ but also because all the ingested water and salts pass through the liver before entering other extracellular departments.

The *hexagonal,* epithelial *liver cells* have multitudinous and most diversified functions. They are the site of the chemical transformations that make body constituents from foodstuffs or their digested breakdown products and which correlate the three main categories of organic body material, so that the totality of the liver cells becomes a great *"metabolic pool"* (see page 36) of the organism. The versatility of this central chemical laboratory of the organism together with the liver's *storage* capacity for glycogen, proteins, fats and vitamins is of utmost

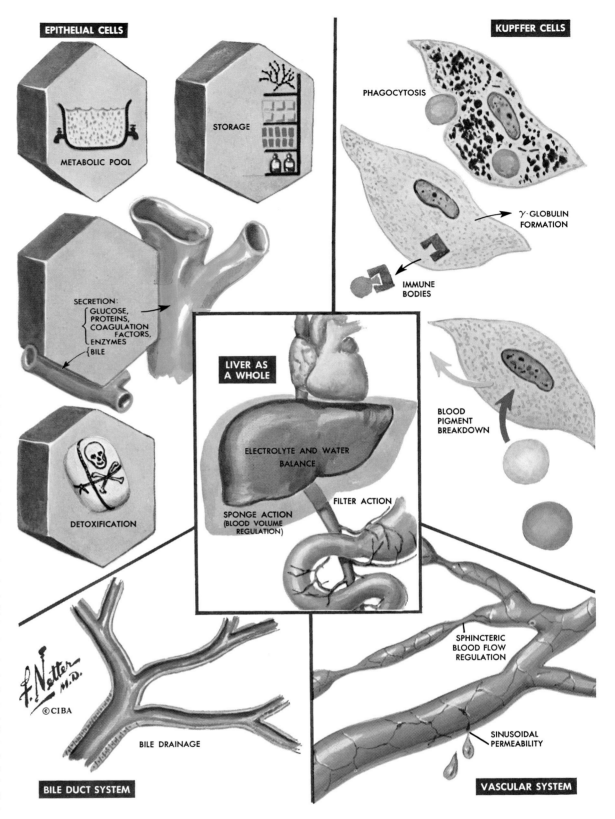

significance for the energy economy of the entire body. The liver stores these organic materials not only for its own need but to satisfy the needs of distant organs. It gives *glucose* to the blood to maintain the sugar level and to supply energy for all vital phenomena. The liver cells form many of the serum proteins to provide forces for the oncotic pressure of the plasma or to be used as a transport vehicle for water-insoluble compounds, or as *coagulating factors* or to fulfill enzymatic functions, etc.

The epithelial hepatic cells, furthermore, protect the organism from injurious agents by a variety of *detoxification processes* (see page 44), which yield substances deprived of detrimental properties.

The bile, also manufactured by the epithelial cells, contains the characteristic bile pigments (see page 47), salts of bile acids, cholesterol and a number of other components. It is excreted into the bile capil-

laries and leaves the liver through the intrahepatic *bile duct system* (see page 11) to reach the duodenum via the extrahepatic bile tract.

The *Kupffer cells,* besides functioning as endothelial cells like others elsewhere in the organism, represent the quantitatively most important part of the reticulo-endothelial system. These cells are concerned with the *breakdown* of *hemoglobin* to bilirubin, participate in the formation of γ-globulin and immune bodies, and act as scavenger cells removing by phagocytosis pigments, bacteria and other corpuscular or macromolecular elements.

The liver's vascular system serves the proper intrahepatic blood distribution by sphincter actions. The two blood supplies (hepatic artery under high and portal vein under low pressure) are harmonized. The hepatic sinusoids differ from other capillaries in that they have a greater permeability for proteins.

THE "METABOLIC POOL"

The liver is the main site of the interchange, synthesis, breakdown and storage of the foodstuffs, their metabolites, the tissue constituents and other substances necessary for the material balance of the body. The following survey, incomplete and inadequate as it must be in view of the manifold facets of biochemical reactions, and the diagrammatic illustration serve only to emphasize the complexity of the organ's metabolic function and to create a prospective understanding of the diagnostic hepatic tests discussed in the following pages.

Carbohydrates or sugars are ingested in the form of polysaccharides, such as starch, or oligosaccharides, *e.g.*, sucrose, the common commercial sugar, or lactose, otherwise called milk sugar. In the intestine the oligo- and polysaccharides are broken down enzymatically into monosaccharides, the hexoses and pentoses, the simple form of the sugars represented by glucose, fructose, galactose, ribose and others. The simple sugars enter the liver via the portal vein and are either transferred directly into the general circulation or are retained by the liver where, with the aid of the enzyme *hexokinase* and adenosine triphosphate (ATP), they are transformed into hexose-6-phosphate. (The number refers to the structural position of the carbon atom to which the phosphate molecule is attached.) Hexose-6-phosphate, in turn, is enzymatically transformed into hexose-1-phosphate, which subsequently loses the phosphate moiety under the influence of *phosphorylases*. The hexose is then, by enzymatic action, incorporated into the branched chain polymer, known as glycogen. *Hepatic glycogen* is the main form of carbohydrate storage. The process of glycogen synthesis is called glycogenesis; the breakdown of glycogen to liberate glucose, thereby maintaining the blood sugar level, is glycogenolysis. In this latter process glycogen is attacked by a *debranching enzyme* and again esterified with phosphate by a phosphorylase. This series of polymerizing and depolymerizing reactions involves a highly interrelated and complex sequence of enzymatically controlled events. For practical purposes glycogenolysis might be considered the reversal of glycogenesis. Both processes, as established by animal experiments, run continuously side by side, glycogen being formed and broken down simultaneously, with one phase or the other predominating in accord with the energy requirements of the organism. Deficiency of one of the enzymes involved in this reciprocal interaction, as, *e.g.*, in Gierke's disease (see page 86), will lead to serious metabolic disturbances, the consequences of which are not restricted to the liver alone. The quantity of glycogen stored in the liver depends on many factors. High carbohydrate intake increases and a prolonged carbohydrate-deficient diet decreases the

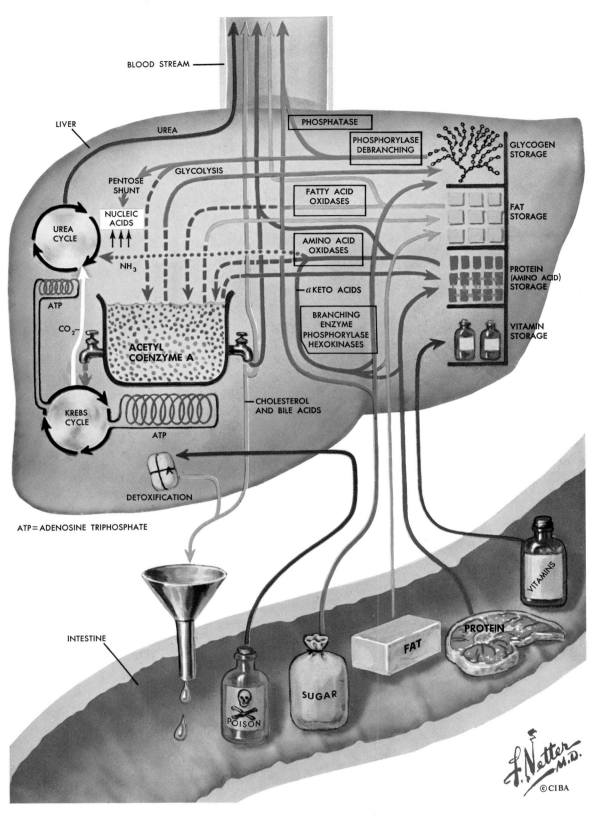

glycogen reserves. Extreme inactivity and exercise have similar effects, respectively. The supply of sugar and the need for it elsewhere in the body determine the amount of glycogen in the liver at a given moment.

Not all glucose arriving in the liver from the intestine or released from the breakdown of glycogen enters the blood stream. Some of the glucose, in the stage of the 6-phosphate ester, is oxidized with the loss of 1 carbon atom. This process, the hexose monophosphate shunt (HMP) (or *pentose shunt*), yields a 5-carbon sugar, a pentose which, besides being broken down for energy purposes over 3-carbon compounds, is used for the biosynthesis of nucleotides and *nucleic acids*. The former consists of a pentose (ribose) or desoxypentose esterified with phosphoric acid and combined with one of two classes of basic substances known as purines and pyrimidines. The nucleotides are polymerized to nucleic acids, which

in combination with certain proteins are designated nucleoproteins, universally present in all cells. The hexose monophosphate shunt, one of the processes for the synthesis of nucleic acids, is not specific for the liver, but it is an important feature of the hepatic metabolic functions, since one of the resulting compounds is *adenosine triphosphate* (ATP). This ribose- and adenosine-containing compound with high-energy phosphate bonds (symbolized in the picture by a heating coil), provides the energy transfer required for many of the biochemical reactions and transformations carried out by the liver.

Another part of the glucose in the liver is directly transformed into compounds with 3 carbon atoms, *e.g.*, pyruvic acid. This is an important intermediate link in a great number of chemical reactions concerning carbohydrate and protein metabolism. A major

(Continued on page 37)

(Continued from page 36)

function of pyruvic acid is its rôle as precursor for the 2-carbon structures, the acetyl radical and acetate ion, connecting links between carbohydrate and fat metabolism. Together with other short-chain carbon compounds, these form the *"metabolic pool"* which is fed by small molecular breakdown products and which supplies "building stones" common to all three classes of body constituents, carbohydrates, proteins and lipids. The acetyl and acetate structures never exist in free form but are coupled with other compounds, of which coenzyme A is of particular importance. The latter is a complex composed of the vitamin pantothenic acid, phosphorylated adenosine and sulfur-containing amine. Bound to the acetyl group, it becomes *acetylcoenzyme A*, the "active acetate" (more correctly "active acetyl") involved in numerous metabolic reactions, among which are those of the tricarboxylic acid cycle or *"Krebs cycle"*. This cycle is the aerobic phase of carbohydrate oxidation and the "final common pathway" of fat and protein metabolism.

Neutral fat, i.e., glycerol esterified with three long-chain fatty acid molecules, is hydrolyzed by intestinal lipases, but whether, as assumed formerly, this hydrolysis is complete, with the split products glycerol and fatty acids going their separate ways (via portal blood or lymphatics, respectively), is a subject now being critically reinvestigated. Perhaps only one third of the neutral fat is completely split into glycerol and fatty acids. The water-soluble glycerol is transported with the portal venous blood to the liver, where, as a 3-carbon compound, it may enter several metabolic pathways. The fatty acids, according to recent but not definite evidence, may enter into water-soluble complexes with bile salts and may enter the intestinal wall in such form. This explains the disturbance of fat digestion in biliary obstruction, the appearance of fatty acids as soap in the feces, etc. The fatty acids, according to one theory, are subsequently released in the intestinal wall and may be resynthesized to neutral fat with glycerol. This neutral fat is probably transported via the lymphatics to the peripheral fat depots, as well as to the fat reservoirs of the liver. The neutral fat in the periphery can be transported to the liver if the depots of that organ are exhausted. In general, fat utilization is much the same in the liver as elsewhere. After hydrolysis, glycerol may be consumed in the manner described above. Fatty acids are broken down by specific *oxidases* through gradual shortening of the long fatty acid chain yielding 2-carbon metabolites which join the "metabolic pool" and may contribute to the formation of acetylcoenzyme A, thus providing one of the connecting links between fat and carbohydrate metabolism. By a reversal of fatty acid degradation, the liver can synthesize fatty acids and also neutral fat by subsequent esterification with glycerol. Under normal conditions these anabolic and catabolic processes, as well as the storage and release of liver fat, are in equilibrium. This equilibrium can be displaced in one direction or another in various ways, as, *e.g.,* by fat consumption, by a deficiency of the so-called lipotropic factors or by an imbalance between lipogenic factors and lipotropic factors. Included among the lipogenic factors are the sugars, alcohol and increased metabolic needs, as they are manifest during the period of growth or in pregnancy, when the requirements for lipotropic substances are increased. Contrariwise, the need for lipotropes is reduced with lowered metabolic needs, as in a cold climate or subsequent to a strongly restricted total caloric intake. The lipotropic substances, an

example of which is choline, favor fat removal from the liver by a mechanism not yet completely understood. Evidence points to the possibility that choline supports the hepatic oxidation of fatty acids. Another hypothesis is that choline, as a part of the phosphatid lecithin, is essential for the transport of fatty acids from the liver to the blood. The lipotropic action of protein rests mainly, but not entirely, upon those amino acids in the protein molecule which supply methyl groups for the formation of choline, such as methionine and serine. The dependence of lipotropic function on adequate carbohydrate metabolism is seen in various conditions, *e.g.,* in diabetes and starvation when the exhaustion of hepatic glycogen impedes fat removal from the liver. However, insulin deficiency, as in diabetes, exerts also a specific effect upon fat oxidation, and in starvation fat depots are transported to the liver. This delicate integration of protein, carbohydrate and lipid metabolism explains the pathologic features of the liver, as seen after periods of inadequate or unbalanced nutrition (see pages 77 and 78).

In the course of the oxidative degradation of the fatty acids by specific oxidases, a 4-carbon compound, aceto-acetic acid and its reduced derivative, β-hydroxybutyric acid, appears, particularly when the degradative process is accelerated under abnormal conditions. These compounds, known as ketone bodies, with which the decarboxylated derivative, acetone, is associated, are utilizable in the periphery, especially by muscular tissue but not by the liver which releases them to the blood. The liver, however, is the only place where they are formed as products of certain anabolic and catabolic reactions involved in the oxidation of fatty acids and their synthesis. The most important circumstances under which the ketone bodies rise over their normal low value in the blood are those which force the body to fall back on its energy reserves stored in fat, owing to insufficient carbohydrate reserves in the liver. Starvation and diabetes are typical examples. Similarly, low sugar and high fat intake favor fat utilization, with resultant ketonemia.

Though structurally quite different from the neutral fats, the phospholipids and steroidal compounds are classified under the lipids of the body because of some common physical characteristics, especially their solubility behavior, and to some extent because of their physiologic relationships. The synthesis of *cholesterol*, a compound with the steroid nucleus and a long carbon side chain, occurs predominantly though not exclusively in the liver. According to the best evidence presently available, its synthesis is the result of the condensation of 2-carbon residues involving acetylcoenzyme A. This points to the participation of the "metabolic pool" in steroid synthesis. Esterification of cholesterol with fatty acids takes place also in the liver, which also maintains a fairly stable ratio between free and esterified cholesterol. Variation of this ratio and of the absolute amount of cholesterol circulating in the blood has proved to be a sensitive index for functional deficiency of the liver (see page 42). Associated with hepatic cholesterol synthesis is, apparently, the formation of those specific liver products, the *bile acids*, which also contain the steroid nucleus and belong, together with cholesterol, to the main constituents of the bile.

Little is known about the synthesis and the metabolic fate of the phospholipids or phosphatides, other than that the liver probably plays a major rôle in the genesis and turnover of the serum phospholipids. Choline, a lipotropic factor (see above), is a structural component of leci-

thin. Transmethylation from methyl donors, necessary for the formation of choline and its joining with glycerophosphate and fatty acids to yield lecithin, occurs in the liver. With cephalin, another phospholipid, the situation is similar.

Proteins are broken down by intestinal enzymes to amino acids which are brought to the liver via portal venous blood. A part of the amino acids serve as constituents for specific cell proteins of the various peripheral tissues. Another portion may be retained in the liver or resynthesized into proteins, which either remain in the liver or proceed into the general circulation as plasma proteins. While all tissues form proteins, the plasma albumin, α-globulin and fibrinogen production seems to be a task reserved for the liver cells. Gamma globulin appears to be the product of the reticulo-endothelial system. Of the synthesis of other specific serum proteins we know little. The fate of some amino acids has been successfully investigated. It has been established that amino acids can be attacked by amino acid oxidases, which remove the amino group. The resulting deaminated products enter the "metabolic pool", where they are utilized in various ways; *e.g.,* the deamination product of glutamic acid is α-ketoglutaric acid, which can be utilized as a "building stone" for hexoses or fatty acids. Such an α-*keto acid* may also be reaminated. By a process called *transamination*, amino groups can be transferred from nitrogenous to nonnitrogenous compounds. Pyruvic acid in this manner becomes the amino acid alanine. The amino radical removed from amino acids can be carried away as ammonium salts, but to a greater extent, owing to the omnipresent *transaminating enzyme systems* and to the amino group acceptor quality of α-*keto acids,* they are re-utilized to form a variety of new amino acids. These interactions — only examples of many anabolic and catabolic processes involving amino acids — are not exclusive liver functions. However, the formation of urea, main end product of protein metabolism, seems to be entirely a function of the liver, which engages for this purpose a series of reactions known as the Krebs-Henseleit or *urea cycle*. The term "cycle" indicates that the urea production is performed in a continuous operation which starts and ends with one and the same compound, namely, the amino acid ornithine. The necessary energy for this process derives from adenosine triphosphate, the same energy source that plays a dominant rôle in the "metabolic pool". Failure of this exclusively hepatic synthesis of urea, as in liver diseases, leads to a diminished urea and increased amino acid level in the blood and in the urine (see pages 40 and 51).

The *detoxification* function of the liver is performed by a variety of chemical reactions, such as oxidation, methylation, acetylation, esterification and conjugation with glucuronic acid or glycine, of which especially the last has been utilized in the functional diagnosis of liver disease (see page 44). The inactivation of the steroid hormones (androgens, estrogens, progesterone and corticoids) by oxidation and esterification belongs also to this type of liver function.

Besides storing carbohydrate, fats and protein, the liver supports the economy of the organism by serving as *depot for vitamins*. Over 90 per cent of vitamin A is deposited in the liver (see page 7). The hepatic reserve for other vitamins in the liver is less impressive and to a great extent is shared with other tissues.

In recent years the emphasis, in metabolic study, has shifted from the biochemical pathways of the liver as a unit, to those of its individual cells (see page 172).

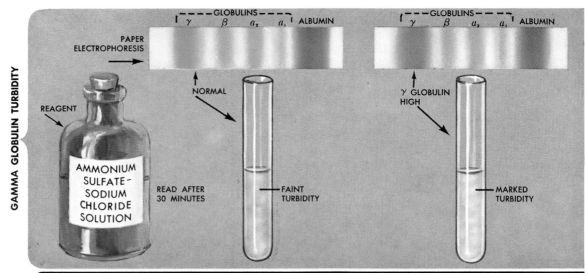

TESTS RELATED TO PROTEIN METABOLISM

Flocculation, Turbidity and Fractionation Tests

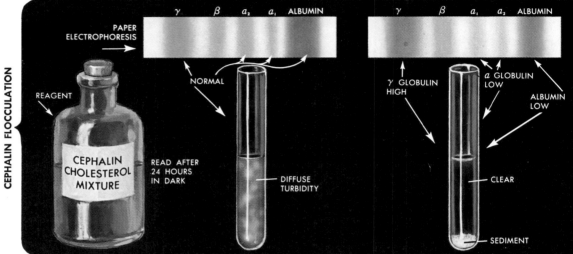

The metabolism of the three chief classes of body constituents being interwoven as it is (see page 36), one cannot expect that the examination of specific serum or plasma constituents with the so-called hepatic tests will disclose an isolated hepatic deficiency restricted to the protein metabolism. Abnormalities of serum proteins almost always reflect a far more general disturbance of liver functions in spite of the fact that the liver has a monopoly to manufacture albumin, fibrinogen, prothrombin and the greater part of the globulins. For many years in the past, flocculation and turbidity tests have been employed to determine alterations of the serum proteins. But these tests do not indicate directly a change in the liver; they only give evidence that the colloidal state, the solubility characteristics of the serum proteins, the ratio of large and small protein molecules, etc., are normal or abnormal.

After adding to small amounts of serum a solution containing ammonium sulfate and sodium chloride, a turbidity develops, the degree of which is read, either optically or spectrophotometrically, after an interval of 30 minutes. The obtained values are interpolated on a standard curve which has been calibrated with γ-globulin or with a serum, the γ-globulin content of which is known. The results of this method check satisfactorily with γ-globulin determinations performed chemically or electrophoretically on sera from patients with hepatic or chronic infectious diseases. Normally, γ-globulin ranges between 0.7 and 1.25 gm. per 100 ml. serum. As a rule, γ-globulin is elevated in hepatic disorders of any type, but especially in chronic hepatitis and cirrhosis. The highest values are observed in postnecrotic cirrhosis. In uncomplicated biliary obstruction the elevation is slight but becomes more marked when infection intervenes. Because high turbidity values are obtained also in nonhepatic chronic infections, such as tuberculosis, sarcoidosis and myeloma, as well as in collagen diseases, nor-

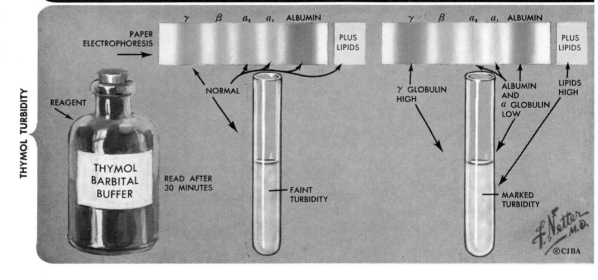

mal γ-globulin values are often of greater diagnostic significance than an elevated γ-globulin.

The zinc sulfate turbidity test also mirrors the amount of γ-globulin in serum, but it is also influenced by a depression of the albumin amount in serum.

A colloidal suspension of a *cephalin-cholesterol mixture becomes diffusedly turbid* when normal serum is added but exhibits distinct flocculation, resulting in sediment formation, when the serum stems from patients with liver damage. The increased tendency to flocculate depends upon changes of the plasma proteins, namely, reduced or altered albumin or diminished α- and, less so, augmented γ-globulin. A reduction of the unstable α-lipoproteins overshadows the increase in γ-globulin. Cephalin flocculation is, therefore, a sensitive test for hepatocellular dysfunction, reflecting, mainly, defective formation of the electrophoretically slowly moving protein frac-

tions. After standing in the dark for 24 hours, the intensity of the flocculation is estimated arbitrarily from 0 to "4 plus". A "1 plus" flocculation is considered abnormal, but only "2 plus" or more is significant for the diagnosis of hepatobiliary disease. Because some protein alterations may balance themselves mutually, a higher or lower degree of flocculation does not necessarily imply a more or less progressed cellular damage. In general, the cephalin-cholesterol flocculation test yields abnormal results in hepatitis, except in mild forms, infectious mononucleosis and in cirrhosis, except in an arrested stage. Hardly any flocculation is observed in noninfected extrahepatic biliary obstruction, even in the presence of an associated hepatic damage, and this makes the test a valuable aid for the differential diagnosis of "medical" and "surgical" jaundice (see pages 50 and 51). With prolonged obstruction or

(Continued on page 39)

(Continued from page 38)

superimposed bacterial infection, the flocculation becomes more pronounced. Sometimes abnormal results are encountered in patients with hepatic tumor metastases, with chronic congestion or with nonhepatic disease, *e.g.*, pulmonary tuberculosis or gastro-intestinal disturbances.

Addition of a thymol-barbiturate buffer to serum causes normally a faint turbidity, which is determined 30 minutes later and recorded in arbitrary units varying from laboratory to laboratory. Decrease or alteration of serum albumin and increase of γ-globulin tend to augment the turbidity. The main alteration is sometimes the increase in γ-globulin, as in late viral hepatitis, and in other instances, *e.g.*, in acute hepatitis, the changes in albumin and α-globulin. In severe cholestasis the serum contains a factor which tends to depress the turbidity, and a rise in serum lipids increases it. The results of the *thymol turbidity test* concur essentially with those of the cephalin flocculation test, though differences may be met sporadically. As with cephalin-cholesterol flocculation, the greatest diagnostic value of the thymol turbidity test lies in its behavior in noninfected extrahepatic obstruction, in which condition the turbidity remains only faint in contrast to the marked turbidity in hepatitis and cirrhosis, with the exception of intrahepatic cholestasis (see page 97).

Ammonium sulfate precipitation, the earliest method to separate albumins and globulins by "salting-out" techniques, is now being displaced by the use of sodium sulfate, introduced by Howe. Both procedures rest upon the different solubility characteristics of the serum proteins. In more recent years physical methods, especially ultracentrifugation and *electrophoresis,* have come to the fore; these separate the components according to their molecular size and shape. When mixed with buffer solution in a glass chamber and exposed to electric current, the smallest plasma proteins migrate faster than larger ones, so that boundaries between the fraction develop which are registered photographically, yielding a curve with peaks, the heights of which are in proportion to the quantity of the corresponding component. An *electrophoretic pattern of plasma proteins* is also obtained *on filter paper* on which the separated fractions can be stained, *e.g.*, by bromphenol blue and quantitated by elution or photometry. The electrophoretically separated fractions of the proteins in serum are attributed to *albumin* and *globulin,* the latter producing more than one peak, permitting the subdivision into α-, β- and γ-*globulins* and even further resolution into α_1- and α_2- and, occasionally, γ_1- and γ_2-*globulins*. These electrophoretic fractions are by no means chemically homogeneous, and they do not quite concur quantitatively with the "salting-out" fractionations, because, in the latter, part of the α-globulin remains with the albumin fraction, thus calling forth a higher albumin-globulin ratio than the one determined electrophoretically.

The total amount of proteins varies

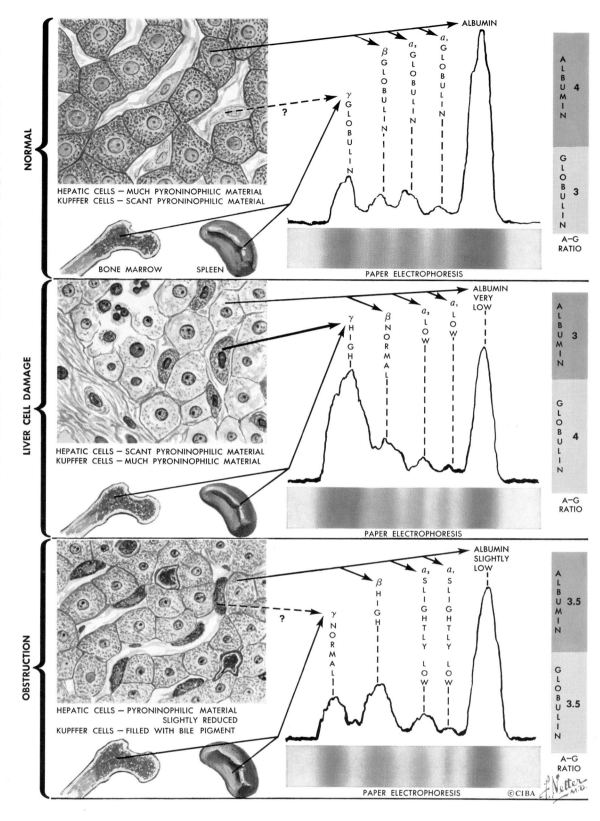

between 6 and 8 gm. per 100 ml. serum. Albumin, the largest fraction, and α-globulins are formed by the liver cells. The α- and β-globulins contain proteins conjugated with carbohydrates (glycoproteins) and lipids (lipoproteins). The origin of β-globulin which is especially rich in lipoprotein has not been established. The slowest-moving γ-globulins contain the antibodies and are formed by plasma and reticuloendothelial cells, under normal circumstances primarily in bone marrow and spleen and to a small degree, if any, by Kupffer cells and wandering mononuclear cells in the portal triads of the liver. Since the cytoplasmic basophilic granules stained by pyronine are said to reflect protein formation, the normal distribution of pyroninophilic material in the liver reflects the serum protein formation. It is possible to correlate, at least tentatively, the marked *pyroninophilia* of liver cells with the formation of albumin and

α-globulin and the scant pyroninophilia of the Kupffer cells with low or no globulin formation.

Liver cells with decreased and Kupffer cells with increased pyroninophilia are observed in *hepatocellular damage,* which would be in harmony with the reduced serum albumin and α-globulin, the elevated γ-globulin and the inverted albumin-globulin ratio (=1 or lower), as observed especially in cirrhosis. In biliary *obstruction,* the albumin reduction is slight but more marked in chronic cases, and β-globulin is distinctly elevated, whereas γ-globulin only slightly so, even in the presence of severe liver cell injury. The electrophoretically determined A-G ratio approaches 1. This serum protein distribution can again be hypothetically correlated with pyroninophilia, reduced in liver cells and absent in Kupffer cells, which are heavily bile pigmented so as to possibly prevent γ-globulin formation.

PROTHROMBIN FORMATION, COAGULATION TEST, AMINO-ACIDURIA

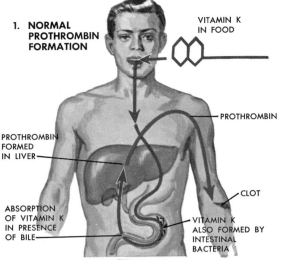

1. NORMAL PROTHROMBIN FORMATION

VITAMIN K IN FOOD

PROTHROMBIN

PROTHROMBIN FORMED IN LIVER

ABSORPTION OF VITAMIN K IN PRESENCE OF BILE

CLOT

VITAMIN K ALSO FORMED BY INTESTINAL BACTERIA

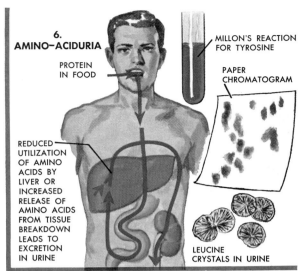

6. AMINO-ACIDURIA

PROTEIN IN FOOD

MILLON'S REACTION FOR TYROSINE

PAPER CHROMATOGRAM

REDUCED UTILIZATION OF AMINO ACIDS BY LIVER OR INCREASED RELEASE OF AMINO ACIDS FROM TISSUE BREAKDOWN LEADS TO EXCRETION IN URINE

LEUCINE CRYSTALS IN URINE

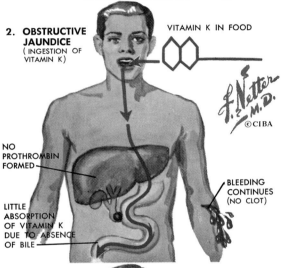

2. OBSTRUCTIVE JAUNDICE (INGESTION OF VITAMIN K)

VITAMIN K IN FOOD

NO PROTHROMBIN FORMED

LITTLE ABSORPTION OF VITAMIN K DUE TO ABSENCE OF BILE

BLEEDING CONTINUES (NO CLOT)

F. Netter M.D. ©CIBA

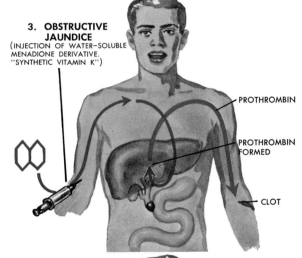

3. OBSTRUCTIVE JAUNDICE (INJECTION OF WATER-SOLUBLE MENADIONE DERIVATIVE, "SYNTHETIC VITAMIN K")

PROTHROMBIN

PROTHROMBIN FORMED

CLOT

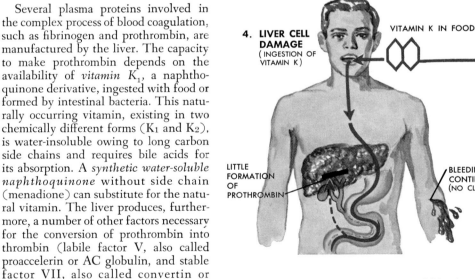

4. LIVER CELL DAMAGE (INGESTION OF VITAMIN K)

VITAMIN K IN FOOD

LITTLE FORMATION OF PROTHROMBIN

BLEEDING CONTINUES (NO CLOT)

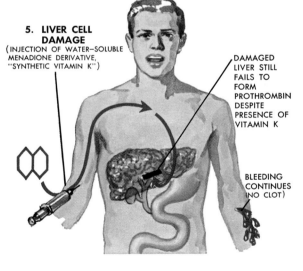

5. LIVER CELL DAMAGE (INJECTION OF WATER-SOLUBLE MENADIONE DERIVATIVE, "SYNTHETIC VITAMIN K")

DAMAGED LIVER STILL FAILS TO FORM PROTHROMBIN DESPITE PRESENCE OF VITAMIN K

BLEEDING CONTINUES (NO CLOT)

Several plasma proteins involved in the complex process of blood coagulation, such as fibrinogen and prothrombin, are manufactured by the liver. The capacity to make prothrombin depends on the availability of *vitamin K₁*, a naphtho-quinone derivative, ingested with food or formed by intestinal bacteria. This naturally occurring vitamin, existing in two chemically different forms (K_1 and K_2), is water-insoluble owing to long carbon side chains and requires bile acids for its absorption. A *synthetic water-soluble naphthoquinone* without side chain (menadione) can substitute for the natural vitamin. The liver produces, furthermore, a number of other factors necessary for the conversion of prothrombin into thrombin (labile factor V, also called proaccelerin or AC globulin, and stable factor VII, also called convertin or cothromboplastin). Deficiency effects of these factors in *liver disease* parallel those of prothrombin lack.

Prothrombin formation is impaired in *obstructive jaundice* as well as in conditions with liver cell damage, in the former because the absence of bile prevents vitamin K absorption and in the latter not only because of a deficiency in bile acid production but more so because of a fundamental loss in the faculty of the liver to create prothrombin. Accordingly, *parenteral administration* of menadione restores prothrombin formation and therewith normalizes "prothrombin time" but does not, or does so only temporarily, if the liver cells are damaged.

Many laboratory techniques have been devised to determine disturbances of blood coagulation, of which the "one-stage" method of Quick, establishing the prothrombin clotting time, is probably the most important test for the evaluation of bleeding tendencies, for the management of jaundiced patients and for guiding vitamin K therapy. In this test the minimal time necessary for the formation of a grossly visible clot is measured after addition of excess thromboplastin and calcium to blood or plasma. The more elaborate "two-stage" method, measuring the prothrombin concentration, is somewhat more efficient for the separation of obstructive jaundice from hepatocellular disease, but, being rather cumbersome, it is not widely applied. One of the two methods should always be used preoperatively in jaundiced patients, even before biopsy.

In view of the liver's central rôle in protein metabolism, it is not surprising to find alterations in the level of nitrogenous substances in blood and urine when hepatic function is disturbed. Reduction of the blood urea is frequently observed, but renal failure may act as an overcompensating factor, so that an increase in the total blood nitrogen occurs. Reduced hepatic utilization of amino acids or increased tissue breakdown in the organ causes elevated amino acid level in the blood and excessive *amino-aciduria*, which denotes an alarm signal for massive liver necrosis, or in fulminant hepatitis (see page 94). With paper chromatography one can demonstrate almost all amino acids; it is easier, however, to look for leucine crystals or to observe the appearance of a red precipitate upon boiling the urine with a few drops of Millon's reagent. Amino-aciduria is a characteristic sign in Wilson's disease (see page 87) and in Fanconi's syndrome, a congenital renal disturbance, which may involve the liver too.

BLOOD SUGAR REGULATION, GALACTOSE TOLERANCE TEST

The discontinuity of food intake, characteristic of all animals, stands in contrast to the unbroken continuity of the energy need of the entire organism. A variety of complex mechanisms serve to compensate for this disparity — mechanisms such as the transformation of dietary breakdown products into compounds suitable for *storage,* yet readily available for retransformation into substances that can be transported with the blood to those places in the body where energy is needed. The most important transport forms of energy are the monosaccharides, glucose, fructose and galactose, of which the first mentioned holds the predominant rank. Under normal conditions and after 8 hours of fasting, the glucose concentration in the blood varies not more than between 70 and 100 mg. per 100 ml., depending upon the analytical technique used. This concentration is maintained essentially by the liver, which releases glucose when the blood sugar falls below and removes it when the blood sugar rises above a threshold level. The interplay of hepatic *glycogenesis* and *glycogenolysis* (see page 36) is instrumental in this delicate adaptive arrangement necessary to satisfy the widely varying requirements of the body. This blood sugar maintaining and stabilizing function of the liver is regulated by integrated actions of hormones. *Epinephrine,* secreted in the adrenal medulla, promotes glycogenolysis in the liver (and muscle), whereas *glucagon,* produced by the α-cells of the pancreatic islands, furthers hepatic glycogenolysis and raises therewith the blood sugar, justifying the name hyperglycemic-glycogenolytic factor. Though known longer, the second hormone of the pancreas, *insulin,* manufactured by the β-cells, reduces the blood sugar by a mechanism or mechanisms still not fully understood but which are in some way connected with an increased utilization of glucose. It facilitates the entry of glucose into the hepatic cells as into any other cells and stimulates fatty acid synthesis in the liver (see page 37). From the anterior lobe of the pituitary is derived the insulin-antagonistic "diabetogenic factor", which has not yet been separated from the growth hormone. Its mechanism has not been established, but evidence points to an inhibition of hexokinase and, therewith, to a restricted conversion of hexoses to glycogen. Adrenal hormones secreted under the influence of the pituitary (ACTH) enhance glucogenesis from noncarbohydrate sources, as well as hepatic synthesis of glycogen. The *thyroid,* finally, has a stimulating effect on glycogenolysis and

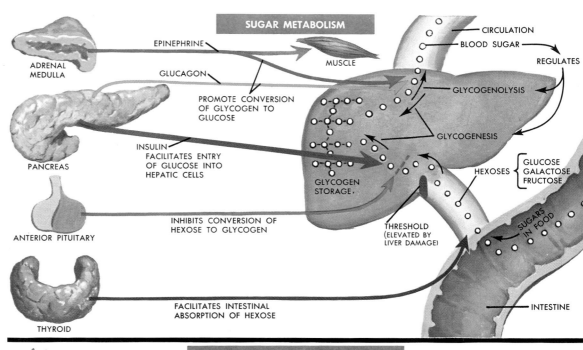

SUGAR METABOLISM

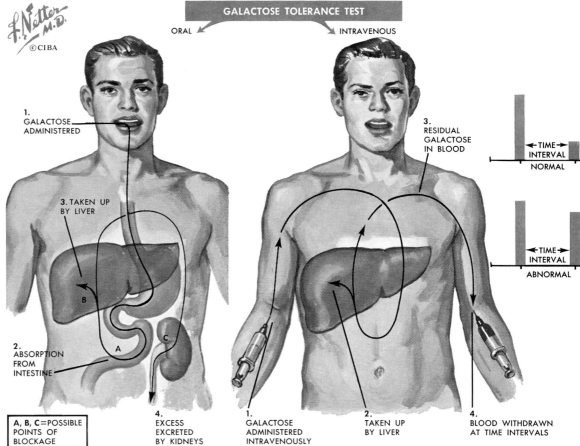

GALACTOSE TOLERANCE TEST

A, B, C=POSSIBLE POINTS OF BLOCKAGE

facilitates intestinal glucose absorption.

Though the liver is not the only organ involved in carbohydrate metabolism, it certainly assumes a central position. Hepatic functions concerned with carbohydrate metabolism are altered when the liver is damaged, but the all-important formation of blood sugar is maintained to the utmost and at times when the damaged liver cells can no longer fulfill many other functions. The hypoglycemia characteristic of the hepatectomized dog is seldom found in clinical hepatic failure. More readily is glycogen formation disturbed. In glucose tolerance tests a diabetic sugar curve is obtained in hepatic disease. Because the fate of glucose is dependent upon too many extrahepatic factors, the *galactose tolerance test* is preferred to determine the liver's efficiency to store glycogen. It rests upon galactose uptake by the liver and the hepatic conversion to glucose. The normal liver trans-

forms so much of 40 gm. galactose administered orally that not more than 3 gm. appear in the urine after 5 hours. Provided intestinal absorption is not increased as in hyperthyroidism or decreased as in deficiency diseases, and provided renal insufficiency does not interfere, a large amount of galactose in the urine may be considered an indication of liver injury. To eliminate sources of error, galactose has also been injected intravenously, and its blood level is determined at appropriate intervals. In liver injury galactose remains longer in the blood than under normal circumstances. However, abnormal results are found not only in primary hepatocellular damage but also in prolonged extrahepatic biliary obstruction, so that the tolerance or the clearance test (expressed, *e.g.,* as galactose removal constant) has no advantage over other methods in differential diagnosis of jaundice, some of which are simpler and less time-consuming.

70% ESTERIFIED 30% FREE CHOLESTEROL IN BLOOD STREAM

PHOSPHOLIPIDS GO FROM LIVER STOREHOUSE TO BLOOD STREAM

STORAGE AND FORMATION OF PHOSPHOLIPIDS IN LIVER

CHOLESTEROL ESTERIFIED, STORED AND FORMED IN LIVER

ABSORPTION OF CHOLESTEROL AND PHOSPHOLIPIDS FROM GUT

EXCRETION OF CHOLESTEROL AND PHOSPHOLIPID IN BILE

GUT

CHOLESTEROL AND PHOSPHOLIPID RELATIONS

NORMAL
PHOSPHOLIPIDS
ESTERIFIED CHOLESTEROL — 70%
FREE CHOLESTEROL — 30%

LIVER CELL DAMAGE
PHOSPHOLIPIDS — 20%
ESTERIFIED CHOLESTEROL — 80%
FREE CHOLESTEROL

OBSTRUCTION
PHOSPHOLIPIDS
ESTERIFIED CHOLESTEROL — 60%
FREE CHOL. — 40%

OBSTRUCTION PLUS LIVER CELL DAMAGE
PHOSPHOLIPIDS
ESTERIFIED CHOLESTEROL — 30%
FREE CHOL. — 70%

CHOLESTEROL AND PHOSPHOLIPID BLOOD LEVELS

Cholesterol belongs to the steroids and occurs in the body either as free alcohol or as *fatty acid ester*. The liver forms cholesterol from small hydrocarbon compounds; it esterifies free cholesterol and stores both the alcohol and esters coming from the intestine. The liver is the chief site of cholesterol degradation, excretes the chemically related bile acids with small amounts of free cholesterol in the bile and releases cholesterol and its esters into the serum, where their solubility is influenced by phospholipids, serum bile acids and proteins, all three produced by the liver. Although the liver is the main source of serum cholesterol, its level is, of course, influenced by a great number of other factors, such as age, diet, hormones, etc.

Phospholipids or phosphatides, a large group of heterogeneous substances, are extractable by fat solvents, yield on complete hydrolysis inorganic phosphates and are constituents of every body cell. The liver, a dominant site of their synthesis and an important organ for their storage, excretes them with the bile but is also, together with the diet, the main supplier of the serum phospholipids.

Under normal circumstances the total serum cholesterol ranges between 130 and 250 mg. per ml., with an occasionally unexplained value above and below this range in healthy individuals. The level is high in obesity, the last trimester of pregnancy, nephrosis and hypothyroidism. It is low in malnutrition, infec-

tions and hyperthyroidism. Of the total cholesterol, 70 per cent is normally esterified, and a drop of the cholesterol ester-cholesterol ratio below 50 is definitely abnormal. Phospholipids normally range from 8 to 12 mg. per 100 ml. serum.

The *cholesterol ester ratio* decreases when the liver is damaged. Values below 20 per cent become manifest only in severe injury, whereas in milder injuries values just below 50 per cent are observed. Reduced serum levels of total cholesterol require severe and those of the phospholipids slightly less severe hepatic damage.

Partly because of inhibited excretion, partly because of increased hepatic formation, the total cholesterol and, to a lesser degree, the phospholipids in the serum rise in biliary obstruction, though the magnitude of

the rise does not mirror the degree or duration of the blockage. With high total cholesterol levels, the cholesterol ester ratio remains within normal limits in the absence of *hepatocellular degeneration,* but if the obstruction is associated with liver damage, the ratio drops somewhat in proportion to the total cholesterol rise, which may, for unexplained reasons, climb in both *intra-* and *extrahepatic cholestasis* to extremely high levels, so that xanthomas form (see page 97). In the "surgical" type of jaundice, in which the total cholesterol is usually high, the decrease of the cholesterol ester ratio is a far more sensitive sign of liver cell damage than it is in hepatitis and cirrhosis, in which, because of the low total cholesterol level, severe damage is required to reduce the ratio significantly.

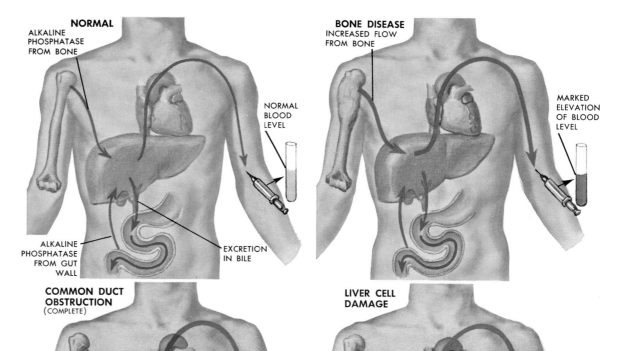

ALKALINE PHOSPHATASE TEST

Phosphatases are esterases which hydrolize reversibly monophosphoric acid esters. These enzymes, especially those with activity for a specific phosphorus compound, play a major rôle in metabolism. Of diagnostic significance are serum phosphatases without established specific substrate but separated by their peak activity in either alkaline (pH 9) or acid (pH 6) buffer media. Alkaline phosphatase is probably formed, but anyway is found, in appreciable amounts in the bone-forming cells, the osteoblasts, which apparently release the enzyme into the blood. The serum alkaline phosphatase activity is elevated with increased osteoblastic activity. It is very high in such bone diseases as rickets, osteomalacia and Paget's disease. It is moderately elevated with most carcinoma metastases to the bone, especially so if they are osteoblastic. In myeloma the activity is not elevated. Alkaline phosphatase is also delivered to the blood from the intestinal wall.

In many hepatobiliary diseases alkaline phosphatase is elevated. Some alkaline phosphatase is normally excreted in the bile, and, therefore, the serum activity of alkaline phosphatase is said to rise as a result of interference with bile flow. Some experimental evidence supports this viewpoint. However, other evidence indicates that under abnormal circumstances, especially intra- or extrahepatic cholestasis, the liver forms excessive alkaline phosphatase and releases it to the blood. Whatever the physiologic basis, in almost all hepatic diseases with

jaundice, including hepatitis and cirrhosis, the alkaline phosphatase activity is slightly elevated, whereas in *extrahepatic biliary obstruction* the activity is markedly elevated. This situation renders the *determination of alkaline phosphatase* a valuable tool in the differential diagnosis of jaundice. However, marked elevation of alkaline phosphatase is also reported in cases of intrahepatic cholestasis either as a component of a hepatic disorder or as cholangiolitis (see page 97). After subsidence of the obstruction, the serum bilirubin drops more rapidly than the phosphatase, which may remain high in the presence of persisting cholangitis, even if the jaundice has greatly declined. This indicates that alkaline phosphatase elevation is a more sensitive index of biliary obstruction than is the bilirubin level. In space-occupying lesions within the liver, such as *carcinoma metastases* or abscesses, the alkaline phosphatase may be elevated even in the

absence of jaundice. Also in *cirrhosis* or primary hepatic carcinoma, the alkaline phosphatase may be high without apparent obstruction.

The alkaline phosphatase activity is measured by incubating a phosphoric acid ester, such as β-glycerophosphate, with buffered serum and measuring the liberated phosphate. It is expressed in arbitrary units which depend on the substrate and method used. Most widely used are the Bodansky and King-Armstrong units. The normal values vary, depending on the techniques used and also on the individual; during the growth period (children and adolescents) they are higher than in adults.

Alkaline phosphatase must be differentiated from acid phosphatase formed in the prostate and released to the blood in carcinoma of the prostate, especially if the latter has metastasized to the bones (see THE CIBA COLLECTION, Volume 2, pages 21 and 56).

DETOXIFICATION

Hippuric Acid Formation

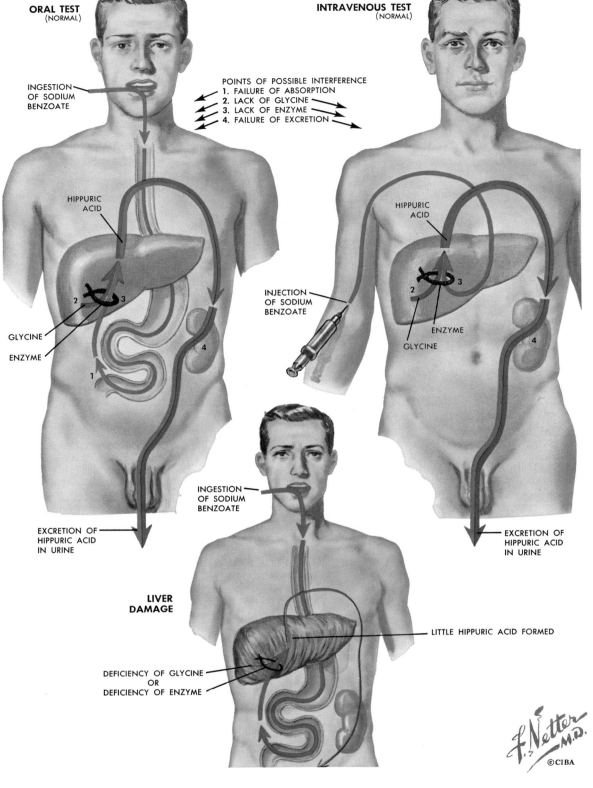

ORAL TEST (NORMAL)

INTRAVENOUS TEST (NORMAL)

INGESTION OF SODIUM BENZOATE

POINTS OF POSSIBLE INTERFERENCE
1. FAILURE OF ABSORPTION
2. LACK OF GLYCINE
3. LACK OF ENZYME
4. FAILURE OF EXCRETION

HIPPURIC ACID

HIPPURIC ACID

INJECTION OF SODIUM BENZOATE

GLYCINE

ENZYME

ENZYME

GLYCINE

EXCRETION OF HIPPURIC ACID IN URINE

EXCRETION OF HIPPURIC ACID IN URINE

INGESTION OF SODIUM BENZOATE

LIVER DAMAGE

LITTLE HIPPURIC ACID FORMED

DEFICIENCY OF GLYCINE OR DEFICIENCY OF ENZYME

Next in importance to the liver's rôle in carbohydrate, protein and lipid metabolism is its function to alter foreign compounds or useless metabolites. For this detoxification of exogenous and endogenous substances, the liver has a variety of chemical processes at its disposal. Some alkaloids, such as quinine or the barbiturates, are degraded by the liver, essentially by oxidation. Inactivation and preparation for appropriate elimination are performed partially by reduction, partially by oxidation and, finally, by conjugation. Halogenated benzines, phenols or indoles react with cysteine or sulfates to form mercapturic acids or sulfuric acid ester, respectively. Acetylation is another detoxification mechanism, *e.g.,* for sulfonamides or p-aminobenzoic acid. Conjugation with the glycogen derivative glucuronic acid is executed with a great number of compounds. Although conjugation is usually considered a detoxification, it mainly results in the formation of a compound which is more readily excreted in the urine than the nonconjugated material. The same substance may be conjugated via several pathways of different complexities. The conjugation depends in principle on both a conjugating enzyme and the availability of that substance or radical which constitutes the conjugation partner. In hepatic injury both these liver constituents may fail to be present in adequate amounts.

The detoxification processes have been the basis of several hepatic tests, the most popular of which is at present the *hippuric acid test*. The ability of the liver to couple benzoic acid with glycine, yielding hippuric acid, is easily measured, because the latter is readily excreted in the urine. Hippuric acid formation takes place almost entirely in the liver and only to a slight, not significant degree in the kidney. After *oral administration* of a standard dose of sodium benzoate, the urinary excretion of hippuric acid may be reduced in *liver damage* either because of lack of glycine or of the conjugating enzyme. Normally, almost all of the benzoic acid is transformed to hippuric acid and only very little to benzoyl glucuronate. Since in liver injury the conjugation with glycine is readily impaired, a substantial part of the benzoic acid may appear in the urine as glucuronate and can be detected as such by various methods. Intestinal disturbances may interfere with absorption of the benzoate and may, therefore, be misleading when the substance is given orally. To overcome this source of error, the *intravenous hippuric acid test* has been recommended. Though the kidneys' ability to excrete hippuric acid far exceeds the rate of its synthesis by the liver, severe renal insufficiency is a limiting factor, and the results can be considered significant only when the urea clearance or the nonprotein nitrogen values in the serum are normal.

Hippuric acid synthesis is reduced relatively early in liver damage resulting from biliary obstruction, so that both the oral and intravenous tests are of little value in the differential diagnosis of jaundice. The test's significance is furthermore curtailed by the fact that several nonhepatic conditions, *e.g.,* senility, cachexia and anemia, impair hippuric acid formation and that the determination procedure is fraught with technical errors. The test is useful mainly to ascertain roughly the degree of hepatic injury. Various modifications have been proposed, such as administration of p-aminobenzoic acid and estimation of p-aminohippuric acid in the serum rather than the urine to eliminate complication from faulty renal excretion.

Dye Excretion Test

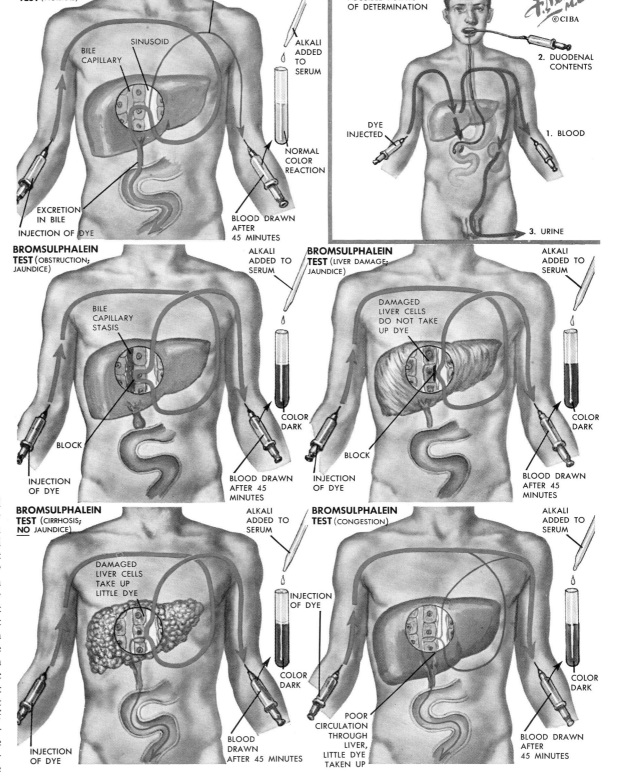

Most dyes brought into the blood stream are excreted either by the kidney through the urine or by the liver through the bile. Minor changes in the chemical structure may determine the predominant pathway of excretion. If either the kidney or the liver is damaged, the other organ takes over the excretion in compensatory fashion. Formerly, it was thought that the Kupffer cells take up the dyes, but now it has been shown that many of them enter directly into the hepatic cells. The uptake of dye, being fairly rapid from blood circulating through the hepatic sinusoids, depends, therefore, to a great degree on circulation, so that in heart failure dye excretion is impaired out of proportion to the degree of the accompanying hepatic failure as reflected in the results of other hepatic tests. Local disturbance of the blood flow through the sinusoids also impairs dye excretion. Supposedly, the swelling of the hepatic cells, as in fatty metamorphosis, accounts for impaired dye excretion even if hepatic cell function is otherwise not altered. In principle, the hepatic dye elimination can be measured either by clearance of the dye from the blood or by its excretion in the bile and its demonstration in the duodenal contents, or from the compensatory increase in urinary excretion.

A great number of dye tests have been developed; the most popular at present is the *Bromsulphalein®* test. Either 2 or 5 mg. of *Bromsulphalein* per kg. of body weight is injected intravenously, and its disappearance from the blood is determined after 30 or 45 minutes, respectively. The color (after alkalinization)

of serum drawn at these periods is compared with that of serum drawn immediately after distribution of the dye in the circulating blood, or a standard curve prepared with known amounts of dye is used for comparison. Assuming that the plasma volume averages 50 ml. per kg. of body weight, results are recorded as percentage retention in the blood, taking the concentration after distribution of the injected material as 100 per cent. The larger dose of Bromsulphalein is usually preferred, because it increases the burden on the liver and thus permits more reliable testing of its functional ability. In normal persons retention is less than 6 per cent. In jaundice caused by *biliary obstruction,* the bile stasis prevents the uptake of the dye and increases retention. Similarly, *damaged liver cells* take up much less of the dye, which makes the Bromsulphalein test of little, if any, value in the differential diagnosis of jaundice. It is not recommended in

jaundice even though the Bromsulphalein color in jaundiced serum may be adequately measured by spectrophotometry. In the absence of jaundice, Bromsulphalein retention is one of the most sensitive tests for damaged function of the liver and serves well in screening for hepatic injury, for instance after exposure to hepatotoxic drugs or in convalescent viral hepatitis. In cirrhosis without jaundice, the retention permits differentiation from other types of hepatomegaly. It is frequently abnormal also in metastatic carcinoma of the liver without jaundice (see page 115). Although exceptional anaphylactoid reactions occur, especially following serial tests, Bromsulphalein is less toxic and easier to determine than most other dyes, and the test has replaced, for instance, the previously used rose bengal test.

The roentgenologic visualization of the gallbladder is also based upon hepatic dye excretion (see page 54).

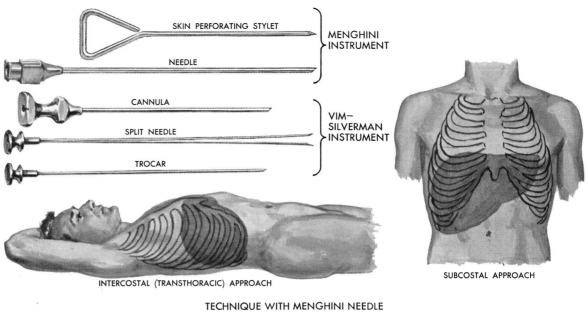

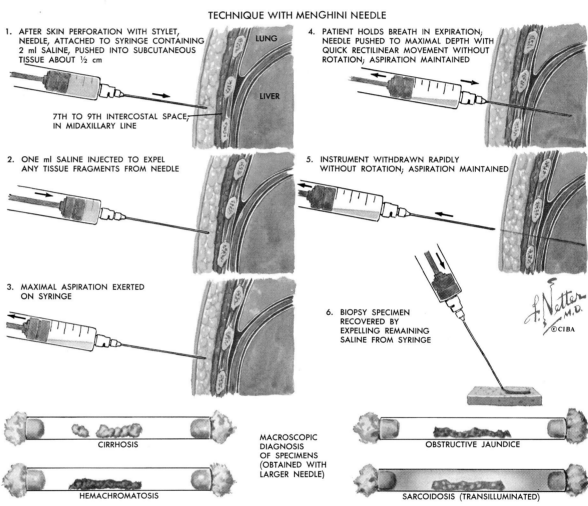

TECHNIQUE WITH MENGHINI NEEDLE

SKIN PERFORATING STYLET

NEEDLE

MENGHINI INSTRUMENT

CANNULA

SPLIT NEEDLE

TROCAR

VIM— SILVERMAN INSTRUMENT

INTERCOSTAL (TRANSTHORACIC) APPROACH

SUBCOSTAL APPROACH

1. AFTER SKIN PERFORATION WITH STYLET, NEEDLE, ATTACHED TO SYRINGE CONTAINING 2 ml SALINE, PUSHED INTO SUBCUTANEOUS TISSUE ABOUT ½ cm

LUNG

LIVER

7TH TO 9TH INTERCOSTAL SPACE, IN MIDAXILLARY LINE

2. ONE ml SALINE INJECTED TO EXPEL ANY TISSUE FRAGMENTS FROM NEEDLE

3. MAXIMAL ASPIRATION EXERTED ON SYRINGE

4. PATIENT HOLDS BREATH IN EXPIRATION; NEEDLE PUSHED TO MAXIMAL DEPTH WITH QUICK RECTILINEAR MOVEMENT WITHOUT ROTATION; ASPIRATION MAINTAINED

5. INSTRUMENT WITHDRAWN RAPIDLY WITHOUT ROTATION; ASPIRATION MAINTAINED

6. BIOPSY SPECIMEN RECOVERED BY EXPELLING REMAINING SALINE FROM SYRINGE

CIRRHOSIS

HEMACHROMATOSIS

MACROSCOPIC DIAGNOSIS OF SPECIMENS (OBTAINED WITH LARGER NEEDLE)

OBSTRUCTIVE JAUNDICE

SARCOIDOSIS (TRANSILLUMINATED)

LIVER BIOPSY

The microscopic examination of liver tissue, obtained by biopsy, is an important tool in the diagnosis of liver disease. It provides important basic information on hepatic structure and changes thereof in such disease, information not available at autopsy because of severe agonal changes.

Liver biopsy can be performed in several ways. Wedge specimens, obtained from the free edge of the liver at laparotomy, are usually unsatisfactory, because subcapsular fibrosis is accentuated on the free edge to the extent that an almost normal liver may appear to be cirrhotic. Specimens should be excised from the anterior aspect of the liver, or a needle biopsy of the more central parts may be obtained. The procedure is best performed at the beginning of the operation, in order to minimize the observation of misleading, nonspecific tissue alterations, particularly focal necrosis with leukocytes, which may result from the operation per se.

Biopsy performed under peritoneoscopic observation, whether with a forceps or, preferably, with a *needle,* is advantageous, since the site of biopsy can be selected. This is especially important in the presence of focal lesions such as tumor nodules. Needle biopsy without visual control is the most widely used technique. The *rapid aspiration method of Menghini* uses a simple thin-walled needle, 70 mm. long and 1.4 mm. in diameter, with a convex sharp tip. After perforating the skin with a stylet, the needle, attached to a syringe containing saline or procaine, is inserted into the subcutaneous tissue. A small amount of fluid is injected to remove tissue fragments from the needle lumen. The plunger is next retracted, creating suction in the syringe, and the needle is advanced into the liver at the end of an expiration or while the breath is held in expiration. The instrument is then withdrawn quickly, aspiration being maintained. The diameter of the specimen is relatively small, but not distorted, and is sufficient in diffuse hepatic diseases such as hepatitis. The technique is readily applied in small children and in other uncooperative persons. Larger specimens, thus obtained, are particularly advantageous in detecting focal lesions such as granulomas or carcinomas. The Terry

modification of the Gillman needle combines punch and aspiration. A cutting effect also produces a wider specimen, but there is some marginal distortion by compression. The *Vim-Silverman needle* is particularly useful for the detection of focal lesions. A split needle is passed through a cannula and advanced into the liver, where the beveled halves punch out a small core. The cannula is subsequently advanced over the needle, so that both halves are brought together, trapping some tissue. Then, the entire instrument is quickly withdrawn.

With any technique the specimen can be extruded from the needle into a glass tube in which it can be inspected with *transillumination,* frequently permitting a macroscopic diagnosis. In *cirrhosis,* nodules can be seen, and the specimen readily breaks into small pieces. In severe *cholestasis* the specimen appears green, in *hemochromatosis* it is brown, and *granu-*

lomas or *tumor metastases* may be recognized as white nodules.

If the liver is large or nodular, a *subcostal anterior approach* is best; otherwise, a *lateral intercostal approach* through the thoracic cavity appears safer.

Contraindications to liver biopsy are hemorrhagic tendencies, infections and prolonged obstructive jaundice, the latter presenting the danger of lacerating a dilated, aberrant bile duct on the surface of the liver. Further risks of lacerating the liver occur with intraperitoneal hemorrhage, bleeding from tumor tissue and fracture of an amyloid-containing liver. Additional hazards concern laceration of an intercostal artery, purulent peritonitis, following the perforation of an abscess, and pneumothorax. Careful consideration of the indications for biopsy and vigilant observation of the patient following the procedure will sharply reduce the chance of dangerous complications.

BILE PIGMENT METABOLISM

Normal and Abnormal

From the quantity of bile pigment excreted, the rate of hemoglobin turnover has been calculated to be 16 to 24 gm. per day under normal conditions. Of the available pathways of hemoglobin breakdown, the one via the bile pigments is the most important. The site of bile pigment formation is the reticulo-endothelial system, of which the Kupffer cells are a part. The excretion of bile pigment, however, is the task of the parenchymal liver cells. Any defect in this excretion process, either because of liver cell damage or because the liver is unable to cope with the quantity of bile pigment, leads to jaundice. The increase of bilirubin in the blood results in its appearance in the urine.

Most of the hemoglobin molecule (96 per cent) for each species is globin, a specific protein to which the pigment radicle, heme, is attached. Heme consists of four pyrrole rings connected by methene (−CH) bridges, forming a ring, inside of which a bivalent iron atom is bound. Hemoglobin is released when red blood cells are destroyed. Its breakdown starts by an opening of the tetrapyrrole ring structure at one of the methene bridges. The resulting biliverdin-iron-globin (verdohemoglobin) loses its iron and globin and becomes biliverdin which, subsequently, is reduced to free or unconjugated bilirubin. This pigment, soluble in lipids but only slightly soluble in water, gives the red diazo reaction (with sodium nitrite and sulfanilic acid) of *van den Bergh;* however, this is possible only after special treatment of the pigment to increase its water solubility, *e.g.,* by the addition of alcohol, caffeine or urea. For this reason the pigment has also been called *indirect-reacting, unconjugated bilirubin* (or heme bilirubin, bilirubin B or bilirubinglobin). Unconjugated bilirubin is taken up by *liver cells* which conjugate it, apparently in the endoplasmic reticulum (see page 170). A water-soluble bilirubin diglucuronide forms, which gives the van den Bergh reaction without pretreatment. This form has been designated as *prompt* (direct)-*reacting bilirubin* (also cholebilirubin, bilirubin A or sodium bilirubinate). Direct-reacting bilirubin can be chromatographically subdivided into two pigments. Some consider the first, or Pigment I, a monoglucuronide, formed also outside the liver, whereas others feel that it is a simple mixture of free bilirubin and bilirubin diglucuronide. Pigment II is bilirubin diglucuronide. Under normal circumstances, very little direct-reacting bilirubin circulates in the blood. The amount does not suffice to give a positive qualitative van den Bergh reaction, although it can be measured by

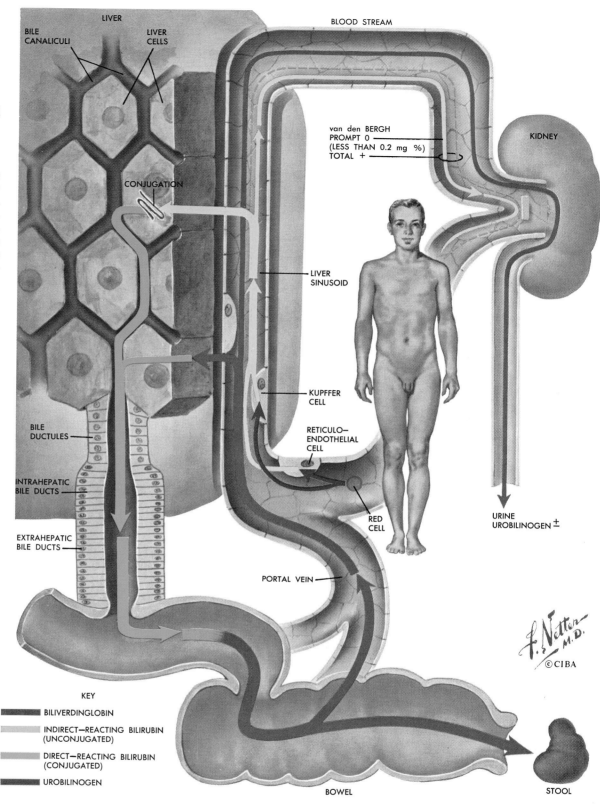

LIVER

BILE CANALICULI

LIVER CELLS

BLOOD STREAM

CONJUGATION

van den BERGH
PROMPT 0
(LESS THAN 0.2 mg %)
TOTAL +

KIDNEY

LIVER SINUSOID

BILE DUCTULES

INTRAHEPATIC BILE DUCTS

EXTRAHEPATIC BILE DUCTS

KUPFFER CELL

RETICULO—ENDOTHELIAL CELL

RED CELL

URINE UROBILINOGEN ±

PORTAL VEIN

KEY

▬ BILIVERDINGLOBIN
▬ INDIRECT—REACTING BILIRUBIN (UNCONJUGATED)
▬ DIRECT—REACTING BILIRUBIN (CONJUGATED)
▬ UROBILINOGEN

BOWEL

STOOL

spectrophotometric techniques. However, it probably is not water-soluble conjugated bilirubin, since none of it appears in the urine; rather, it represents free bilirubin, reacting slightly with diazo reagent because of the presence of bile acids and other solubilizing agents in the serum.

Conjugated bilirubin passes from the liver cells into the *bile canaliculi* and flows from there into the *biliary passages.* If it is retained there for protracted periods, it can be oxidized to *biliverdin.* Under normal conditions, conjugated bilirubin eventually reaches the intestines, where it is reduced by intestinal bacteria into several compounds, mainly the colorless mesobilirubinogen and stercobilinogen, both being designated collectively as *urobilinogen.* Only with the suppression of bacterial flora by antibiotics or with increased peristalsis in diarrhea does bilirubin appear in the feces. The main fecal pigment is uro-

bilin, the intestinal oxidation product of a part of the urobilinogen compounds. Approximately one third of the urobilinogen formed from bilirubin is reabsorbed and returned by the *portal blood stream* to the liver. The bulk of the reabsorbed portion is transformed back into bilirubin, thus completing an enterohepatic circulation.

A very small amount of urobilinogen escapes the liver and appears in the urine, where it can be demonstrated by its red reaction product with Ehrlich's aldehyde reagent (dimethyl-amino-benzaldehyde acidified with HCl).

Oxidizing bacteria may transform urobilinogen into urobilin either in the bladder or, more frequently, in urine which has been left standing too long before examination. One should be mindful that this type of urobilin formation may lead to erroneous diagnostic interpretations.

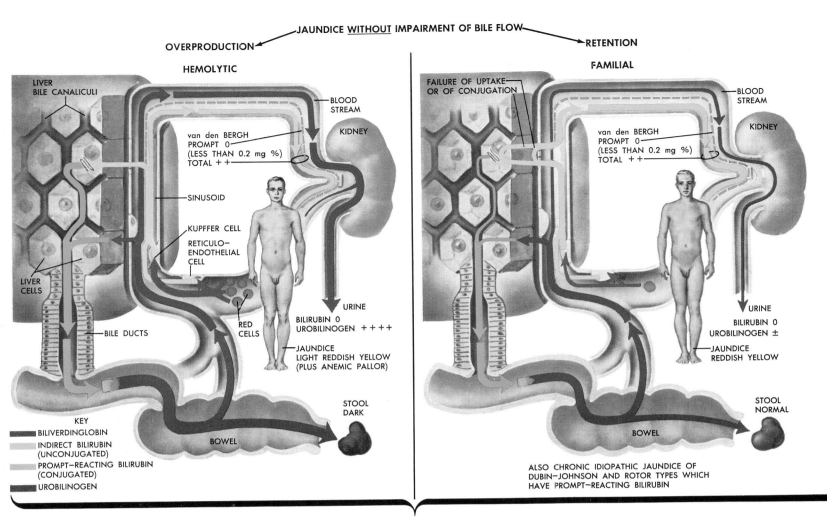

OVERPRODUCTION → ← RETENTION

HEMOLYTIC

FAMILIAL

LIVER BILE CANALICULI

BLOOD STREAM

FAILURE OF UPTAKE OR OF CONJUGATION

BLOOD STREAM

van den BERGH PROMPT 0 (LESS THAN 0.2 mg %) TOTAL + +

KIDNEY

van den BERGH PROMPT 0 (LESS THAN 0.2 mg %) TOTAL + +

KIDNEY

SINUSOID

KUPFFER CELL

RETICULO-ENDOTHELIAL CELL

LIVER CELLS

URINE
BILIRUBIN 0
UROBILINOGEN + + + +
JAUNDICE LIGHT REDDISH YELLOW (PLUS ANEMIC PALLOR)

URINE
BILIRUBIN 0
UROBILINOGEN ±
JAUNDICE REDDISH YELLOW

BILE DUCTS

RED CELLS

STOOL DARK

STOOL NORMAL

KEY
■ BILIVERDINGLOBIN
■ INDIRECT BILIRUBIN (UNCONJUGATED)
■ PROMPT-REACTING BILIRUBIN (CONJUGATED)
■ UROBILINOGEN

BOWEL

BOWEL

ALSO CHRONIC IDIOPATHIC JAUNDICE OF DUBIN–JOHNSON AND ROTOR TYPES WHICH HAVE PROMPT–REACTING BILIRUBIN

ALL THESE OCCUR IN LIVER CELL INJURY

JAUNDICE

Jaundice (icterus) is characterized by pigmentation of the skin, mucous membranes and sclerae. Produced by many conditions, the common denominator is an increase of bilirubin in the blood. The degree of pigmentation varies from very *light yellow* to intense deep *greenish-yellow* or brown. The syndrome may be divided simply into jaundice with or without impairment of bile flow. Increased production or decreased excretion of biliary pigments leads to jaundice *without bile flow impairment*. Hemolytic jaundice is due to *overproduction* of bile pigment. It occurs in septicemia, pernicious anemia, acquired or congenital hemolytic anemia, sickle cell anemia and in other diseases with shortened red cell survival. Exaggerated hemolysis produces excess biliverdin and, subsequently, bilirubin, which raises the serum level of unconjugated bilirubin. The skin has a reddish hue, superimposed on the anemic patient's pale appearance. Conjugated bilirubin is not elevated, and none appears in the urine. More urobilinogen than normal is formed in the intestine, and the *feces are darkly colored.* Reabsorption of urobilinogen is increased proportionally. The liver, probably somewhat damaged by anemia, cannot excrete all the urobilinogen, which thus appears in the urine. A rare form of jaundice without impaired bile flow is *retention jaundice,* in which no hemolysis is evident. Unconjugated bilirubin increases in the blood, because either its uptake therefrom or its conjugation within the liver cells is impaired. The *feces are normal in color,* and urinary urobilino-

gen is not increased. Severe retention jaundice manifests itself by reddish-hued skin. It is often *familial* and warrants further discussion (see page 180). Chronic idiopathic jaundice with prompt-reacting bilirubin also belongs in this group, either with excess hepatocellular pigment deposition (Dubin-Johnson syndrome) or without it (Rotor's disease).

Jaundice with impairment of bile flow is caused by *intrahepatic cholestasis* or *extrahepatic biliary obstruction.* The latter is readily explained on a mechanical basis. Since hemoglobin breakdown is not altered, normal quantities of biliverdinglobin and unconjugated bilirubin are formed. *Complete extrahepatic obstruction* is associated with *great dilatation of the bile canaliculi and intrahepatic bile ducts* (hydrohepatosis), and the bile passages contain bile casts or plugs. The increased biliary pressure interferes with the secretion of conjugated bilirubin into the bile. It accumulates within the liver cells and, to different degrees, in neighboring cells, and the Kupffer cells. It enters sinusoidal spaces and then the blood stream, directly or via lymphatics. Stagnation of bile in liver cells interferes with the uptake and conjugation of unconjugated bilirubin, which, in turn, also increases in the blood. Moreover, conjugated bilirubin may flow back through the bile ductules and ducts into the lymph and blood because of increased pressure in the biliary system. It causes a prompt van den Bergh reaction and appears in the urine. The high total bilirubin level is reflected in deep jaundice with a greenish hue, due to biliverdin. As no bile pigment reaches the intestine, no urobilinogen is formed, and the *feces are acholic or clay-colored.* No urobilinogen appears in the urine.

Incomplete extrahepatic obstruction, in contrast to the complete form, is more frequently caused by stones and strictures than by tumors. It is often intermittent, with *stones* acting as ball valves. Bile stasis, *distention of the biliary passages,* disturbance of hepatocellular bilirubin transport, regurgitation of conjugated bilirubin, and retention of unconjugated bilirubin occur, but to a lesser degree, and bilirubin is excreted in the urine. The skin has a light to medium greenish color. Since bilirubin is excreted in the bile, urobilinogen is formed in the intestine, so that the *feces become light-colored but not acholic.* Urinary urobilinogen increases because the bile stasis produces sufficient liver damage to prevent hepatic uptake and transformation of urobilinogen. Intermittent obstruction is characterized by alternating high and low urinary urobilinogen levels (see page 51).

Atresia of the smallest bile ducts or scarring after an inflammatory process may cause *intrahepatic cholestasis.* This, however, develops more often without an anatomically demonstrable mechanical obstruction.

Cholestasis may occur in all forms of *hepatitis* as well as in *cirrhosis.* Electron microscopic studies indicate damage of the bile secretory apparatus (see page 171) as the cause of the functional alterations. These are identical to changes found in biliary obstruction; however, the lesion is not induced by pressure, but rather by *primary injury to the liver cells.* Impaired biliary excretion of conjugated bilirubin and interference with the uptake or conjugation of unconjugated bilirubin result in increased serum levels of both forms and in a prompt van den Bergh reaction. Bilirubin appears in the urine. Although

(Continued on page 49)

INTRAHEPATIC CHOLESTASIS

HEPATITIS, CIRRHOSIS

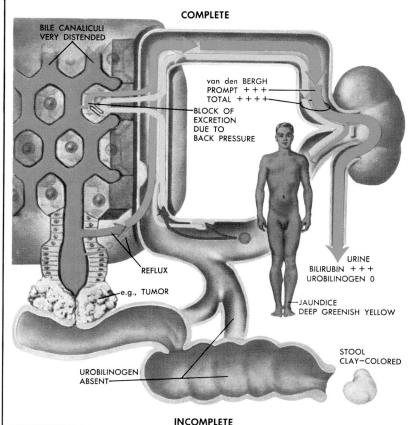

LIVER CELLS DAMAGED

CANALICULI IRREGULAR

van den BERGH
PROMPT +
TOTAL ++

EXCRETION IMPAIRED
(ALSO CONJUGATION AND UPTAKE)

UROBILINOGEN UPTAKE BLOCKED

BILE PLUGS

URINE
BILIRUBIN ++
UROBILINOGEN +++

JAUNDICE DEEP REDDISH YELLOW

STOOL LIGHT

EXTRAHEPATIC OBSTRUCTION

COMPLETE

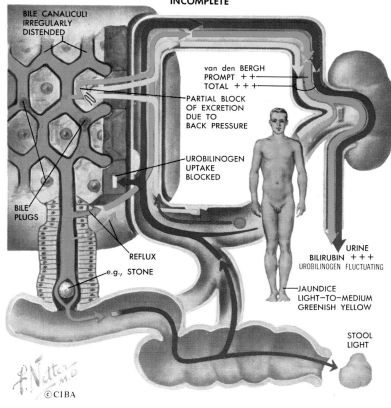

BILE CANALICULI VERY DISTENDED

van den BERGH
PROMPT +++
TOTAL ++++

BLOCK OF EXCRETION DUE TO BACK PRESSURE

REFLUX

e.g., TUMOR

URINE
BILIRUBIN +++
UROBILINOGEN 0

JAUNDICE DEEP GREENISH YELLOW

STOOL CLAY-COLORED

UROBILINOGEN ABSENT

PURE CANALICULAR, DUCTULAR OR DUCTAL

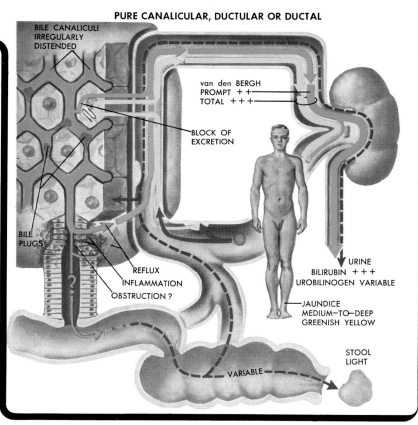

BILE CANALICULI IRREGULARLY DISTENDED

van den BERGH
PROMPT ++
TOTAL +++

BLOCK OF EXCRETION

BILE PLUGS

REFLUX
INFLAMMATION
OBSTRUCTION ?

URINE
BILIRUBIN +++
UROBILINOGEN VARIABLE

JAUNDICE MEDIUM-TO-DEEP GREENISH YELLOW

STOOL LIGHT

VARIABLE

INCOMPLETE

BILE CANALICULI IRREGULARLY DISTENDED

van den BERGH
PROMPT ++
TOTAL +++

PARTIAL BLOCK OF EXCRETION DUE TO BACK PRESSURE

UROBILINOGEN UPTAKE BLOCKED

BILE PLUGS

REFLUX

e.g., STONE

URINE
BILIRUBIN +++
UROBILINOGEN FLUCTUATING

JAUNDICE LIGHT-TO-MEDIUM GREENISH YELLOW

STOOL LIGHT

F. Netter M.D.
©CIBA

(Continued from page 48)

bilirubin excretion in the bile is reduced, causing *light-colored stools,* the uptake of urobilinogen by the damaged liver cells is blocked, thus increasing urobilinogen excretion in the urine.

The intensity of the cholestatic component varies greatly in hepatitis and cirrhosis, as does the contribution of liver cell injury in the individual case. Sometimes, "hepatic tests" indicate strongly that cholestasis may be prominent, but biopsy reveals alcoholic or viral hepatitis. In other instances, only cholestasis is seen, as in

drug-induced hepatitis or, in the absence of a recognizable etiology, in viral hepatitis. The alterations of the bile pigment metabolism are the same as in the preceding form, although usually more severe. Sole involvement of the bile secretory mechanism may become complicated by disorders of the bile ducts and ductules in which possible obstruction or, more likely, inflammation with changed permeability, leads to reflux of conjugated bilirubin and other biliary substances into the blood stream. This form of elevation of conjugated bilirubin, resulting from

regurgitation, cannot be differentiated from the cholestatic form by biochemical tests. In the absence of cholestasis, regurgitation occurs in early primary biliary cirrhosis and, possibly, in early extrahepatic obstruction.

In liver cell injury, all types of jaundice in any combination may occur simultaneously. The determination of urinary bilirubin or urobilinogen assists in their separation, but the ratio between conjugated and unconjugated bilirubin is of little assistance in adults with bilirubin levels above 6 mg. per cent.

EVALUATION AND APPLICATION OF HEPATIC TESTS

The many functions which the liver fulfills, some of which are reflected in characteristic patterns of composition of the serum and urine, raised the hope that liver function tests would be developed which would be diagnostic for alterations of the liver and for specific diseases. Despite continued research and increasing clarification of liver function, tests based on biochemical alterations have not become more helpful and, consequently, are less appreciated. Other techniques, especially liver biopsy and the newer physical methods (see page 179), are increasingly replacing the biochemical tests. One difficulty is that most of the tests in clinical use do not measure a function that is solely of the liver; rather, they measure a function which the liver shares with other organs, or they furnish biochemical data which are altered in the presence of liver cell injury without necessarily being related to liver function. It is for this reason that the term "hepatic test" is preferable to "liver function test". Moreover, a reduction of hepatic function, as such, is only occasionally of diagnostic significance, because some reduction of liver function is found in almost every disorder that is accompanied by fever or other systemic manifestations. In this sense, most tests for liver function proper are too sensitive.

Of the numerous laboratory procedures recommended for the recognition, differential diagnosis and appraisal of liver disease, only a few have been presented in the preceding pages, supplemented by the recently developed use of the type of test which *transaminase* represents (see page 175). This does not indicate that they are the only ones worthy of consideration, or that they can provide all the answers the clinicians desire. Every hepatic test potentially offers some diagnostic clue, provided the results are correlated with the history and the clinical findings. However, no single test replaces any other in settling the diagnostic or prognostic problems. Furthermore, the interpretation of a single result is unreliable, because of the high incidence of false positive and false negative results. Abnormal findings occur often without any significant alteration of hepatic structures. The existence of anicteric viral

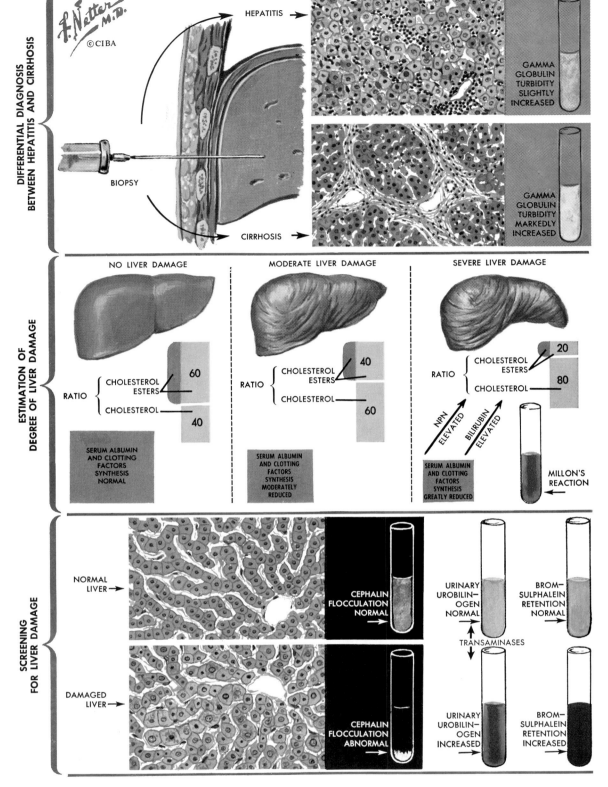

hepatitis with questionable morphologic features contributes significantly to this confusion. In contrast, however, almost all hepatic tests yield normal values in approximately 10 per cent of patients suffering from severe hepatic injury. The imperfections of laboratory diagnostic procedures and of their interpretation are a challenge to clinicians and basic scientists alike; hence, the coordinated use of several tests is recommended. If the results of these tests are charted together, they are called "liver profiles". They are used for the solution of specific clinical problems. Support of the clinical analysis of liver diseases by a methodical evaluation of multiple tests has been most successful, particularly if correlated with biopsy findings. Several such problems, in the order of increasing importance, include the recognition of preceding liver disease in an acute episode, *estimating the degree of liver cell damage, screening for liver*

damage, and the *differential diagnosis* of jaundice.

For the *differential diagnosis between hepatitis and cirrhosis* in the presence or absence of jaundice, only *liver biopsy* is reliable. For the discrimination between hepatitis and cirrhosis or the recognition of preceding liver disease in acute episodes, the results of biochemical tests are of little use except for the *serum γ-globulin* level, as measured by the *turbidity reaction* or, now more frequently, by paper electrophoresis. As a rule, in hepatitis it is only slightly elevated, but the elevation is conspicuous in cirrhosis and is most striking in active postnecrotic cirrhosis. It frequently decreases with steroid therapy.

Even more important is the need to estimate the *degree of liver cell damage* in established hepatic disease, in order adequately to follow its course, to be aware of improvements or deterioration and to deter-

(Continued on page 51)

(*Continued from page 50*)

mine the optimal time for surgical intervention. The determination of the serum albumin level and of such clotting factors as prothrombin and, possibly, the *cholesterol-cholesterol esters ratio* provides acceptable evidence to estimate the degree of hepatic damage. A severe drop of this ratio and/or a sharp decline of serum albumin or a rise in prothrombin time in the presence of vitamin K administration will indicate rapid deterioration of hepatic function, especially if sharp rises of *bilirubin* and blood *urea nitrogen* are observed simultaneously. The latter point to an associated renal injury, and together they represent important alarm signals. In previous years, tests for a reduction of the *hippuric acid synthesis* were similarly applied, but these are now rarely used. A strongly positive *Millon's test* (amino-aciduria) implies very severe hepatocellular failure.

When *screening for liver damage* in apparently healthy persons who have been exposed to viral hepatitis in military or civilian populations, or to hepatotoxic substances in industrial plants, abnormal results of the *cephalin flocculation* test, the appearance of bilirubin in the urine, an increase of *urinary urobilinogen* and *Bromsulphalein® retention* may disclose evidence of damage otherwise not detectable. At present, a test for elevation of the activity of *serum transaminase*, particularly SGPT (serum-glutamic-pyruvic-transaminase) (see page 175), is the most widely used method for such screening purposes. Apparently, this is more sensitive than is the elevation of other similarly used enzyme activities, such as isocitric dehydrogenase.

The thorniest problem regarding the application of "hepatic tests" is the differential diagnosis of "medical" and "surgical" jaundice. This concerns the separation of cases which are likely to be amenable to surgery (because of the interruption of *bile flow* by tumors, calculi, and strictures) from those resulting mainly from hepatitis and cirrhosis, as well as from intrahepatic cholestasis. The clinician, aiming at the recognition of *liver cell impairment* in contrast to *interference with bile flow*, or vice versa, has at his disposal a series of tests such as those listed in Plate 16. The implication of these terms has recently been changed on the basis of electron microscopic evidence, which indicates that interference with bile flow may result from alteration of the bile secretory mechanism of the liver cell (see page 177). Hepatocellular damage may be assumed to be present if the results of at least two of the tests on the left deviate significantly from the normal. Jaundice in patients with liver cell impairment but without bile flow interference is assumed to be "medical" in nature. A small percentage of this group of patients will have to be reclassified if repeated *urinary urobilinogen* analyses detect *fluctuating excretion*, which is a characteristic of incomplete biliary obstruction by calculi. A *palpable mass* in the upper right quadrant overrules a decision based on the results of hepatic tests which favor "medical" jaun-

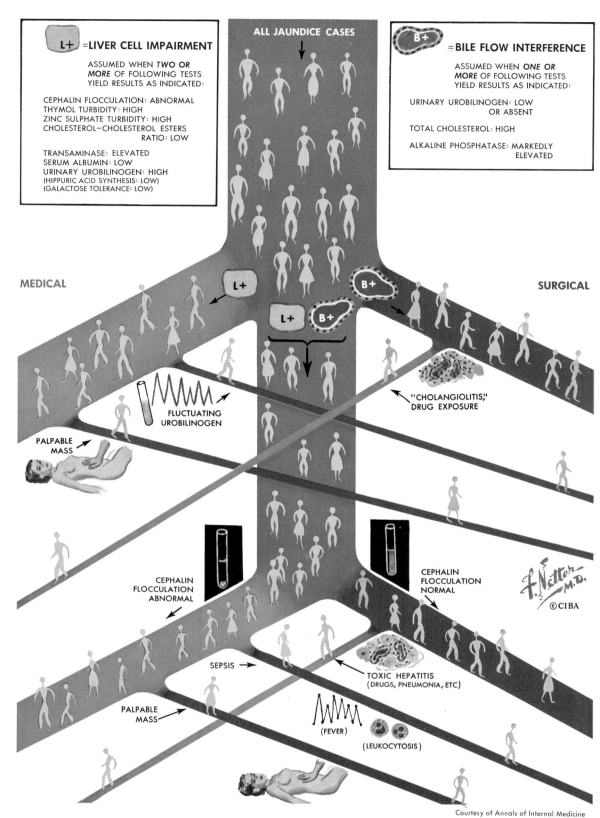

ALL JAUNDICE CASES

L+ =LIVER CELL IMPAIRMENT

ASSUMED WHEN *TWO OR MORE* OF FOLLOWING TESTS YIELD RESULTS AS INDICATED:

CEPHALIN FLOCCULATION: ABNORMAL
THYMOL TURBIDITY: HIGH
ZINC SULPHATE TURBIDITY: HIGH
CHOLESTEROL—CHOLESTEROL ESTERS RATIO: LOW

TRANSAMINASE: ELEVATED
SERUM ALBUMIN: LOW
URINARY UROBILINOGEN: HIGH
(HIPPURIC ACID SYNTHESIS: LOW)
(GALACTOSE TOLERANCE: LOW)

B+ =BILE FLOW INTERFERENCE

ASSUMED WHEN *ONE OR MORE* OF FOLLOWING TESTS YIELD RESULTS AS INDICATED:

URINARY UROBILINOGEN: LOW OR ABSENT

TOTAL CHOLESTEROL: HIGH

ALKALINE PHOSPHATASE: MARKEDLY ELEVATED

MEDICAL

SURGICAL

FLUCTUATING UROBILINOGEN

PALPABLE MASS

"CHOLANGIOLITIS," DRUG EXPOSURE

CEPHALIN FLOCCULATION ABNORMAL

CEPHALIN FLOCCULATION NORMAL

F. Netter M.D. ©CIBA

SEPSIS

TOXIC HEPATITIS (DRUGS, PNEUMONIA, ETC)

PALPABLE MASS

(FEVER)

(LEUKOCYTOSIS)

Courtesy of Annals of Internal Medicine

dice. In such an instance the evidence of liver cell damage results either from secondary hepatic involvement or from false positive responses. These exceptions are indicated in the picture by the narrow bands pointing to the right and downward from the broader stripe, representing those cases recognized as "medical" jaundice. Jaundice with evidence of bile flow interference without liver cell impairment is considered "surgical". However, one will find cases of intrahepatic cholestasis among those patients. Essentially, these exceptions belong to the conditions designated as acute or chronic *cholestasis* (see page 97).

The *cephalin flocculation* test should be a guide for the separation of those not infrequent cases which, according to the results of the tests suggested, show evidence of both hepatocellular damage and interference with bile flow. With abnormal cephalin flocculation, a medical condition complicated by

intrahepatic cholestasis probably exists, although, as discussed above, a *palpable mass* directs the patient to the surgical side. Moreover, signs of *sepsis* (chills, spiking fever, leukocytosis, etc.) should prompt one's reconsideration of conclusions drawn from the cephalin flocculation test, because all laboratory manifestations pointing to the medical type of jaundice can be produced by a purulent hepatitis evolving from infection of an extrahepatic biliary obstruction. If the hepatic tests disclose interference with bile flow, as well as impairment of hepatic function, the latter is assumed to be secondary to prolonged biliary obstruction, provided the cephalin flocculation test has remained normal. This would divert the patient to the surgical side, if no clues point to intrahepatic cholestasis induced by *drugs, pneumonia*, or other forms of *toxic hepatitis*, which account for hepatocellular damage and bile stasis.

FUNCTION OF GALLBLADDER AND CHOLEDOCHODUODENAL SPHINCTER

Under basal conditions, *i.e.*, with no food in the stomach or duodenum, no bile, though continuously secreted by the liver, enters the duodenum, because the *sphincter of Oddi* is contracted. Therefore, the bile piles up in the common bile duct, whence it is directed into the gallbladder when the pressure in the system reaches about 20 cm. H_2O. If food enters the duodenum, the *sphincter relaxes*, the gallbladder contracts and bile enters the duodenum, while the biliary pressure drops to 10 cm. H_2O or less. Then the gallbladder empties slowly and intermittently, being gradually reduced to thumb size. The total evacuation period of the gallbladder varies from 15 minutes to several hours. The pattern of contraction exhibits great individual variation.

The natural stimuli for the release of bile into the duodenum (cholecystokinetic effect), *i.e.*, the co-ordinated *contraction of the gallbladder* and *dilatation of the sphincter of Oddi*, are food ingredients, of which fats are the most potent, followed by proteins. Carbohydrates have, if anything, an inhibitory influence. Proteins are stronger than fats in exerting stimulation of bile production in the liver (choleretic effect), and carbohydrates, again, are inhibitors in this respect. The cholecystokinetic effect is apparently mediated by a hormone, *cholecystokinin,* which the intestinal mucosa releases when fats or some saline cathartics enter the duodenum. Egg yolk and cream, or a mixture of both, or magnesium or sodium sulfate, having a very strong cholecystokinetic effect, are used diagnostically to test the contractibility of the gallbladder by X-rays. The dual (sympathetic and parasympathetic) innervation of gallbladder and sphincter of Oddi (see page 21) also supports a co-ordinated effect. According to Meltzer's law of contrary innervation, sympathetic stimulation causes contraction of the sphincter and dilation of the gallbladder, whereas vagus stimulation relaxes the sphincter and contracts the bladder, as does purified cholecystokinin intravenously (Torsoli), though this does not hold for excessive vagus stimulation, which leads to a contraction of both sites. In general, however, hormonal stimulation induced by cholekinetic food is more important than nervous stimulation.

In individuals with biliary fistulae approximately 1000 ml. of bile per day were produced. Though this figure might not reflect the normal amount of bile, it may be assumed that the gallbladder may accumulate between 200 and 500 ml. of bile between meals. Such a quantity of fluid in a region where liver, intestine,

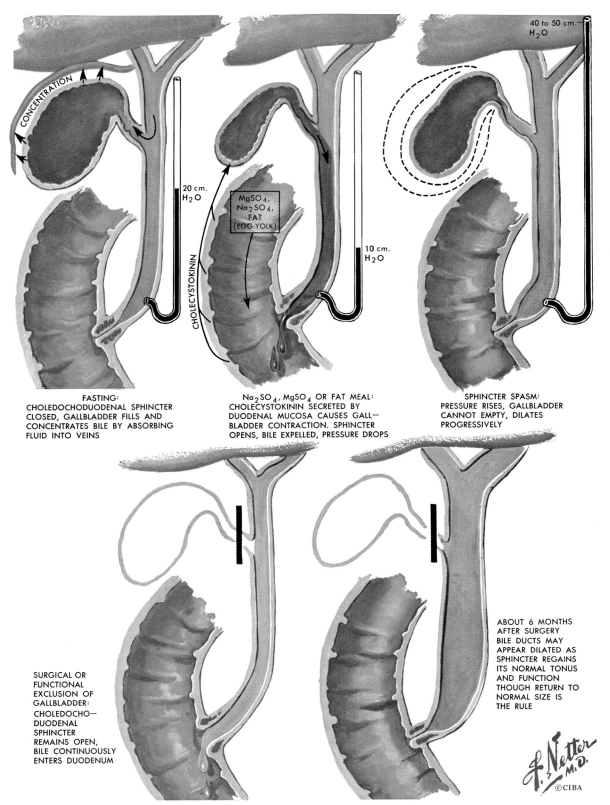

FASTING:
CHOLEDOCHODUODENAL SPHINCTER CLOSED, GALLBLADDER FILLS AND CONCENTRATES BILE BY ABSORBING FLUID INTO VEINS

Na_2SO_4, $MgSO_4$ OR FAT MEAL:
CHOLECYSTOKININ SECRETED BY DUODENAL MUCOSA CAUSES GALL—BLADDER CONTRACTION. SPHINCTER OPENS, BILE EXPELLED, PRESSURE DROPS

SPHINCTER SPASM:
PRESSURE RISES, GALLBLADDER CANNOT EMPTY, DILATES PROGRESSIVELY

SURGICAL OR FUNCTIONAL EXCLUSION OF GALLBLADDER: CHOLEDOCHO—DUODENAL SPHINCTER REMAINS OPEN, BILE CONTINUOUSLY ENTERS DUODENUM

ABOUT 6 MONTHS AFTER SURGERY BILE DUCTS MAY APPEAR DILATED AS SPHINCTER REGAINS ITS NORMAL TONUS AND FUNCTION THOUGH RETURN TO NORMAL SIZE IS THE RULE

kidney and adrenal compete for space would create pressure difficulties were it not for the gallbladder's ability to concentrate the liver bile from four- to tenfold. The gallbladder mucosa can reabsorb water and salts, leaving bile pigment, bile acid and calcium salts in a concentrated solution. This concentrating power may be lost in certain pathologic conditions, or bile acids, which keep cholesterol and bile pigments in aqueous solution, may also be absorbed as in the presence of inflammatory processes. Such functional disturbances may contribute to the formation of gallstones (see page 124).

Another function of the gallbladder is concerned with the regulation of the biliary pressure as it results from the secretion of the liver and the resistance offered by the sphincter of Oddi. The pressure would rise rapidly with spasms of the sphincter if the gallbladder, as an expansile side arm to the biliary system,

would not dilate. If the *gallbladder* is *removed* surgically or is spontaneously eliminated by either cystic duct obstruction or chronic fibrosing cholecystitis, the same situation arises as in rats and horses, which have no gallbladder and also no sphincter of Oddi, so that bile trickles continuously into the duodenum. With the loss of the gallbladder, the regulative influence for the alternating contraction and relaxation is also lost, and the sphincter of Oddi remains permanently open until several months after cholecystectomy, when in some instances the extrahepatic bile ducts dilate and start concentrating bile, substituting in this way for one of the lost gallbladder functions. In time the sphincter regains its tonus, and the normal economy of bile in the intestine is restored. Under these circumstances, however, the common and hepatic ducts may contain concentrated bile and thus become susceptible to stone formation by precipitation of biliary solids.

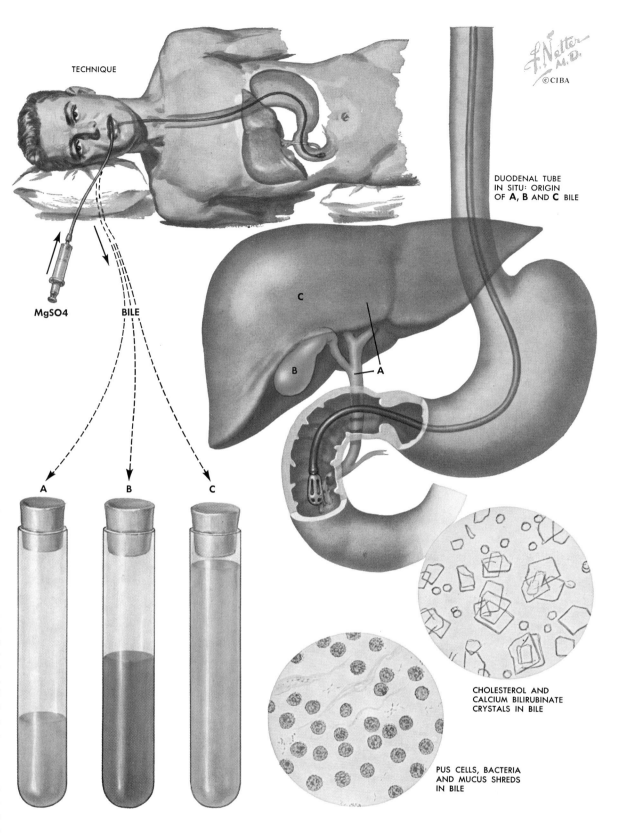

TECHNIQUE

MgSO4   BILE

DUODENAL TUBE
IN SITU: ORIGIN
OF **A**, **B** AND **C** BILE

C

B

A

A   B   C

CHOLESTEROL AND
CALCIUM BILIRUBINATE
CRYSTALS IN BILE

PUS CELLS, BACTERIA
AND MUCUS SHREDS
IN BILE

DUODENAL DRAINAGE OF MELTZER AND LYON

Duodenal drainage of bile, though entailing some technical difficulties and inconvenience to the patient, may procure some valuable information concerning functional and structural alterations of the biliary tract and hepatic function. A rubber tube, 10 to 14 F. (French catheter size) wide and 50 in. long, preferably with a metal tip, is introduced into the empty stomach of the patient in erect or sitting position. When the patient, then lying on his right side, continues to swallow, the tube is supposed to advance through the pylorus. If the tube curls in the stomach, or if the pylorus does not open because of hyperacid stomach content, partial withdrawal will help in the former and sodium bicarbonate instillation in the latter case. Pylorospasm may call for an atropine injection. The proper position of the tube's tip may be established by fluoroscopy or by injection of fluid, which can be almost completely aspirated if the tube is still in the stomach, but not if the tip lies within the duodenum. With the sphincter of Oddi still closed, a light-yellow to gold-brown alkaline fluid can be aspirated, but one frequently obtains immediately a gold-brown *("A") bile,* deriving from the biliary ducts, because the passing of the tube relaxes the sphincter of Oddi. If it does not relax spontaneously, an instillation of 25 ml. of saturated, warm magnesium sulfate solution or of 5 to 10 ml. of olive oil will cause the appearance of "A" bile, which after several minutes becomes darker, indicating the delivery of *"B" bile* from the contracting gallbladder. Eventually, the color changes again from dark brown to golden brown, and this *"C" bile* represents liver bile secreted after the emptying of the biliary ducts and the gallbladder.

Complete biliary obstruction exists if no bile-pigmented fluid can be obtained. Atony of the gallbladder or its failure to concentrate bile or an obstructed cystic duct must be assumed when the color of "A" bile changes to that of "C" bile,

though under said circumstances the liver bile is frequently darker than normal, as it is also in the presence of increased hemolysis. Liver cell function may be judged by intravenous injection of azorubin S, which reddens the bile within 15 minutes. If by that time the dye does not appear, it indicates hepatocellular damage. In this way it is possible to find patients, during recovery from an extrahepatic obstruction, with already adjusted bile secretion but still malfunctioning liver cells.

Samples of all three bile fractions are collected after permitting adequate time for the instilled oil or magnesium sulfate to be drained away. The bilirubin content may be determined and should be found about ten times higher in "B" bile than in "C" bile, with a normal concentrating ability of the gallbladder. Microscopic examination of noncentrifuged and non-stained drops of all three bile portions may uncover

"pus cells" which, if present in "A" and "B" bile, point to gastritis or duodenitis or, provided a distinct pigmentation is recognizable, to cholangitis. Large amounts of pus cells in "B" bile indicate cholecystitis or empyema. *Cholesterol crystals* (square or rhomboid plates with clipped edges) and the lustrous clusters of granular *calcium bilirubinate* indicate tendency for gallstone formation. Excessive amounts of mucus shreds speak for a catarrhal inflammation. Appearance of blood in the bile suggests a carcinoma in the major duodenal papilla of Vater. Rapidly neutralized specimens may be centrifuged, and malignant cells in the stained smear of the sediment are indicative of carcinoma of the major papilla or pancreas or biliary tract. Parasites and bacteria may also be diagnosed. To establish the specific offender in cases of cholecystitis or cholangitis, special precautions for the sterile collection of the bile are required.

CHOLECYSTOGRAPHY—ROUTES OF DYE
AND POSSIBLE POINTS OF BLOCKAGE:
1. FAILURE OF ABSORPTION
2. FAILURE OF EXCRETION BY LIVER
3. BILE DUCT OBSTRUCTION WITH BACK
   PRESSURE ARRESTING SECRETION
4. CYSTIC DUCT OBSTRUCTION
5. FAILURE OF GALLBLADDER (DISEASED)
   TO CONCENTRATE

INTRAVENOUS ROUTE

ORAL ROUTE

CHOLECYSTOGRAM

CHOLECYSTOGRAPHY,
CHOLANGIOGRAPHY,
PORTAL VENOGRAPHY

CHOLANGIOGRAM (THROUGH BILIARY FISTULA)

PORTAL VENOGRAM (INTO SPLEEN THROUGH ABDOMINAL WALL)

CHOLANGIOGRAM

CHOLANGIOGRAM (INTO GALLBLADDER THROUGH LAPAROTOMY OR PERITONEOSCOPE)

PORTAL VENOGRAM (INTO MESENTERIC VEIN THROUGH LAPAROTOMY)

PORTAL VENOGRAM

ROUTES FOR CHOLANGIOGRAPHY AND PORTAL VENOGRAPHY

Radiopaque substances can be introduced into the gallbladder and the biliary tract by various means. Plain, routine X-ray photography of the abdomen may reveal radiolucent gallbladder stones (see also page 124) or can be supplemented to receive valuable diagnostic information by *cholecystography*. With this technique, known also as Graham-Cole test, the patient receives either orally or intravenously an iodine-containing organic substance such as tetra-iodophenolphthalein or similar compounds. When this radiopaque medium reaches the liver, it is excreted with the bile, enters the bile tract system and accumulates in the gallbladder, where normally it is being concentrated to produce a contrast shadow 12 to 14 hours after administration. By taking X-ray pictures at 10-minute intervals and feeding the patient a fatty meal or egg yolks, the motility of the gallbladder can be checked. Normally, the shadow shows a gradual diminution in size to a narrow tubular form. Using the oral route, intestinal disturbances, diarrhea, obstruction in the upper gastro-intestinal tract, etc., may interfere with the absorption of the contrast medium. Thus, in such instances, the intravenous route promises advantages, but failure of gallbladder visualization may have other reasons. Premature emptying of the gallbladder on account of inadequate preparation of the patient, *e.g.*, a fatty meal before or food intake after administration of the contrast medium, inability of the liver to excrete the radiopaque matter because of cellular damage, retardation or blockage of the transport to the gallbladder owing to obstruction of the hepatic, common or cystic ducts, loss of concentration power by an inflammatory process of the gallbladder — all these factors interfere with the production of shadow or permit only a faint one to develop. This list of interferences also explains why, in moderate and severe jaundice of any type, cholecystography is usually unsuccessful.

Recently, contrast media with an iodine content high enough to produce a shadow without requiring concentration in the gallbladder have been introduced. This development led to the visualization of the biliary ducts in patients after cholecystectomy and is helpful also with undisclosed or unobtainable history of previous surgery of the biliary tract.

A more direct method to visualize radiographically the bile duct system is *cholangiography,* in which radiopaque material is introduced into the gallbladder either through an existing biliary fistula or during operation, or without laparotomy with the aid of peritoneoscopy. In a cholangiogram one can recognize the extra- and intrahepatic biliary pathways and stones anywhere in the system and even within the liver. This method, which would visualize the patency of the ductal system even in jaundice, has so far not been in wide use.

Transcutaneous cholangiography is acquiring increasing interest (see page 176).

Another recent development is the demonstration of the portal venous system by injection of Diodrast® either during operation into tributaries of the superior mesenteric vein or without laparotomy by the percutaneous route into the spleen. Such a *portal venogram* is useful in the visualization of the portal tree, for instance, for selection of a proper shunt operation (see page 73) and also in the demonstration of space-occupying lesions such as abscesses or tumors in the liver. See further discussion on page 179.

The cholecystogram, cholangiogram and portal venogram are reproduced by the courtesy of Drs. G. G. Kopstein, D. D. Kozoll, and O. C. Julian, respectively.

NORMAL SECRETORY FUNCTIONS OF PANCREAS

Pancreatic secretion is subject to both neurogenic and hormonal control. Stimulation of the vagus (in animal experiments or by the administration of cholinergic drugs) increases the enzymatic activity but not the volume of the secretion. Vagotomy and parasympatholytic drugs (atropine) conversely decrease enzymatic activity. The volume of the pancreatic secretion is raised by the injection of secretin, a hormone now isolated in crystalline form but postulated ever since stimulation of pancreatic flow was observed after injection of an acid extract of duodenal mucosa (Bayliss and Starling). *Secretin* increases also the concentration of bicarbonate and sodium and decreases that of chloride and potassium, but only slightly, so that in view of the larger volume the total amount of these ions is still greater than without secretin stimulation. Enhancement of enzymatic activity of the pancreatic juice under secretin influence may be an effect of this hormone but more probably of a second intestinal hormone, pancreozymin, accompanying not adequately purified secretin preparations.

Though the figures for the composition of the nonsecretin-stimulated pancreatic juice, as obtained by duodenal drainage or in patients with an external pancreatic fistula, vary to a great extent in the literature, the following, expressed in mEq. per liter, may be taken as averages: bicarbonate 22, chloride 110, sodium 106, potassium 12.3 (with a total pancreatic secretion of 1500 ml.). Other inorganic and organic components are probably also present.

The components of the pancreatic juice of greatest functional and clinical interest (see pages 56, 57 and 58) are the enzymes: lipase, amylase, carboxypeptidase, trypsin and chymotrypsin, of which the last three mentioned are secreted as inactive enzyme precursors to be activated when they have entered the duodenum. The pancreatic *trypsinogen* is rapidly converted to *trypsin* by the enzyme *enterokinase*, secreted by the duodenal mucosa and also autocatalytically by trypsin itself. Trypsin splits chiefly those peptide bonds in which the NH group is combined with the CO group of L-arginine or L-lysine. Chymotrypsinogen, the second proteolytic precursor formed in the acinar cells, is activated by trypsin but not by enterokinase nor by chymotrypsin itself. It is possible that several chymotrypsins result

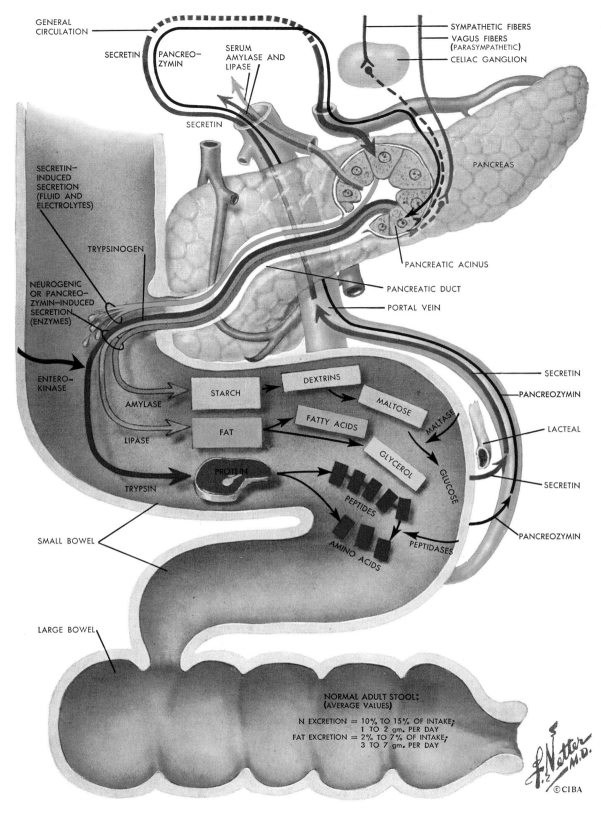

from the activation of one trypsinogen and that each of the chymotrypsins is capable of specific actions on different types of CO-NH linkages. The inactive precursor of carboxypeptidase is transformed by catalytic amounts of trypsin to the active form, which hydrolyzes the CO-NH linkages adjacent to the carboxyl end, in both proteins and peptides. For the optimal activity of these proteolytic enzymes, a slightly alkaline medium (pH 7 to 9) is necessary.

The pancreatic *lipase* or lipases hydrolyze the ester linkages of the ingested triglycerides into the component fatty acids and glycerol also at pH 7 to 9. Pancreatic *amylase* acts on glycogen, starch and its components (amylose and amylopectin, and certain degradation products originating from these polysaccharides) to form fermentable sugars, chiefly maltose, and reducing nonfermentable dextrins.

Fat and nitrogen content of the feces are strongly

related to pancreatic function. The *ranges of the daily fecal fat*, escaping hydrolysis and/or absorption (see page 37), as well as the *total fecal nitrogen*, representing incompletely digested proteins and peptides and nitrogenous products resulting from bacterial action on the large intestine, appear in the accompanying diagrammatic picture.

When fat excretion is expressed as a percentage of the intake, excessive excretion is revealed more readily than when it is described as a fraction of the fecal dry weight. Much has been made of the relative fractions of esterified and free fats in feces as a guide in differentiating between pancreatic and other types of steatorrhea, but evidence for this criterion is poor. With increasing fat or nitrogen intake, the corresponding fecal components increase on an absolute basis but decrease slightly when expressed as percentages of intake.

BIOCHEMICAL CHANGES IN ACUTE PANCREATITIS

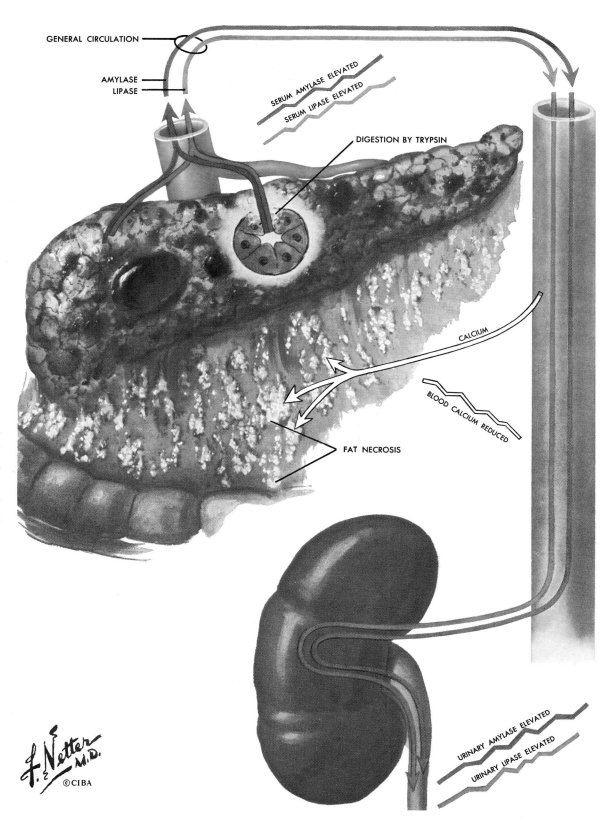

The most characteristic changes in acute pancreatitis (see page 143) and the most useful in diagnosis are the *elevations of amylase and lipase in serum* or plasma (see also page 58). These pancreatic enzymes are present in plasma under normal circumstances, but the exact mechanism by which they enter the blood stream is not known. It may be assumed that the enzymes pass from the secretory cells of the acini to the capillaries in the reticular connective tissue (see page 26). Back pressure by ligation or obstruction of the ducts or injury to the acini seems to augment the passage into the circulation. In approximately 90 per cent of the cases with acute pancreatitis, the amylase values are definitely above the norm (185 units, see page 58), and over 1000 units are found in 30 to 50 per cent, but these levels of activity may change greatly from day to day and even from hour to hour. For example, the activity may drop precipitously from levels of 2000 to 3000 units at the height of attack to normal values within 24 to 48 hours.

The serum lipase values in acute pancreatitis may be as high as six to seven times the upper limit of the normal range (1.5 Cherry-Crandall units, see page 58), particularly in the early course of the disease. For unknown reasons the lipase may rise when the amylase decreases. Both *amylase and lipase* are excreted *in the urine*. The urinary amylase concentration varies greatly from individual to individual and in the same individual during the day, it is usually about two- to sixfold the concentration in the blood. In spite of these fluctuations, the occurrence of a high blood amylase, due to acute pancreatitis or other pancreatic injury, is reflected in a high urinary amylase. Indeed, high excretion in the urine may persist for 24 hours after the blood amylase concentration has receded toward normal levels, and this persistence of urinary amylase

excretion may serve as a diagnostic aid. Because of methodological difficulties, urinary lipase has received little study, but recent studies indicate that more sensitive methods will reflect changes similar to those for urinary amylase. Lately, it has also been shown that the antithrombin titer of the blood is greatly elevated early in the course of acute pancreatitis. This titer is defined as the capacity of a patient's plasma to delay the clotting of a normal plasma by thrombin. The antithrombin titer is elevated in about 90 per cent of the cases with acute pancreatitis and in those cases of gastro-intestinal disease in which the pancreas may be involved as, *e.g.*, gallbladder disease and peptic ulcer. Elevations in antithrombin titer may be produced experimentally in animals by injection of trypsin, a fact which gives reason to believe that the elevated antithrombin titer is another manifestation of the passage of the pancreatic

enzymes into the blood.

Digestion and necrosis of the interstitial and the surrounding extrapancreatic tissue result when, as is typical in acute pancreatitis, the enzyme-rich juice leaks from the secretory cells and from the ductules. The regional fatty necrotic tissue becomes the seat of calcification. The calcium concentration of the pancreatic tissue, normally ranging between 5 and 6 mg. per 100 gm., may in such instances be raised to 500 mg. per 100 gm. The extensiveness of the *calcium deposition* depends in large measure on how long the patient lives after the episode of acute pancreatitis and the resultant necrosis. Such a diversion of the body's calcium stores to the pancreas is reflected by a slight but definite *lowering of the serum calcium*, frequently between about the third and eleventh days of illness, to values less than 9 mg. per 100 ml. and, occasionally, to as low as 5 or 6 mg. per 100 ml.

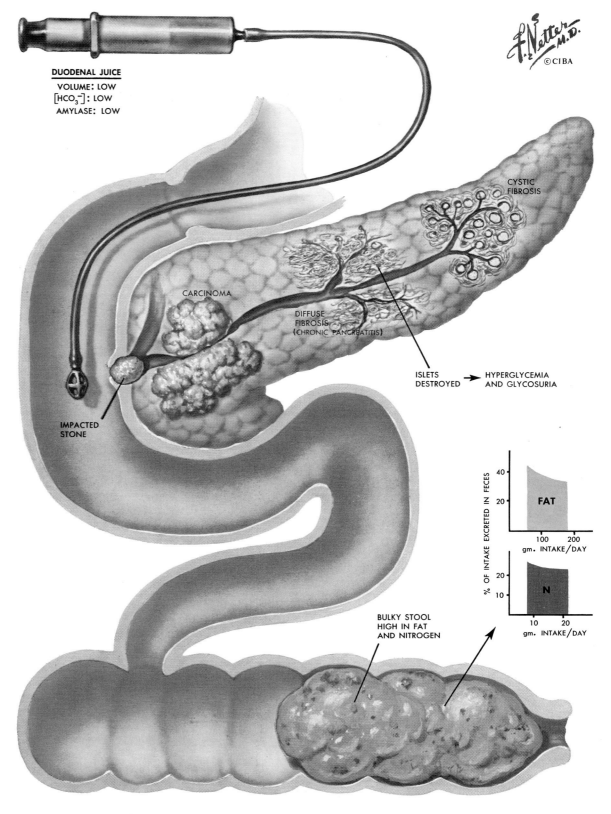

DUODENAL JUICE
VOLUME: LOW
[HCO₃⁻]: LOW
AMYLASE: LOW

CYSTIC FIBROSIS

CARCINOMA

DIFFUSE FIBROSIS (CHRONIC PANCREATITIS)

ISLETS DESTROYED → HYPERGLYCEMIA AND GLYCOSURIA

IMPACTED STONE

BULKY STOOL HIGH IN FAT AND NITROGEN

FAT

100   200
gm. INTAKE/DAY

% OF INTAKE EXCRETED IN FECES

N

10   20
gm. INTAKE/DAY

BIOCHEMICAL CHANGES IN PANCREATIC OBSTRUCTION

A number of biochemical derangements ensue when the pancreatic secretion fails to be delivered to the duodenum or when it lacks a sufficient amount of enzymes. Such deficiencies occur during the course of several diseases, the most typical being *fibrocystic disease* of the pancreas (see page 142), which is a manifestation of a systemic disorder and more properly termed mucoviscidosis. *Chronic pancreatitis* (see page 144), with development of a diffuse fibrosis, is also associated with deficient external secretion, which may be observed also as a result of a *carcinoma of the pancreas* head (see page 148) and, to a lesser or negligible extent, of carcinoma of the body or tail. *Pancreatic calculi,* until recently considered comparatively rare but more frequently recognized nowadays, may vary from pinpoint size to several centimeters in diameter and may cause interruption of the external pancreatic secretion. In all these conditions the internal secretion may also suffer, and *diabetes* may develop when the *islets of Langerhans* become *involved.*

The pancreatic secretion normally increases from about 2 to 3 ml. per hour in children of 1 or 2 weeks of age to about 15 ml. at 5 years and 45 ml. per hour at 7 years of age. In children with cystic fibrosis, even if a child reaches the age of 9 years, the secretion amounts to less than 5 ml. per hour. The enzyme activity per unit of volume is also greatly decreased. Trypsin and lipase activities are most profoundly affected and usually average 1 to 2 per cent of the normal values. Similar findings are also obtained in the other mentioned conditions, *e.g.,* in about 70 per cent of the patients with carcinoma of the head of the pancreas or of the ampulla of Vater, very low values for duodenal trypsin and amylase have been observed.

The decreased delivery of enzymes into the duodenum is reflected, of course,

in a diminution of intestinal digestive functions. The ingestion of casein, gelatin or other proteins by children with pancreatic cystic fibrosis is followed by a much smaller rise in blood amino-nitrogen than occurs in normal children. That this does not indicate an absorption deficiency per se may be concluded from normal rises in blood amino-nitrogen when predigested protein or amino acid mixtures or protein with pancreatin are fed. If adults with carcinoma of the pancreas or with chronic pancreatitis are fed starch, the rise in blood glucose is much smaller than after the ingestion of an equivalent amount of glucose, a difference not observed in patients without pancreatic disease.

Bulky, fatty and foul-smelling *stools* are characteristic of obstructive pancreatic disease, though chronic steatorrhea is seen also in other conditions with disturbed fat digestion and absorption, of which the poorly understood celiac syndrome makes its appear-

ance in the same age group as fibrocystic disease. In the former, however, pancreatic excretion is normal. In the latter, *fat in the feces* may *rise* to between 15 and 40 per cent of the intake. In chronic pancreatitis or with a pancreatic carcinoma, an even higher percentage (30 to 50) is found. Fat excretion, however, varies according to the individual patient and at different times in the same patient. The tendency to excrete less percentagewise at higher levels of intake than at lower levels remains the same in pancreatic disturbances as in normal individuals. The *fecal nitrogen* is also *increased, e.g.,* three to four times in pancreatic cystic fibrosis over that of normal children. The nitrogen may rise to between 4 and 5 gm., or about 20 to 25 per cent, sometimes even 50 to 60 per cent, of the intake, depending upon the severity of the obstruction in cancer or obstruction and secretory failure in chronic pancreatitis.

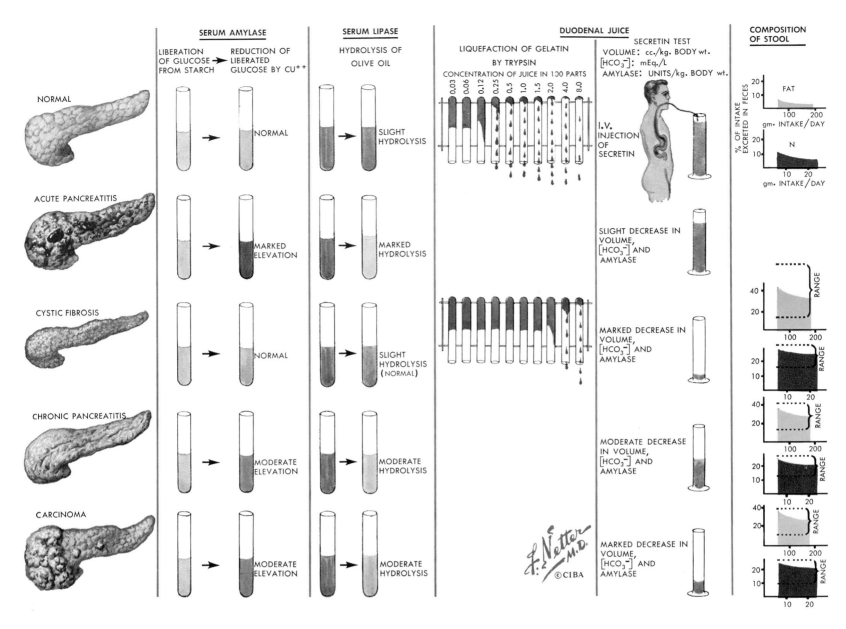

LABORATORY AIDS IN DIAGNOSIS OF PANCREATIC DISEASE

The most helpful laboratory tests for the diagnosis of a pancreatic disease and the evaluation of its severity are tabulated above. Of the several methods to determine *serum amylase,* Somogyi's has found widest use. Plasma or serum is added to a starch solution, and the glucose content over and above the reducing power of the serum before it was incubated with starch is determined. The amylase activity is expressed in units or milligrams of glucose liberated by 100 ml. of serum. The normal values vary greatly in the literature. Widely accepted is 105 units, with a standard deviation of 26 units, as reported in a study of 170 normal individuals (Somogyi). This means that values lower than 50 units or greater than 160 units are *possibly* abnormal, and values lower than 25 or greater than 185 units are *probably* abnormal. Values below 50 units are encountered in 30 to 40 per cent of patients with diseases of the liver and bile ducts, acute cholecystitis, pneumonia, cardiac failure and thyrotoxicosis, and in 60 to 75 per cent with

severe diabetes mellitus or diabetic coma. The characteristic elevation of serum amylase in acute pancreatitis has been discussed on page 56, but less drastic increases (between 200 and 700 units) may be found in peptic ulcers perforating or penetrating into the pancreas; in acute infections of the parotid gland, including mumps; in calculous obstruction of the salivary ducts; in renal insufficiency due to acute and chronic glomerulonephritis; in nephrosis of various types; in nephrosclerosis; etc. In chronic pancreatitis, the serum amylase is within normal limits, but, with a relapse, the level may rise markedly when previously unaffected pancreatic tissue is suddenly involved. The serum amylase activity is of little use as a diagnostic aid in cancer of the pancreas for it is moderately elevated in only about 10 per cent of the cases.

The *serum lipase* is determined by exposing an olive-oil emulsion to the hydrolyzing effect of the enzyme under standardized conditions (Cherry and Crandall) and titrating the liberated fatty acids with a diluted NaOH solution. In general, the lipase activity parallels that of the serum amylase. While substantially elevated in acute pancreatitis (see page 56), the lipase is only moderately increased in chronic pancreatitis and carcinoma. In the latter it sometimes reaches abnormal values when serum amylase is normal.

Estimation of the enzymatic activity of duodenal fluid obtained through a tube may be of value in differentiating between obstructions of

the common bile duct (stone or stricture, see pages 126 and 133) and those from a cancer of the papilla (see page 137) or of the head of the pancreas (see page 148). A practical method to determine *trypsin* activity has been proposed (Andersen and Early) as follows: A gelatin-bicarbonate gel is liquefied under standardized conditions by 0.12 to 0.25 part of normal duodenal juice per 100 parts of reaction mixture but requires much higher concentrations of juice in pancreatic deficiency, e.g., 4 to 8 parts per 100 in pancreatic cystic fibrosis.

In the *secretin test* a patient, intubated after a 12-hour fast, receives 1 unit secretin per kilogram of body weight, intravenously. The duodenal fluid is collected for 80 minutes, yielding mean normal values of 3.2 ± 0.6 ml. per kilogram of body weight for volume, 108 ± 8 mEq. per liter of bicarbonate and 14 ± 2 units amylase per kilogram of body weight (Dreiling). In acute pancreatitis these values are decreased about 20 per cent. About 95 per cent of the patients with chronic pancreatitis have low (40 per cent of the normal mean) bicarbonate concentrations, 60 per cent have low amylase activity and only 40 per cent produce slightly reduced (70 per cent) volume. In diffuse carcinoma of the pancreas, the reduction of all values is very marked, and still lower figures are obtained in cystic fibrosis.

The changes of the composition of the stool as a parameter of pancreatic function have been discussed on page 57.

Section XVII

DISEASES OF THE LIVER

by

FRANK H. NETTER, M.D.

in collaboration with

HANS POPPER, M.D.
Plates 1-8, 10-12, 15-56

VICTOR M. SBOROV, M.D.
Plates 9, 13 and 14

CONGENITAL ANOMALIES

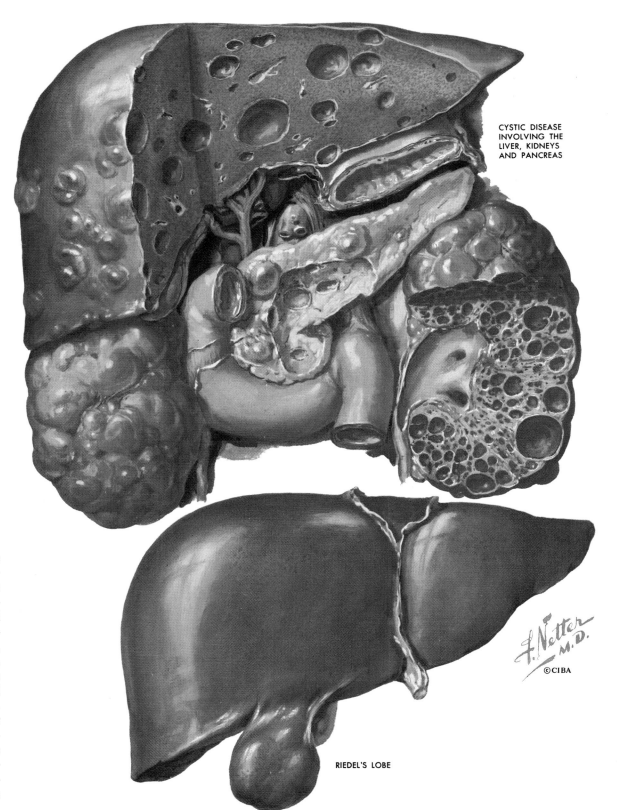

CYSTIC DISEASE INVOLVING THE LIVER, KIDNEYS AND PANCREAS

RIEDEL'S LOBE

The development of ductules and bile ducts depends upon organizing influences (see page 2). Disturbances of this development lead to an irregular arrangement of the ducts, resulting in solid nodules or in cysts. Small irregular proliferations of ductules and bile ducts, surrounded by excessive fibrotic tissue, appearing as small white nodules, are a frequent incidental finding in biopsy and autopsy specimens (see also page 111). The narrow cavities form an irregular plexus, usually connected with the biliary system and often containing small bile calculi. The significance of these hamartomas, also called multiple bile duct adenomas, lies in their differentiation from inflammatory lesions.

The same embryologic disturbance leads to cyst formation when the hamartomatous cavities become large or communicate with each other. The large ones are found mostly in adults, indicating their growth during life. Occasionally, single large cysts are observed, which cause pressure symptoms. More frequent is the *polycystic disease* of the liver which is, in at least half of the cases, associated with polycystic disease of the kidney and, though not so regularly, with pancreatic cysts. Sometimes other anomalies, such as aneurysms of the cerebral arteries, are encountered simultaneously. The lesion is often familiar. Exceptionally, this hepatic involvement may produce upper abdominal pain and a feeling of fullness, without functional impairment. This mostly occurs in the fourth and fifth decades. Malignant degeneration seems to be rare. The health of the patient is primarily influenced by the renal involvement. The hepatic cysts are lined by a cuboidal epithelium which is often desquamated. Their lumen contains a clear yellow fluid. Other hepatic cysts are parasitic (see page 104) or, less commonly, caused by accumulation of blood, lymph and bile. Ciliated cysts derive from misplaced intestinal endoderm, or they may be teratoid.

Riedel's lobe is a tonguelike extension of the right lobe, projecting from the anterior margin around the gallbladder. This projection, as a rule 1 to 2 in. long, is irregularly shaped and frequently narrow at its neck. Exceptionally, it is very long and extends into the pelvis. Sometimes the neck is thinned to a freely movable pedicle, consisting mainly of fibrosed tissue. The liver tissue in the lobe itself is mostly normal, but sometimes it exhibits fibrosis or bile stasis, if blood supply and bile drainage in the pedicle are compromised. The Riedel lobe is either a congenital anomaly or an acquired deformity caused particularly by tight lacing, as suggested by its greater frequency in women and by its apparent decrease in incidence in recent years. The extension may cause a kinking of the cystic duct, which would explain its fairly common association with gallbladder disease. The main clinical significance of the Riedel lobe lies in unusual palpatory findings in the area of the gallbladder, readily mistaken for a distended gallbladder, a tumor in the omentum or a pancreatic cyst.

MALPOSITIONS

COMPLETE
SITUS INVERSUS

PARTIAL
SITUS INVERSUS

Though encountered only on very rare occasions, congenital malpositions of the liver may create diagnostic problems. Transposition of the liver, *i.e.,* the large lobe with gallbladder lying on the left and correspondingly the small lobe on the right side, is usually accompanied by a connatural transposition of at least the other intraperitoneal organs. In such instances the pylorus lies to the left of the midline, while the fundus of the stomach, the descending colon and the sigmoid colon, as well as the spleen, are found on the right side, and the appendix and cecum, of course, on the left. This situation, in which the positional anomaly is restricted to the intra-abdominal organs, is called *partial situs inversus* in contrast to the more frequent *complete situs inversus* in which the chest organs present the same mirror-image transposition. In such cases the pulsation of the apex of the heart may be felt on the right side. The aortic arch extends to and the aorta descends on the right side; the right

lung has two lobes and the left three. Sometimes only the chest organs are transposed, while the abdominal organs, including the liver, are in normal position. Absence of the normal hepatic dullness on auscultatory percussion may lead to wrong diagnosis, particularly in gallbladder diseases, but these and other diagnostic difficulties arising from complete or partial situs inversus are readily resolved by roentgenologic examination.

The causes of situs inversus have not been established, and the explanations offered are all hypothetical. In complete situs inversus, the reversal of right to left and left to right must have been determined during the very first phases of structural organization in the embryo. Alteration of the normal rotation of the intestine has been offered as explanation of the

partial situs inversus, with differences in the width of the vitelline and umbilical veins playing a determining rôle. Rotation of the stomach from the primitive median position to the right rather than to the left has been considered a causative factor for the transposition of the liver.

Other congenital malpositions (not illustrated) include ectopia of the liver, resulting from an inherited defect of the muscles of the abdominal wall, and hepatic hernias at the umbilicus, which produce a peculiar mass near the navel. Bulging of the thin membranous part of the diaphragm into the cavity of the thorax permits herniation of part of the liver; this presents characteristic radiologic findings but, nevertheless, may pose problems of differential diagnosis of intrathoracic or subdiaphragmatic masses.

FEATURES OF DEGENERATION

Liver cell degeneration may be brought about by nutritional deficiencies, chemical agents, lack of oxygen, viral and bacterial infections and metabolic disturbances. Whatever the etiologic factors may be, the same textural picture of degeneration is seen, though it should be kept in mind that more types may exist which cannot be differentiated with the presently available morphologic techniques. Independent of the causes, the degenerative process is associated macroscopically with an enlarged organ, a tense capsule, a rounded anterior edge, reduced consistency and an obscured architecture, provided that passive congestion does not accentuate it. A brownish-red hue conveys the impression that the organ has been cooked. On microscopic examination one finds swollen liver cells associated with edema and Kupffer cell mobilization, a picture frequently found at autopsy and designated as *cloudy swelling*. Though this state has been attributed to altered protein metabolism, altered water content of the liver cells and derangement of the protoplasmatic organization, it is questionable to what degree these morphologic changes seen at autopsy reflect premortal or postmortal autolytic processes.

Biopsy specimens permit more subtle differentiation. Apparently the first morphologically recognizable but relatively mild change is concerned with the cytoplasmic nucleoproteins, most frequently of the centrolobular zone, which lose their basophilism and become acido- or *eosinophilic*. A more severe degree of degeneration is characterized by variations in size and staining qualities of nuclei as well as of cytoplasm of the neighboring liver cells. This *diffuse* change results in a polymorphous irregularity of the liver cell plates ("disarray", "unrest").

Progression of eosinophilic cytoplasmic degeneration leads to formation of acidophilic clumps around the nuclei. They are found in various types of hepatic injuries, though *Mallory*, describing these *bodies*, first considered them originally characteristic of alcoholic cirrhosis. Diffuse clumping of the cytoplasm may induce a homogeneous appearance of the latter; the nucleus, becoming pyknotic, eventually disappears. These cell remnants are then expelled from the liver plate and lie in the tissue spaces as acidophilic masses, the so-called *"Councilman bodies"*, named because of the fact that similar formations were discovered by Councilman in yellow fever. The nonpigmented bodies are encountered also in viral hepatitis (see page 93).

The appearance of ballooned cells, with central but relatively small nuclei, rarefied cytoplasm and sharp borders, remindful of plant cells, represents another type of liver cell degeneration,

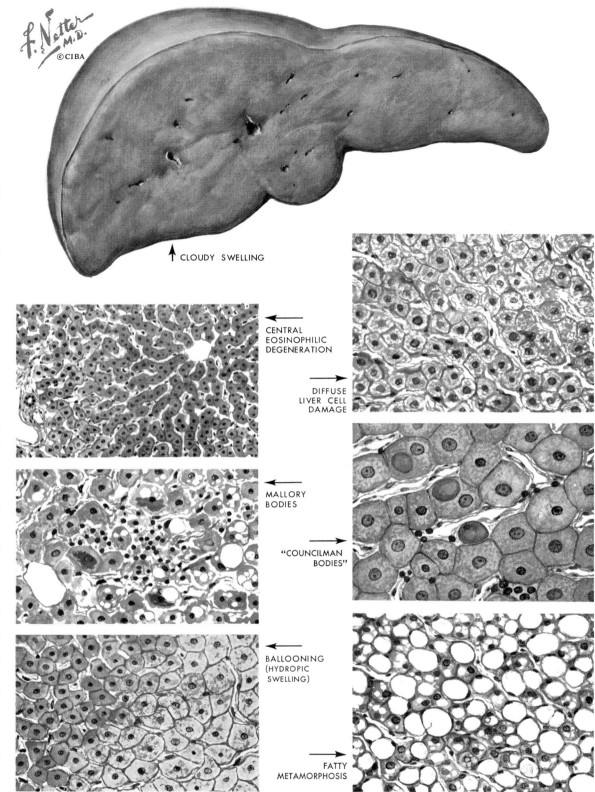

CLOUDY SWELLING

CENTRAL EOSINOPHILIC DEGENERATION

DIFFUSE LIVER CELL DAMAGE

MALLORY BODIES

"COUNCILMAN BODIES"

BALLOONING (HYDROPIC SWELLING)

FATTY METAMORPHOSIS

the *hydropic swelling,* which has been found in individuals exposed to low atmospheric pressure but is observed also in intoxications or conditions causing local interference with respiratory cellular processes.

Imbalance of the fat transport to and from the liver (see pages 67 and 78) leads to excessive fat accumulation. This accumulation, when assumedly traceable to increased storage, has been called "fatty infiltration" in contrast to the *"fatty degeneration"* ensuing from functional alterations as produced by toxic, anoxic or circulatory disturbances. Such sharp differentiation, however, can no longer be maintained, because excessive storage is potentially both the cause and the consequence of disturbed hepatic function. The morphologic separation, which assigned large fat droplets to infiltration and small ones to degeneration, also had to be abandoned, because in fatty degeneration of the lobular center as seen in passive

congestion, or all over the liver in various intoxications (see page 91), one may observe either multiple small droplets in one and the same cell or large fat drops replacing almost entirely the cytoplasm and pushing the nucleus aside.

Another form of liver cell degeneration produced by bile imbibition is called "feathery degeneration" (see page 83). The functional significance of all types of degeneration depends less upon the intensity of the degeneration in circumscribed parts of the lobule than upon the extent of alteration throughout the lobule. Morphologically, relatively inconspicuous but diffuse changes are functionally more important than a circumscribed, very conspicuous degeneration or necrosis (see pages 64 and 65).

Electron microscopic observations (see page 171) provide better understanding of the changes seen with the conventional microscope.

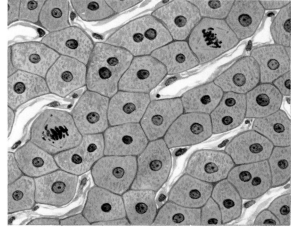

TWO-CELL-THICK PLATES

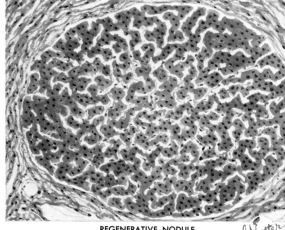

REGENERATIVE NODULE

FEATURES OF HEPATIC REGENERATION AND ATROPHY

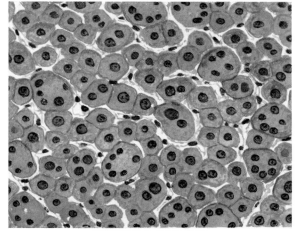

MULTINUCLEAR GIANT CELLS

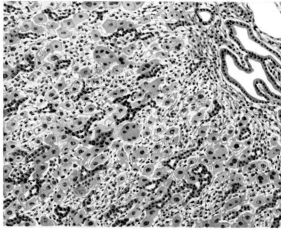

PROLIFERATION OF BILE DUCTULES

Cells of the liver plates constantly disappear and are replaced by new cells by either *mitotic* or *amitotic division*. *Binucleate cells* are, therefore, seen under normal circumstances. This regenerative activity is accentuated if liver cells are lost by disease or trauma. After successive partial hepatectomies the liver restores itself, and eventually the amount rebuilt exceeds by far the weight of those portions which the liver has lost. The regeneration takes place not only close to areas of extirpation or spontaneous necrosis but also in parts remote from the area of lost liver tissue. A stimulating humoral effect must be assumed to explain this phenomenon and is supported, *e.g.*, by the intensive regeneration of the intact liver in a rat living in parabiosis with a rat whose liver has been partially excised.

Local, as well as remote, liver regeneration occurs in hepatic diseases whenever degeneration and necrosis of hepatic tissue occur. Regenerated hepatic tissue may make up, and thus mask, the loss of function, and it is for this reason that hepatic tests sometimes yield normal values in spite of widespread hepatic disease. The regenerative processes are also responsible for the often perplexing variety of morphologic pictures in hepatic diseases.

Regeneration reveals itself in various structural forms and stages. Lost parts of a liver cell plate are replaced by liver cells growing into the empty meshes of the framework (see pages 66 and 67). Mitosis of singular cells or binucleate cells without mitotic figures may appear, or the entire liver cell *plate* may increase from a thickness of one cell to that of *two cells*, simulating the appearance of the liver in lower animals or in the embryo. Liver cells or liver cell groups which become isolated during necrosis of the surrounding tissue or during the development of cirrhosis (see pages 68 and 69) may transform themselves into independent *regenerative nodules*. Active regeneration in these nodules is usually most marked in the periphery where several-cell-thick plates are found in contrast to one-cell-thick plates in their

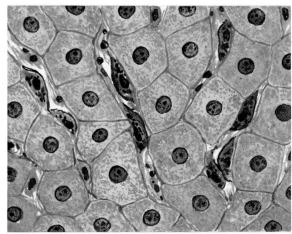

KUPFFER CELL REACTION

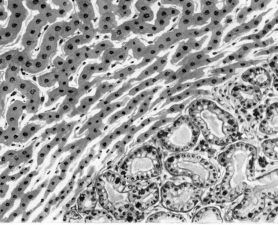

PRESSURE ATROPHY (DUE TO METASTATIC TUMOR)

center. The plates converge toward the center, indicating blood drainage from the center, although a central vein usually is not formed.

Sometimes, especially in infants, the division of liver cells does not keep pace with the division of the nuclei, so that *multinuclear giant cells* form, in which biliary inclusion may be found.

The so-called *proliferations of bile ductules* accompanying degenerative and necrotizing processes are mainly, but not solely, located in the periphery of the lobule. They have often been interpreted as an attempted liver cell regeneration from bile ducts and ductules. Electron microscopic and radioautographic evidence indicates that the proliferated bile ductules derive from ductules and not from liver cells, apparently in contrast to what occurs in the embryo (see page 2). However, regenerated liver cells might resemble bile ductules.

The reticulo-endothelial system and, consequently, the Kupffer cells respond to injury with more extensive regeneration than any other system of the body. *"Kupffer cell reactions"* may, therefore, be elicited by injuring stimuli such as bacteria, liver cell breakdown, intoxications, etc., or by agents which only cause phagocytosis. Most endothelial cells of the liver sinusoids exhibit Kupffer cell character. Their cytoplasm bulges into the lumen and contains engulfed material.

Atrophy of the liver cells may be the result of starvation (see page 77), but it may come forth also as the result of pressure in the vicinity of space-occupying lesions such as tumors, abscesses, granulomas or amyloidosis. The liver cells in such instances become stretched and may eventually lose their cytoplasmic basophilia, indicating focal functional insufficiency. Hardly ever is a focal loss significant enough to be reflected in the over-all function of the liver.

HEPATIC NECROSIS

Necrosis implies not only death of cells but also the phenomena following cell death, namely, the disappearance of cells and frequently also the environmental reactions to and the vanishing of dead cells. The final and irreversible stage of degeneration, hepatic necrosis, in most forms involves only the liver cells, whereas Kupffer cells and stroma remain intact. The Kupffer cells respond to most types of hepatocellular degeneration and necrosis with reactive proliferation. Suppression of this proliferation and necrosis of the Kupffer cells, as well as breakdown of the connective tissue stroma, is observed mainly when the blood supply has been interrupted. In necrosis attributable to anoxia, the entire hepatic structures appear homogeneously eosinophilic. The nuclei of the connective tissue elements have lost their affinity for stains. Changes of this kind are seen, for instance, in anemic infarcts (see page 107) or as results of arterial diseases (see page 109) or in areas with severed blood supply following trauma (see page 116).

Of greater significance is the necrosis restricted to the liver cells alone and instigated by a variety of etiologic factors. Chemical poisons (see page 91) interfering with the oxidative enzyme system in the liver may have the same effect as hypoxia (see page 90). Other chemical poisons increase the need for hepatic metabolites, which are required for their detoxification. An example is bromobenzene which is combined with cystein to be excreted as mercapturic acid and raises, therewith, the need for this amino acid. Compounds of this kind create a relative deficiency of metabolites similar to nutritional deficiency (see pages 77 and 78). Infections either impair the hepatocellular enzyme system or may increase the local need for oxygen or metabolites. In general, under circumstances such as those just mentioned, the damage in the liver is zonal except in infections, which tend to cause more scattered injuries, depending upon the spread of microorganisms or their products, and thus set up focal necrosis. Localization of necrosis in the lobule and the extent of the necrotic process determine the morphologic or structural manifestations, whereas the pathophysiologic consequences of hepatic necrosis depend not on the localization of the necroses but mainly on the total number of hepatic cells, the function of which has been lost.

Necrosis may be focal, i.e., single cells or a small group of cells have been injured, have disappeared and are replaced by scavenger cells, usually by neutrophilic segmented leukocytes but occasionally also, especially in viral infections, by histiocytes and lymphocytes. This chemotactic accumulation of scavenger cells makes the lesion more conspicuous than is diffuse liver cell damage (see page 62). Focal necroses may also be the result of focal obstruction of the sinusoidal blood flow, e.g., by cellular debris or fibrin thrombi. Obstructing proliferations of the Kupffer cells may operate in the same way. In typhoid fever, Hodgkin's disease (see page 110) or tuberculosis (see page 100), focal necrosis may thus become the initial stage of granuloma formation. Only rarely do focal necroses enlarge, and then sizable necrotic areas coalesce without specific relation to lobular arrangement.

Zonal necrosis, in contrast to focal, is characterized by its lobular distribution. In central necrosis the destructive process takes place around the central vein, whence it may extend toward the periphery of the lobule. The lobular architecture appears exaggerated and, were it not for a usually reduced consistency of the liver, the differentiation from acute passive congestion (see page 106) would be difficult. Depending upon the intensity of the damage and the age of the lesions, either liver cell fragments are still recognizable or the liver cells have entirely disappeared, and red cells engorge sinusoids as well as tissue spaces. In more progressed stages the framework is collapsed, and only a few scavenger cells are found intermixed with Kupffer cells and red cells. Necrosis of the liver cells in the center of the lobule is mainly the result of a failure of intralobular hepatic circulation (as seen in passive congestion or shock), of oxygen want (low atmospheric pressure) or of both. Since the blood brought by portal vein and hepatic artery reaches the center of the lobule after it has given up some oxygen to the peripheral and intermediate zones, anoxemia makes itself felt primarily and mainly in the central zone.

Periportal or peripheral necrosis indicates loss of the liver cells of the limiting plate and in the adjoining peripheral zone of the parenchymal lobule. Inflammatory exudate accumulates and usually merges with similar exudate in the portal triads. Proliferation of bile ducts and cholangioles is also frequent. Periportal necrosis, as a rule, results from inflammation in the portal triads which extends into the peripheral zone and is thus seen in infections involving the portal triads, in chronic biliary obstruction (see page 83) or in chronic viral hepatitis (see page 96). Midzonal necrosis is rare in human beings.

Extensive zonal, mainly central, necrosis results from exposure to various chemical poisons but is also observed following infections or shock. Since it is also produced or aggravated by cardiac failure, it is sometimes difficult to decide to what degree primary damage of the liver cells accounts for the hepatic necrosis and to what degree vascular factors, including agonal circulatory insufficiency, have contributed. Many examples of so-called toxic hepatic necrosis are hence probably not a primary hepatic disease.

If central necrosis becomes more extensive, bridges develop connecting the central zone, thus reversing the lobular pattern in that the intact portal zone appears surrounded by a necrotic periphery. This may proceed further to almost complete loss of liver cells in a lobule, i.e., to massive necrosis. It may be caused by any etiologic factor but is, in this country, probably most frequently produced by viral hepatitis, trauma or vascular occlusion. Experimentally, it has been produced in rats which were fed a yeast diet, low in cystine and vitamin E. Massive necrosis of isolated lobules may not be reflected as such in functional impairment, which depends on the capacity of the surrounding, still-functioning parenchyma. Massive necrosis in a considerable part of the liver produces hepatic insufficiency, sometimes fatal, which, on historical grounds, is called acute yellow or red atrophy of the liver. The liver cell fragments in massive necrosis are usually hardly recognizable, especially so in the fulminant form of viral hepatitis (see page 94). The liver cells are initially replaced by a large number of scavenger cells between which only a few proliferating ductules can be found. Subsequently, the scavenger cells disappear and the framework, emptied of liver cells, collapses.

In massive collapse the central and portal canals are closely approximated, but their relative position is not disturbed. Since all liver cells of a respective plate have been lost, regeneration leading to re-expansion does not take place, and a scar persists as a permanent indication of a massive collapse. Sometimes it happens that the vast majority of, but not all, liver cells of a lobule become necrotic (submassive necrosis). The remaining liver cells, sometimes fragments of one lobule or sometimes fragments of several adjacent lobules, undergo regeneration and may form nodules of various sizes and shapes, in some of which intact portal triads and central canals can still be recognized. The parenchyma surrounding the areas of collapse is, as a rule, also involved, essentially because break fissures develop around areas of collapse which are filled out by connective tissue membranes (see pages 66 and 67).

The appreciation of the functional significance of hepatic necrosis and degeneration has been promoted by recent experiences with liver biopsy. The former efforts to correlate between morphologic lesions seen in autopsy specimens and functional alterations, as reflected in the results of the hepatic function tests, led to erroneous conclusions, owing to the marked changes which the liver undergoes in the agonal and postmortal periods. Comparison between the picture in biopsy specimens and that in specimens obtained at autopsy shortly afterward has demonstrated that the liver undergoes the following changes: The liver cells lose their glycogen and, therefore, their normal vacuolated appearance of the cytoplasm, which appears dense in the autopsy specimen. Furthermore, the continuity of the liver cell plates is disturbed, and isolated liver cells have broken away and lie in the tissue spaces. These spaces themselves, hardly visible in biopsy specimens, become widened markedly and are filled with proteinic debris which apparently has escaped from the sinusoids because of increased permeability of the capillary wall, caused by anoxia. Finally, centrolobular necrosis may be found, which is not seen in the biopsy specimen. Most probably, all these changes develop mainly because of disturbed hepatic circulation. However, even the correlation between the morphologic picture of the biopsy specimen and the indications of functional changes is frequently hazy. Marked alteration of the liver cells may be the reflection of regeneration rather than degeneration, and the functional capacity of regenerating cells is but poorly understood. Degenerative changes may be morphologically inconspicuous but functionally very significant. In general, a diffuse lesion, even if not impressive, has greater significance functionally than a circumscribed severe alteration. Hepatic failure may be present with almost intact-appearing liver cells, while, on the other hand, all liver cells may appear altered, with hardly any functional impairment. Despite such discrepancies in individual cases, statistically a fairly good correlation exists between the presence and degree of diffuse hepatocellular degeneration or necrosis and the results of hepatic tests, especially those of cephalin flocculation and thymol turbidity and with a decreased serum albumin.

The center picture of the illustration on the opposite page is reproduced through the courtesy of The American Journal of Medicine *(16:98 [January] 1954).*

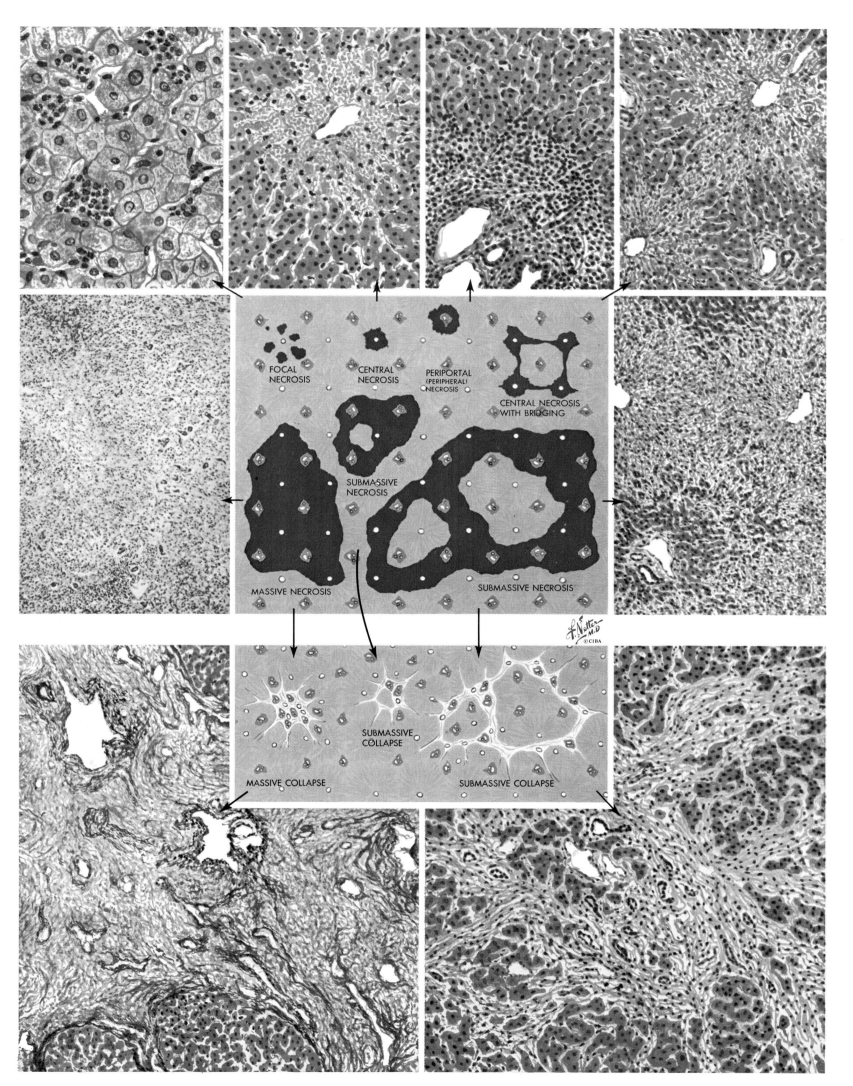

FOCAL
NECROSIS

CENTRAL
NECROSIS

PERIPORTAL
(PERIPHERAL)
NECROSIS

CENTRAL NECROSIS
WITH BRIDGING

SUBMASSIVE
NECROSIS

MASSIVE NECROSIS

SUBMASSIVE NECROSIS

SUBMASSIVE
COLLAPSE

MASSIVE COLLAPSE

SUBMASSIVE COLLAPSE

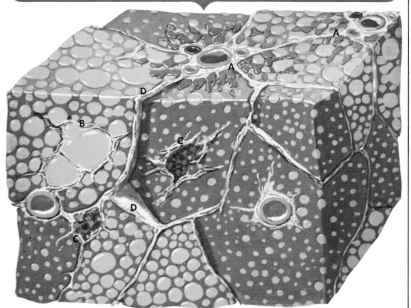

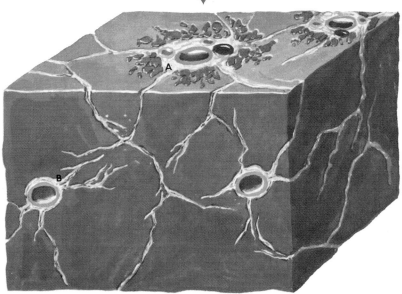

MICROMEMBRANES DEVELOP, RADIATING FROM PORTAL TRACTS (A), AROUND FATTY CYSTS (B), IN NECROTIC AREAS (C) AND IN "STRESS FISSURES" BETWEEN AREAS OF IRREGULARLY DISTRIBUTED FAT (D). SIMULTANEOUSLY REGENERATION (PURPLE) STARTS DIFFUSELY AROUND LOBULAR PERIPHERY

MICROMEMBRANES RADIATE DIFFUSELY THROUGH PARENCHYMA – OFTEN ORIG-INATING AT PORTAL TRIADS (A) AS RESULT OF IRRITATION (GRANULOMATOUS DISEASE, HEMACHROMATOSIS, VIRAL HEPATITIS?); OR FROM CENTRAL FIELDS (B) (PASSIVE CONGESTION, INTOXICATIONS). REGENERATION STARTS (PURPLE)

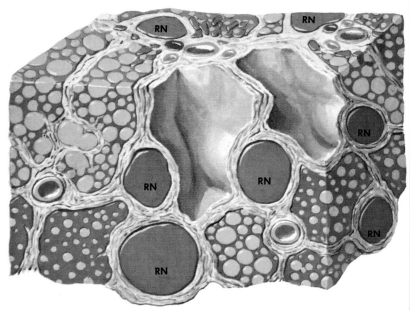

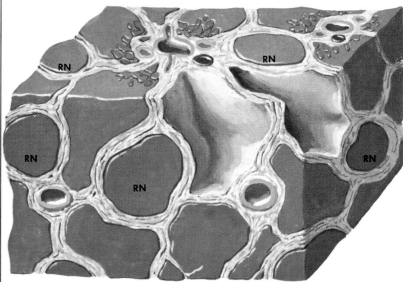

MICROMEMBRANES AGGREGATE INTO THICKER TWO–DIMENSIONAL IRREGULARLY RADIATING SHEETS OR SEPTA, WHICH DISSECT THE LOBULES. REGENERATIVE NODULES (RN) FURTHER ALTER THE ARCHITECTURE

AS IN FATTY TYPE, MEMBRANES AGGREGATE INTO DISSECTING SEPTA AND REGENERATIVE NODULES (RN) DEVELOP. NOTE SEPTA CONNECTING PORTAL TRIADS AND CENTRAL VEINS

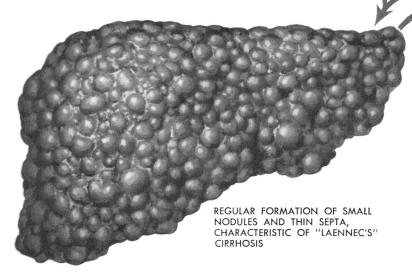

REGULAR FORMATION OF SMALL NODULES AND THIN SEPTA, CHARACTERISTIC OF "LAENNEC'S" CIRRHOSIS

SECTION XVII — PLATE 6

CIRRHOSIS I

Pathways of Formation

The definition of cirrhosis has been much debated by pathologists. To best correlate the well-defined clinical picture of cirrhosis (characterized by the cardinal functional manifestations of portal hypertension, reduced hepatic function, tendency to progression and ascites with structural changes), any increase in connective tissue without disturbance of the lobular architecture should be called "hepatic fibrosis", and fibrotic processes associated with alterations of the lobular structure and the presence of regenerative nodules and vascular anastomoses should be called "cirrho-

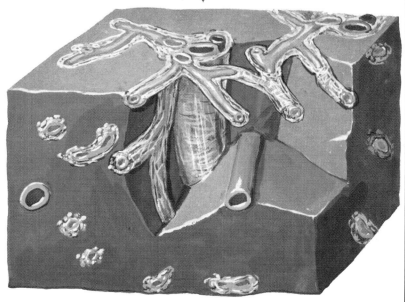

IN INFECTED OR PROLONGED EXTRAHEPATIC BILIARY OBSTRUCTION OR IN PRIMARY DUCTAL DISEASE, FIBERS FORM AROUND DISEASED BILE DUCTS AND MAY ALSO EXTEND AROUND INTRALOBULAR DUCTULES. STRANDS, NOT SHEETS, TRAVERSE THE LOBULES AS A NETWORK (PSEUDOCIRRHOSIS)

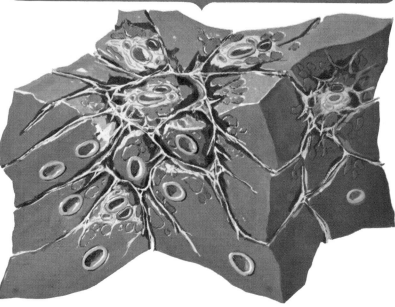

CIRCUMSCRIBED COLLAPSE AFTER MASSIVE OR SUBMASSIVE NECROSIS CAUSES STRESS IN SURROUNDING TISSUE, AND FISSURES APPEAR. SEPTA DEVELOP IN THESE AS WELL, AS A RESULT OF LESS SEVERE INVOLVEMENT OF SURROUNDING PARENCHYMA. REGENERATION STARTS (PURPLE)

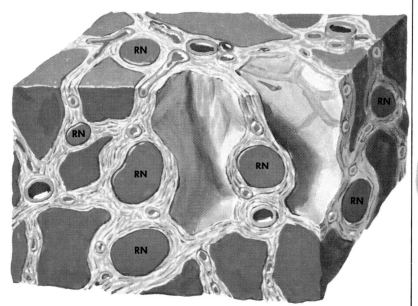

IN LATER STAGES, AS RESULT OF INFLAMMATION OR OTHER IRRITATION, SEPTA FORM, PARTLY BETWEEN STRANDS, IN PART INDEPENDENTLY, DISSECTING LOBULES AND COMPROMISING THE CIRCULATION. REGENERATIVE NODULES (RN) APPEAR

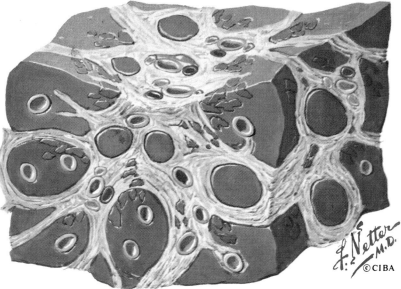

BROAD BANDS OF CONNECTIVE TISSUE RESULT FROM MASSIVE COLLAPSE, WHEREAS SURROUNDING TISSUE IS SUBDIVIDED INTO SMALL AND MULTILOBULAR NODULES OWING TO DEVELOPING MEMBRANES, WHILE REGENERATION TAKES PLACE IN NODULES AND IN LOBULES

MASSIVE OR RELENTLESS PIECEMEAL NECROSIS AND EXTENSIVE REGENERATION

sis". Thus the term cirrhosis indicates, in effect, an alteration of hepatic circulation, with or without manifestations of underlying chronic hepatitis.

Many hypotheses have been offered to explain the forces that transform a normal liver into a cirrhotic one. One pathway leading to cirrhosis starts in the presence of and is, in part at least, caused by steatosis of long standing. The *fat droplets* gradually enlarge and then coalesce to form *fatty cysts* (Hartroft), often more numerous in the central zone. Eventually, the fat disappears from the cysts, and the condensed connective tissue framework converges and develops into sheetlike structures or *septa*. Moreover, throughout the lobules, territories with severe *fatty metamorphosis* occur with fat-free ones, and irregular areas of regeneration alternate with those of degeneration as well. This results in zones of different parenchymal tissue turgor within the lobules, so that *fissures develop in planes of stress*. Fine connective tissue membranes are laid down in these fissures. They aggregate to form *straight septa* with no specific relation to lobular

(Continued on page 68)

IRREGULAR DISTRIBUTION OF VARIABLE—SIZED NODULES, MANY MULTILOBULAR, AND OF SEPTA, MANY OF WHICH ARE BROAD BANDS; POSTNECROTIC CIRRHOSIS

(Continued from page 67)

topography. However, the formation of connective tissue membranes around the portal tracts, as a result of inflammatory reactions partially secondary to liver cell injury, are more important. These membranes extend from the tracts into the parenchyma and produce a stellate shape. The membranes condense finally to become typical septa. While these complex patterns of septa expansion evolve, regenerative processes start. These lead to the formation of two-cell-thick plates and a complete rearrangement of the original plates, especially on the lobular periphery, and, eventually, to *regenerative nodules.* The septa fuse eventually to connect portal tracts and central fields. These connections contain vessels which become portal vein-hepatic vein anastomoses. Liver cells in those parts of lobules that have been separated from the rest of the parenchyma also start to multiply, and this regenerative effort results in cell plates directed toward the middle of the separated portion. This creates a regenerative nodule which, by compression of the adjacent connective tissue, contributes further to the formation of septa. In time, this series of associated events, with progressive formation of new nodules and septa, obscures the lobular architecture and replaces it with a nodular one. The final result is a *diffusely nodular liver,* which may have shrunk to one half or less of its original size when the fat disappears.

In man, fat accumulation is not the only factor responsible for the formation of a cirrhotic liver. Clinical experience verifies that persons may have a fatty liver for many years without developing cirrhosis. The mechanism characterized by *stress fissures* may be set up by variations in fat content within the liver, but it may also be stimulated by circumscribed hepatocellular damage. Intralobular and periportal types of septa development are elicited by hepatic necrosis, implying that septa formation in human fatty cirrhosis is largely caused by hepatocellular necrosis, to which the fatty liver is apparently predisposed.

Septa formation associated with regenerative nodules may emerge also in the absence of steatosis. Hepatic granulomas such as tuberculosis (see page 100) and sarcoidosis (see page 101), iron deposition in hemochromatosis (see page 89) or some types of portal inflammation, possibly resulting from viral hepatitis (see page 96), can initiate the formation of membranes and septa. These are around areas of intralobular necrosis and also extend from portal tracts, which then become stellate. Eventually, septa radiate from portal tracts into the lobular periphery, where a rearrangement of the liver cell plates takes place, associated with regeneration culminating in fully developed regenerative nodules. Membrane formation may also begin in the lobular centers, especially when liver cells in the central zone become necrotic and disappear, as in prolonged passive congestion (see page 106). The lobular parenchyma is gradually dissected by these septa, radiating either from the central zones or from the periphery. When the septa eventually reach portal tracts or central fields, respectively, they establish vascular anastomoses, and the process continues just as in fatty cirrhosis.

In diseases of *intrahepatic bile ducts,* either primary or secondary to extrahepatic biliary obstruction, *fibers* form around the ducts. In contrast to septa, however, these strands do not disturb the lobular architecture and, thus, do not interfere with hepatic blood flow. In this stage of biliary *pseudocirrhosis,* with a smooth surface and severe jaundice, regenerative nodules are seldom present, and no portal hypertension develops. Eventually, the ductules proliferate, and fibers accumulate around them, sometimes resulting in an increase of the intralobular connective tissue without significant disturbance of lobular architecture. *Septa do form* in later stages, however (owing to irritation from the sustained jaundice or other inflammatory stimuli), starting in the portal tracts or from the intralobular strands and leading to cirrhosis, as described above. In some instances, usually after many years, a nodular liver develops which, in its final stage, is indistinguishable from other types of far-advanced cirrhosis.

Another pathway to cirrhosis starts with *massive* or *submassive collapse* following *extensive* necrosis, either acutely, as in viral hepatitis and toxic injuries, or developing gradually from relentlessly progressing *piecemeal necrosis.* With *collapse of the framework,* portal tracts and central fields become approximated, and a postnecrotic scar develops. In these scars, some sinusoids are transformed into venous channels shunting blood from portal veins to central veins, and the rest are obliterated. Postnecrotic scars, as encountered in syphilitic hepar lobatum (see page 99) or in circumscribed atrophy, do not imply cirrhosis. Only if the scars accompany changes in the surrounding parenchyma can cirrhosis be assumed. Owing to the collapse and irregular tissue stresses, break fissures form, as massive necrosis progresses. In these fissures, as described in fatty cirrhosis, *membranes condense to septa,* in which capillaries are transformed into *venous channels.* In submassive necrosis the framework between the persisting lobular fragments collapses and is converted into *broad septa.* The effect of these forces is a separation of portions of the lobular parenchyma, with exceedingly active regenerative qualities. In contrast to fatty and nonfatty septal cirrhosis, alterations of the lobular pattern and the nodule formation, as well as the development of broad connective tissue bands, are very irregular throughout the liver, even in moderately advanced postnecrotic necrosis. Either because of the persistence of the original disorder or of processes inherent in the cirrhosis formation itself, even multilobular nodules become subdivided, so that sometimes diffuse small nodular cirrhosis, instead of the coarse nodular form, presents itself.

All pathways may lead to a uniformly *small nodular liver* with *narrow septa.* However, continued massive collapse of cirrhotic parenchyma, stimulating accentuated regeneration and the formation of new lobules, may transform the regular liver into an irregular organ with *large multilobular nodules* and *broad septa* corresponding to postnecrotic cirrhosis. This, rather than *Laennec's cirrhosis,* may be the final stage of all pathways, if the patient lives long enough to reach it. The same disease may thus initiate different pathways and end stages.

SECTION XVII—PLATE 7
(Illustration on opposite page)

CIRRHOSIS II

Fundamental Vascular Changes

Two distinct features, the regenerative nodule and the connective tissue septa, account for the main pathophysiologic sequelae of cirrhosis, whatever its etiologic starting point may have been. Both together are also the determining factors for the morphologic characteristic, namely, the nodular reconstruction of the originally lobular parenchyma, as described above and illustrated on pages 66 and 67.

Regenerative nodules may originate from parenchymal remnants persisting after massive or submassive necrosis or from parenchymal tissue parts which have been separated from their indigenous environment by connective tissue septa (see above). The nodules may even be the offspring of small liver cell islands entrapped in the septa. Whatever their origin, the regenerative nodules, after the concentrical rearrangement of the cell groups, expand and compress the surrounding tissue, including the vessels of the liver, but especially the septa, which become increasingly dense. The branches of the hepatic artery and of the portal vein are surrounded by a thick coat of connective tissue in the portal triads and are, therefore, less exposed to this compression, in contrast to the tributaries of the hepatic veins which lack in their thin walls adequately protective tissue elements. The *narrowing of the hepatic vein* branches has been actually demonstrated in injection preparations of cirrhotic livers. Naturally, the compression of the hepatic vein branches interferes with the drainage of blood from the liver and is thus one of the main causes of portal hypertension (see page 72). The number and size of the regenerative nodules have been found to have some relationship to the degree of portal hypertension in cirrhosis. The smaller and more numerous the nodules are, the greater is their compression effect, and the portal hypertension is correspondingly more severe.

During the formation of septa, irrelevant whether they start from collapse after massive or submassive necrosis or as an aggregation of collagenous membranes around necroses or fat accumulation (see pages 66 and 67), the liver sinusoids become included within the septa and some of them widen, assuming the appearance of veins. Having lost contact with the liver cells, they become *short cuts* between *branches of the portal vein* and *tributaries of the hepatic vein,* shunting blood so as to by-pass the parenchyma. In addition, they no longer equilibrate the dif-

(Continued on page 69)

(Continued from page 68)

ference between the blood pressures in the hepatic arteries and portal veins but act rather as short anastomoses between the two vascular systems of the liver. When, in the course of the fibrotic process, the smaller branches of the portal vein become compressed and in part even obliterated, the share of hepatic blood coming from the artery increases relatively to the amount of blood from the portal vein system, so that the ratio of portal and arterial blood is quite different in the cirrhotic from that in the normal liver. The arterial pressure, being at least partly transmitted into the portal vein branches by the anastomoses in the septa, increases the pressure in the portal vein. The arteriovenous anastomoses are, thus, the second main cause of portal hypertension in cirrhosis. The fibrotic compression of the intrahepatic venous system represents possibly a third cause.

As the *portal vein pressure rises* from the norm of 10 to 20 or 30 mm. Hg or more (as measured directly during operation or indirectly by percutaneous insertion of a needle into the spleen, or by determining the wedge pressure in the hepatic veins by transcardiac catheterization), a variety of collaterals between portal vein and caval systems come into existence (see also pages 18, 72 and 73). Some of them are clinically of minor importance, but others are of eminent significance (see page 179).

Retroperitoneal and diaphragmatic veins become more and more dilated but are seen only at operation or autopsy. The veins in the anterior abdominal wall dilate as a result of collaterals developing around the remnants of the fetal circulation in the round ligament. They become especially marked in the Cruveilhier-Baumgarten syndrome, in which the umbilical vein itself has either persisted or become patent. Veins at the gastroesophageal junction and the anus dilate at a site where glandular gastro-intestinal epithelium meets squamous epithelium. Bleeding hemorrhoids are frequent in portal hypertension, but far more important are the *varices at the lower end of the esophagus* and at the cardia of the stomach. Esophageal varices, which are demonstrable radiologically, develop in many liver diseases, occasionally, however, without any alteration of the liver or portal vein system, but they are the most frequent and also most serious attendant complications of all types of cirrhosis. They are fed by the *coronary vein*, which under normal circumstances is an affluent of the portal vein, and are drained by the *azygos vein*. The submucosal veins of the esophagus also receive blood from the spleen through the *short gastric vein*, which normally empties into the splenic vein but permits the blood to flow in the opposite direction when the pressure in the portal vein and its tributaries increases. The incongruence between the affluent blood stream and the restricted possibilities to release the blood to the vena cava, and also the thinness of the venous walls, bring about a dilatation

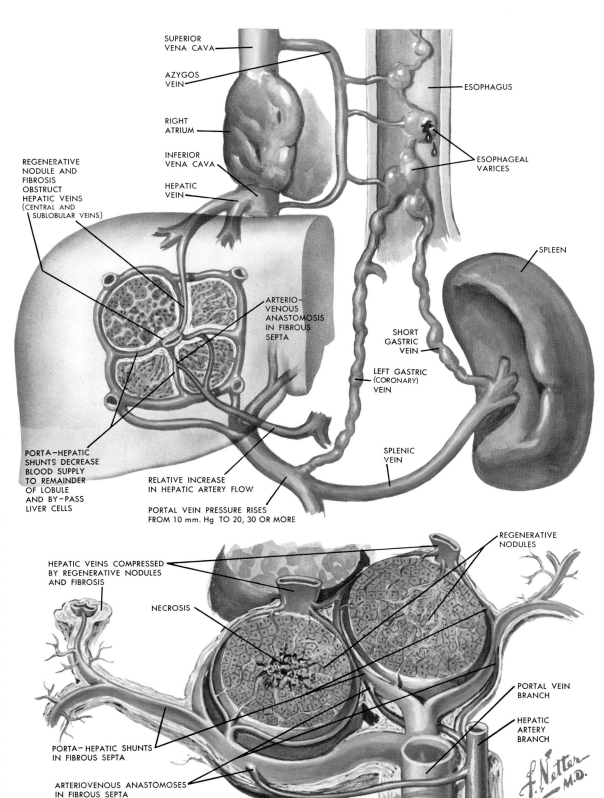

of the vessels and the development of varices in the lower third of the esophagus and in the cardia of the stomach. The developmental process of these varices, however, is not fully understood, especially when no hydromechanic reasons are apparent. The varices finally rupture, probably as result of peptic digestion. This leads to hemorrhage, the most frequent cause of death in portal hypertension.

These extrahepatic venous anastomoses have also another effect. They combine with the intrahepatic anastomoses, which shunt the blood from the portal vein to the hepatic vein, in depriving the lobular or nodular hepatic parenchyma of portal blood. This has serious consequences for the entire organism, which gradually loses the vitally important functions of the liver cells and will inevitably suffer from a "hepatocellular failure". Though this condition may be the end result of almost all kinds of liver disease, cir-

rhosis represents certainly the most common cause.

The effects of the *intrahepatic and extrahepatic shunts* can explain also the hepatic insufficiency in cirrhosis without jaundice and without evidence of severe liver cell damage. The shunts are a link in a sort of vicious circle, considering their origin within the septa of a damaged liver (fatty metamorphosis, collapsed necrotic liver lobules) and their disadvantageous effect upon the remaining as well as the regenerated parenchyma. Stemming from degenerative processes, they are also the cause of the centronodular or centrolobular necroses, so frequently observed in every type of cirrhosis. These necroses, in turn, lead to additional fibrosis and cirrhotic transformation and maintain liver cell damage and the cirrhotic process, even if the original cause of the cirrhosis, such as malnutrition, virus infection or exposure to hepatotoxic agents, has long since vanished.

CIRRHOSIS III

Clinical Manifestations

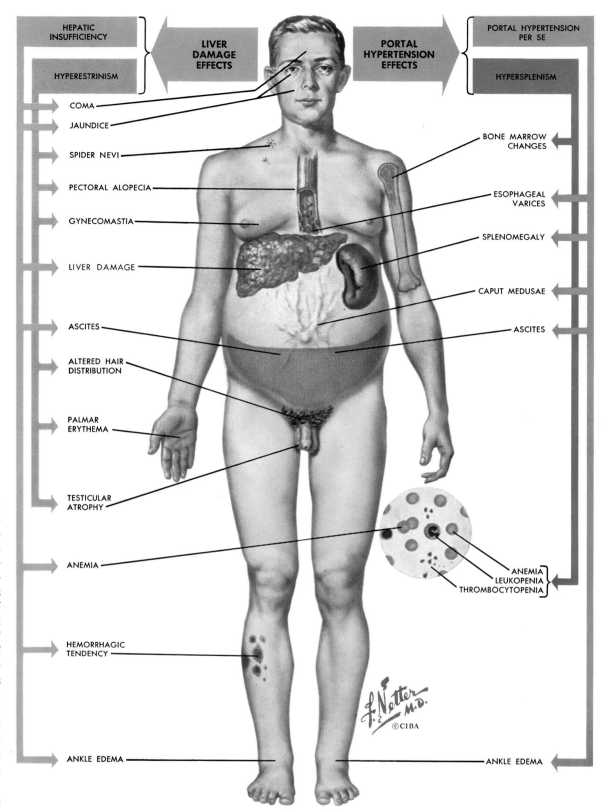

The *clinical manifestations of cirrhosis* vary with its different forms. Chills, high fever and leukocytosis are induced by an infected extrahepatic biliary obstruction and are observed in secondary biliary cirrhosis (see page 84). Peripheral neuropathy, as a symptom of malnutrition, is encountered in the nutritional type of cirrhosis. Hepatic insufficiency, the result of liver cell damage, and/or loss of hepatic functions due to diversion of blood by extrahepatic portacaval collaterals and intrahepatic portahepatic venous anastomoses (see page 69), explain many clinical symptoms. Palpation and percussion uncover a sometimes enlarged, sometimes shrunken liver, depending upon the stage of the disease. The organ, in most cases, is firm, and the granular character of the surface is rarely palpable.

Severe jaundice is seen only in the minority of instances; a subicteric hue is extremely frequent. Central nervous manifestations vary from somnolence to precomatous manifestations (reflected in flapping tremor, mental confusion and electro-encephalographic changes) to frank *coma* (see page 75). The *hemorrhagic tendency* is caused by a defect in the hepatic formation of serum proteins active in the processes of blood coagulation, especially prothrombin, and of the coagulation factor VII (see page 40). Capillary damage also may be important. Fibrinogen formation is usually not decreased in cirrhosis but may be increased. Hypoproteinemia and a pressure upon the inferior vena cava by ascites may

explain the appearance of ankle edema. Liver cell damage produces *anemia* of the macrocytic and normochromic type by hypersplenism as well as probably by a nonspecific toxic effect upon the bone marrow. *Testicular atrophy, gynecomastia,* a *female escutcheon, pectoral* and axillary *alopecia,* and a marked reddening of thenar and hypothenar (*palmar erythema*) are all considered to eventuate from an excess of circulating estrogen, which escapes its inactivation (see page 37) because of the hepatic insufficiency. Hyperestrinism also induces cutaneous *spider nevi,* which are found mainly in the upper half of the body, mostly on the neck, forearm and dorsum, and sometimes on mucous membranes. They consist of a central arteriole from which many small vessels radiate. Most manifestations of hyperestrinism are more mani-

fest in the male. In the female, mainly hair loss and spiders are seen, but also some masculinizing effects, even hirsutism, are noted.

The hepatic failure, combined with the effects of portal hypertension (see pages 69 and 72), leads to *ascites, esophageal varices* and the dilatation of abdominal veins (*caput medusae*). Leukopenia, thrombocytopenia and anemia are the resultants of the *enlargement of the spleen* and signs of hypersplenism. The change in the blood components is associated with alteration of the bone marrow, which may show increased hematopoietic activity and, thus, a *red marrow.* Usually, the erythroblastic activity is more marked, possibly as a reflection of the hemolysis, and the myeloid-erythroid ratio is decreased or even reversed.

PHYSICAL DIAGNOSIS OF LIVER DISEASE

The clinical diagnosis of liver disease is not difficult in advanced hepatic decompensation. A history of deepening jaundice, dark urine, light stools, progressive increase in girth of the abdomen and subjective symptoms of weakness, anorexia and other digestive difficulties focuses the attention of the clinician upon the liver.

Icterus, i.e., more or less deep staining of the skin, sclerae and mucous membranes, may be present in extrahepatic obstructive jaundice as well as in hepatocellular injury. The icterus present in prehepatic (hemolytic) jaundice (see page 48), however, usually does not stain the tissues as deeply as in the other forms. In hepatic and posthepatic jaundice the *urine* is *dark* and the *feces* are *light,* particularly if the jaundice is deep. In prehepatic jaundice, on the other hand, bilirubin does not appear in the urine, but the urine may be dark owing to increased amounts of urobilin. For the same reason, the feces in prehepatic jaundice are also dark. It is important to remember that in certain advanced cases of liver disease little or no jaundice may be apparent.

The appearance of *spider nevi* or telangiectasia, *gynecomastia, palmar erythema, testicular atrophy,* fine skin, sparsity of body hair and prostatic atrophy is generally believed to be due to hyperestrogenism (see pages 37 and 70). Despite the fact that these changes are secondary, their appearance frequently helps to establish the diagnosis.

The detection of an *enlarged* or tender *liver* is the most striking indication of some disease, either primary or secondary, of that organ. In patients with a relaxed abdominal wall or in thin individuals with low diaphragms, the liver may be palpable even in the absence of hepatic disease. In patients with biliary cirrhosis (see page 84) or fatty metamorphosis (see pages 79 and 80) or with a primary or secondary hepatic neoplasm, the liver may be massively enlarged and nodular. In congestive heart failure (see page 106) or constrictive pericarditis (see page 72), it may also be enlarged and tender. In some patients with far-advanced or rapidly progressing liver disease, the organ may be very small and not palpable. An atrophic liver incapable of regeneration is usually a very ominous finding in patients with known hepatic disease.

The presence of *splenomegaly, ascites* and *caput medusae* raises the suspicion of portal hypertension (see page 69), though the spleen may be enlarged in patients with parenchymal liver disease without

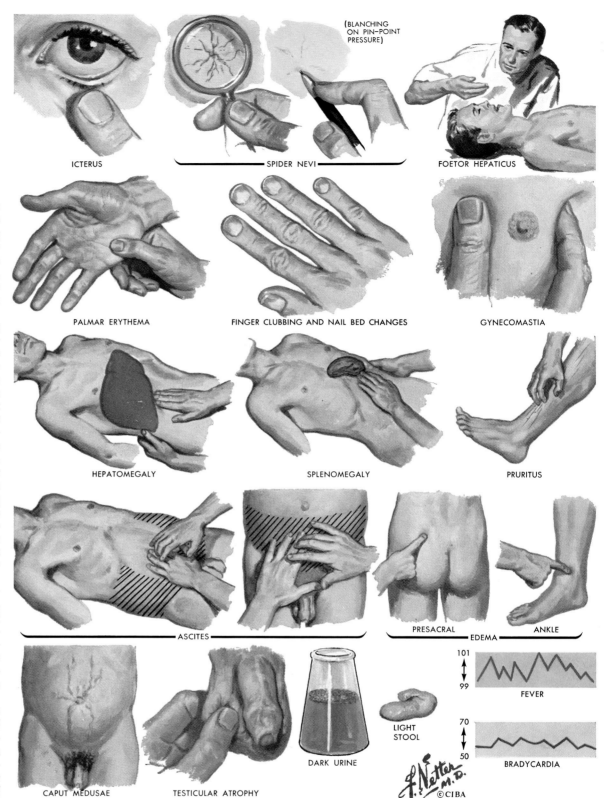

ICTERUS — SPIDER NEVI (BLANCHING ON PIN-POINT PRESSURE) — FOETOR HEPATICUS

PALMAR ERYTHEMA — FINGER CLUBBING AND NAIL BED CHANGES — GYNECOMASTIA

HEPATOMEGALY — SPLENOMEGALY — PRURITUS

ASCITES — PRESACRAL — EDEMA — ANKLE

CAPUT MEDUSAE — TESTICULAR ATROPHY — DARK URINE — LIGHT STOOL — FEVER — BRADYCARDIA

portal hypertension, *e.g.,* in congestive heart failure.

In moderately severe and advanced cases of hepatic disease, particularly when hepatic coma has supervened, a *foetor hepaticus* is often discerned by the trained clinician. This odor is distinctive but difficult to describe. It is a musty, sweetish odor, not unpleasant, which at times is more easily detected by the physician upon entering the sickroom than when he is close to the patient. Although it may disappear following enemas or drastic bowel movement, and though observed sometimes in mild or chronic forms of liver disease, foetor hepaticus is mostly to be considered of grave prognostic significance.

Clubbing of the fingers and *whitening of the nail beds* are seen in some patients with cirrhosis of the liver. These signs are not specific for hepatic disease, but they serve to confirm the diagnosis. Severe *pruritus,* with or without jaundice, may be the outstanding

symptom in patients with the cholangiolitic type of liver disease and is frequently present in posthepatic jaundice. The pruritus is thought to be due to an increased concentration of bile salts in the blood stream. Elevated alkaline phosphatase and serum cholesterol are frequently seen in association with the pruritus, comprising the outstanding features of the so-called primary biliary cirrhosis (see page 84).

Presacral and *ankle edema,* often notable in patients with advanced liver disease, are primarily the result of lowered serum albumin, although sodium retention (see page 74) is considered a contributive factor.

Worthy of mention is the *irregular fever* seen in patients with cirrhosis of the liver. This febrile reaction is noted in about 25 per cent of the reported cases of chronic liver disease. Although its exact cause is not yet established, it is believed to be connected with intrahepatic necroses.

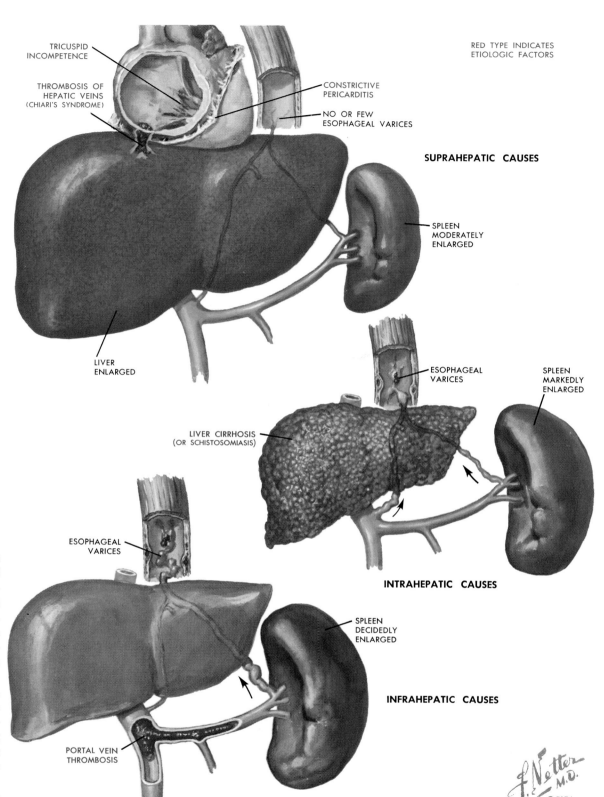

TRICUSPID
INCOMPETENCE

THROMBOSIS OF
HEPATIC VEINS
(CHIARI'S SYNDROME)

CONSTRICTIVE
PERICARDITIS

NO OR FEW
ESOPHAGEAL VARICES

SUPRAHEPATIC CAUSES

SPLEEN
MODERATELY
ENLARGED

LIVER
ENLARGED

ESOPHAGEAL
VARICES

SPLEEN
MARKEDLY
ENLARGED

LIVER CIRRHOSIS
(OR SCHISTOSOMIASIS)

INTRAHEPATIC CAUSES

ESOPHAGEAL
VARICES

SPLEEN
DECIDEDLY
ENLARGED

INFRAHEPATIC CAUSES

PORTAL VEIN
THROMBOSIS

PORTAL HYPERTENSION I

Causes

The portal venous pressure rises above the norm of approximately 20 cm. of water because of (1) block in the intrahepatic portal vein tree, (2) impaired outflow of blood from the liver, (3) excessive flow of either splanchnic or hepatic arterial blood to the liver or (4) transmission of hepatic arterial pressure into the portal vein branches.

Portal hypertension is associated in the early stages with dilatation of the splenic capillary sinuses and is subsequently followed by fibrotic thickening of the sinus walls and atrophy of the splenic follicles (fibrocongestive splenomegaly).

The *suprahepatic* form of portal hypertension is induced either by heart failure with passive congestion or by obstruction of the main hepatic veins. In heart failure, portal hypertension parallels increased systemic venous pressure, and hepatic involvement represents no specific problem. Only in *tricuspid incompetence* or *constrictive pericarditis*, particularly if it involves the entrance of the vena cava inferior, a special problem arises in view of the fact that the emptying of the hepatic vein is impaired. Occlusion of the hepatic veins, leading to *Chiari's syndrome,* a rare condition, results from tumors or abscesses in the vicinity of the entrance of the hepatic veins into the vena cava inferior, but syphilitic or rheumatic vascular diseases,

spontaneous thrombosis and congenital defects may also play an important rôle. A rapidly developing acute condition is differentiated from a slowly developing occlusion. In suprahepatic portal hypertension the *liver* is *large* and tender; ascites develops; the *spleen* is only slightly to *moderately enlarged.* Because of an equally elevated pressure in the portal and caval systems, esophageal varices do not develop.

The most frequent type, *intrahepatic* portal hypertension, is, of course, caused by *cirrhosis,* for reasons described earlier (see pages 68 and 69). But syphilitic hepar lobatum (see page 99), primary hepatic carcinoma (see page 112), schistosomiasis (see page 105) and, occasionally, even fatty liver may also create portal hypertension, the degree of which does not necessarily parallel the degree of liver shrinkage.

The *spleen* is *markedly enlarged,* and *esophageal varices* are well developed.

In *infrahepatic portal hypertension* the *liver* is of *normal size,* the *spleen* is *decidedly enlarged* and so are the *esophageal veins.* This form occurs more frequently in younger age groups. The most important cause is portal vein thrombosis (see page 108). But portal vein compression, by tumors or inflammatory masses, or congenital anomalies of the portal vein (see page 19) may also represent causative factors. On rare occasions severe portal hypertension has been observed in children without detectable anatomic alterations.

The modern measurements of portal pressure have added new understanding to the problems of portal hypertension (see page 179).

PORTAL HYPERTENSION II
Relief by Surgery

Cirrhosis of the liver is considered, in principle, an alteration of hepatic circulation, and surgical procedures have been applied specifically to correct the resulting portal hypertension. Measures used in acute esophageal hemorrhages include esophageal tamponade with the Sengstaken-Blakemore tube and balloons, ligation of the varices (transthoracically or transabdominally) and attempted reduction of blood flow in the varices either by intraluminal cooling or Pitressin®. Obliteration of the varices by sclerosing agents, or resection of the lower esophagus or of the gastric antrum has been recommended after bleeding has been controlled. These procedures are now supplemented by correction of the circulatory condition, either by the diversion of portal blood into the systemic circulation to bypass the liver, or by the reduction of blood passing through the hepatic sinusoids. The oldest, simplest, but not very efficient, surgical procedure, patterned after the spontaneously developing anastomoses in the peritoneum, is the Talma-Morison *omentopexy*. Anastomoses between the portal and caval venous systems are more efficient. The *splenorenal shunt* links the splenic vein and the left renal vein, and the *portacaval shunt,* Eck's fistula, diverts splanchnic blood from the liver, either by an end-to-side insertion of the portal vein into the vena cava, or by a side-to-side anastomosis. To avoid the disadvantages of either of these anastomoses, a double-barreled shunt has been introduced in which both ends of the divided portal vein are connected with the inferior vena cava. Other shunts, such as those using the mesenteric veins with the left renal or the inferior vena cava, are seldom effective. Shunt operations were initially associated with a very high mortality rate (approximately 66 per cent) but today it is below 10 per cent. The splenorenal shunt, sometimes difficult, frequently becomes occluded by thrombi, but it is the operation of choice if the main portal vein stem is obstructed or malformed. The portacaval shunt is more effective in portal decompression, because the blood of the main source of the esophageal varices, the coronary vein (see page 18), is diverted directly. For portal vein decompression the end-to-side anastomosis is preferred. It is also technically easier. The side-to-side shunt, being incomplete, does not interrupt the total portal blood flow to the liver but it does decompress the splanchnic system also, since, with the blood potentially flowing backward, the portal vein is drained. The double-barreled shunt, by decompressing both the liver and the splanchnic systems, therefore is particularly recommended in the treatment of intractable ascites. The various theoretical and practical advantages of these shunt procedures are not yet agreed upon, but, usually, preopera-

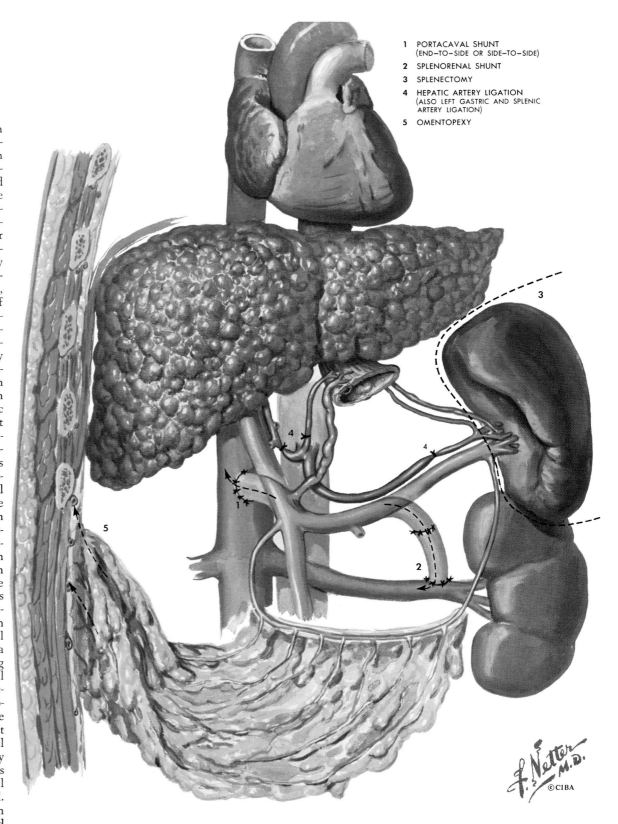

1 PORTACAVAL SHUNT (END-TO-SIDE OR SIDE-TO-SIDE)
2 SPLENORENAL SHUNT
3 SPLENECTOMY
4 HEPATIC ARTERY LIGATION (ALSO LEFT GASTRIC AND SPLENIC ARTERY LIGATION)
5 OMENTOPEXY

tive or intra-operative portovenography (see page 54) determines the selection of the type of anastomosis.

The diversion of blood from the liver is potentially dangerous for the hepatocytes, and transient functional impairment always follows the operation; this may become critical with pre-existing hepatocellular damage. The results of shunt operations are best in patients with normal serum albumin levels, bilirubin levels below 2 mg. per cent, without ascites and neurologic manifestations and with excellent nutrition. In general, therefore, the prognosis is much better in schistosomiasis or portal vein thrombosis without parenchymal involvement than it is in most forms of cirrhosis. The operation is sometimes performed as an emergency procedure. However, even when shunt operations are clearly indicated, undesirable sequelae may develop. These include neurologic manifestations, especially portosystemic encephalopathy (see

page 75) and peptic ulcer. Rarer complications are hemochromatosis, diabetes mellitus and even myelopathy. For this reason the question of whether a prophylactic shunt operation is justified, when esophageal varices are roentgenologically demonstrated but no hemorrhage has occurred, cannot be answered lightly.

Splenectomy was once widely used to relieve hypersplenism and to reduce blood flow to the portal vein and esophageal varices. Now it is thought to be contraindicated unless combined with a splenorenal shunt, which is not feasible, however, once the splenic vein has been obliterated after splenectomy.

Ligation of the hepatic artery reduces the blood flow to the liver and, supposedly, the pressure in the portal vein branches, when extensive intrahepatic anastomoses exist. The results are questionable, however, because definite proof that the portal pressure drops, in survivors of this operation, has not been cited.

Ascites

Pathogenesis

Fluid exchange between intraperitoneal fluid and blood plasma is subject to the same forces which regulate the distribution of fluid between interstitial and intravascular departments. Under normal conditions the serum water, which filtrates through the semipermeable wall of the arterial capillary limb, where the blood pressure is higher than the oncotic pressure, is reabsorbed as interstitial fluid by the blood in the venous capillary limb, where the oncotic pressure exceeds the blood pressure. Disturbance of this mechanism results in accumulation of tissue fluid, *i.e.*, edema. If more fluid passes into the peritoneal cavity than is reabsorbed, ascites develops in analogy to the formation of edema in peripheral areas.

A general rise of venous pressure tends to cause edema. Similarly, *portal hypertension* tends to facilitate ascites formation, though ascites is by no means an obligatory sequela of portal hypertension. Partial experimental obstruction of the portal vein has not led to ascites, and the operative relief of portal hypertension does not necessarily reduce it. Ascites may also disappear despite undiminished portal hypertension.

Diminished serum protein concentration, especially of albumin, its smallest and, therefore, osmotically most potent fraction, reduces the oncotic pressure of the blood and induces edema and/or ascites formation, because filtration through the capillary wall is increased and reabsorption of tissue fluid is impaired. If hypoproteinemia complicates portal hypertension, a rapid development of ascites may be expected and occurs promptly, *e.g.*, after hemorrhage from ruptured esophageal varices. Ascites is well correlated with diminished albumin synthesis in all types of cirrhosis, but, setting up a vicious circle, the albumin loss into the ascitic fluid also increases the hypo-albuminemia.

Sodium retention, as it may be brought on by *heart failure, renal congestion* or an *excess of hormones* regulating reabsorption of water and serum in the renal tubules, is nowadays considered a main causal factor in ascites formation. The increased hormone activity is possibly caused by liver damage. An *antidiuretic principle* released *from the posterior*

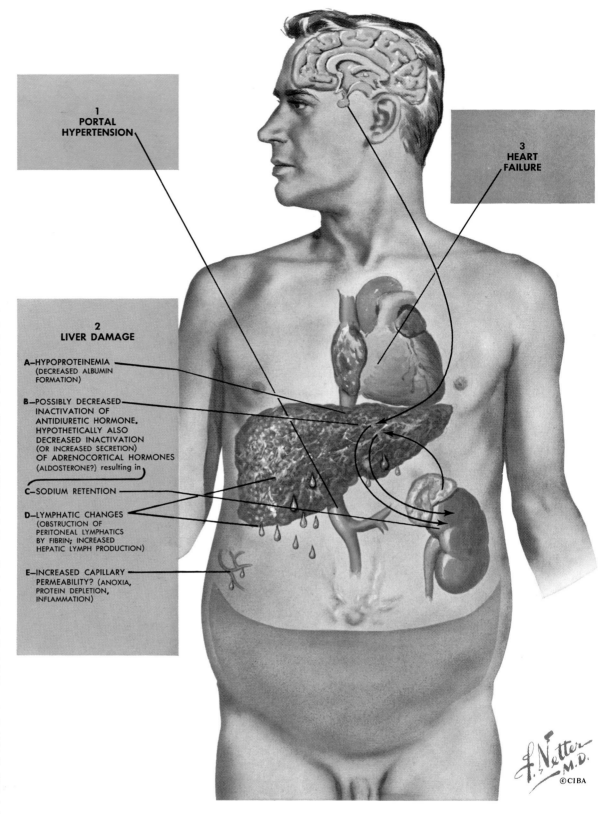

pituitary is supposedly inactivated by the liver. Faulty inactivation has been claimed as a cause of water retention in cirrhosis, but the experimental evidence for this hypothesis is at best equivocal. Faulty inactivation of *aldosterone*, the recently isolated, sodium-retaining *adrenal* hormone, in the cirrhotic liver may also explain the salt retention correlated with ascites. Another possibility is that aldosterone excretion is stimulated by the reduction of the plasma volume brought about by ascites and accelerated by paracentesis, although, in cirrhosis, the plasma volume may be high, normal or low. Speculative as the explanation of the sodium retention in ascites still is, its rôle and relation to liver injury are well established by clinical experience.

Excessive *hepatic lymph flow* into the peritoneal cavity, incited by alterations of hepatic circulation and by liver damage, has been considered a major

source of ascites. *Oozing of lymph* from the hepatic surface and high protein concentration in the ascitic fluid have been observed when the inferior *vena cava* was experimentally *constricted*. Other factors which can emanate from liver injury, such as fibrinous obstruction of peritoneal lymphatics or excessive protein filtration through *anoxic* or *inflamed peritoneal capillaries,* may contribute to ascites formation.

The rôle of *heart failure* and, especially, its contribution to ascites in cirrhosis are well established clinically. Essentially, two factors are involved: (1) increase of venous pressure in the vena cava inferior and (2) sodium retention by disturbance of the glomerular filtration and tubular reabsorption in congestive heart failure. They might be complicated by lowered plasma protein as a consequence of edema in other parts of the body, malnutrition or diminished protein synthesis in the liver.

HEPATIC COMA

Progression of liver disease over a variable period of time finally results in a deep stupor which, if not interrupted by appropriate therapy, leads to the death of the patient. This end stage of decompensated hepatocellular failure and its neurologic complications, *the hepatic coma,* may have several causes. It may result from gradual or acute deterioration of hepatic function. The most frequent predisposing factor, however, is hemorrhage, usually from bleeding esophageal varices (see pages 72 and 73) or peptic ulcer. It is an accepted observation that massive hemorrhage from any site is not tolerated as well by patients with hepatic disorders as by those with other conditions. Infections, sometimes even mild ones, ensuing in the course of acute or chronic liver disease, may precipitate hepatic coma; in some patients a simple cellulitis may prompt a sudden worsening in those who had appeared to be doing well. Morphine, other opiates, barbiturates or even milder sedatives have been known to precipitate hepatic coma, perhaps because of the liver's failure to metabolize and therewith inactivate the drugs (see pages 36 and 37). Recently, it has also been noted that a high protein diet, or one high in nitrogenous substances, may bring about signs of coma, which disappear when the increased levels of blood ammonia can be lowered by decreased intake of protein or other nitrogen sources.

Although it is admitted that blood ammonia and certain organic acids may play a rôle in its appearance, hepatic coma cannot be adequately defined in the biochemical sense. It is, in most instances, difficult to predict which patient will develop hepatic coma. In general, the comatose state will follow when the manifestations of the disease worsen, when the serum albumin reaches low values (see page 39), when the prothrombin time increases (see page 40) and when the total cholesterol and the percentage of cholesterol esters fall. In some patients, however, liver function, as measured by laboratory tests, seems stable, while lethargy and confusion gradually progress to complete stupor.

In the first of the four stages, which may be recognized in the clinical manifestations of hepatic coma, the patient may appear perfectly rational, but with careful observation he will be found somewhat lethargic and tending to sleep

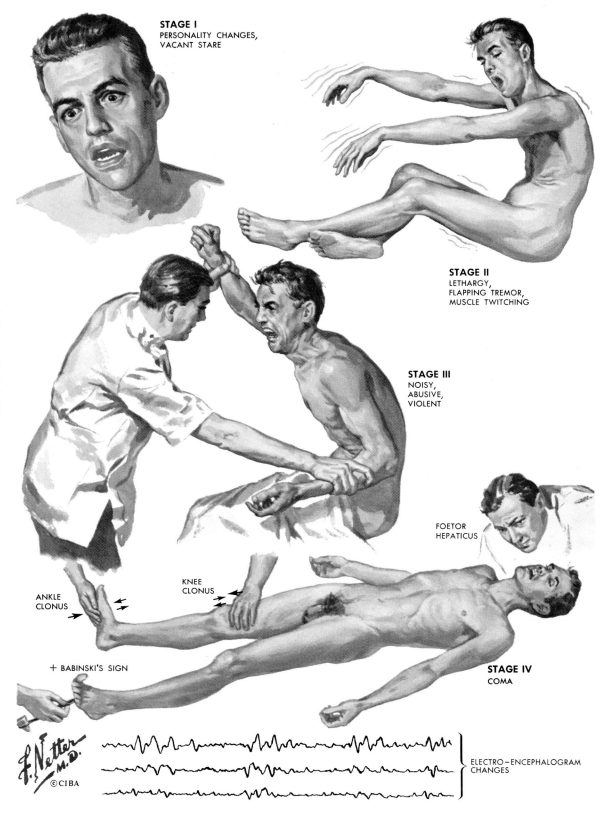

STAGE I
PERSONALITY CHANGES, VACANT STARE

STAGE II
LETHARGY,
FLAPPING TREMOR,
MUSCLE TWITCHING

STAGE III
NOISY,
ABUSIVE,
VIOLENT

FOETOR
HEPATICUS

ANKLE
CLONUS

KNEE
CLONUS

+ BABINSKI'S SIGN

STAGE IV
COMA

ELECTRO–ENCEPHALOGRAM
CHANGES

more than he did in earlier periods. Certain *personality changes,* at times a lack of co-operation or of respect for the attending physician or nurses and an inclination to use abusive language, may be noticed. In the more distinct second stage, *lethargy* is more pronounced, though at times the patient may be quite awake and appear normal, but yawning is frequent and a coarse, *flapping tremor,* particularly of the hands but occasionally involving the entire body, with a generalized muscular *twitching,* will be noticed. In the third stage the patient becomes definitely unco-operative, *noisy* and *abusive,* so that it is frequently necessary to *restrain him forcibly* and to apply heavy sedation. In the fourth stage he fades into *unconsciousness* from which he cannot be aroused and with which *knee* and/or *ankle clonus,* hyperactive reflexes and a positive Babinski's sign appear. *Electro-encephalographic changes* (described as "high voltage,

slow waves in the range of 1 or 1½ to 3 per second superimposed on relatively normal waves"), which are, however, neither specific nor useful to differentiate hepatic coma from other comas, may be recorded in any stage.

It may be assumed that a great number of enzymatic functions have become deficient in the hepatocellular failure which accompanies coma, so that a single therapeutic measure is unlikely to reverse the changes. This would, in part at least, explain the varied regimen (adrenal steroids, low nitrogen intake, oxygen, vitamin E, glutamic acid, antibiotics, support of fluid and electrolyte balance, etc.) that has been recommended for treatment and found successful by some and unsuccessful by others.

Advances in knowledge of ammonia metabolism (see page 178) make the problem of hepatic coma understandable.

RENAL COMPLICATIONS OF LIVER DISEASE

Renal shutdown, with azotemia and hyperkalemia, occasionally complicates the course of failing liver disease. This has been called the "hepatorenal syndrome", a term first used about 20 years ago to describe the series of events which took place in some patients following surgery for obstructive jaundice. With jaundice continuing or recurrent after operation, fever, oliguria or anuria developed without apparent cause and usually resulted in uremia and the death of the patient. More recent experience indicates that these events following biliary tract surgery are exceedingly rare with modern techniques and appropriate pre- and postoperative care. According to the present concept the term "hepatorenal syndrome" is not warranted in the sense that severe liver disease will cause renal failure or that renal disease will cause liver failure. Such a designation may be used, however, when hepatic and renal failure coexist and when they are caused, as in most instances, by the same etiologic factors, e.g., by carbon tetrachloride intoxication. As demonstrated experimentally, certain relationships do exist between the liver and kidney. Administration of a choline-deficient diet, e.g., leads to pathologic changes in both organs (acholinopathy, Hartroft). Another hepatorenal relationship has been postulated in view of the mutual antagonism of the vasoexciting and vasodepressing material (VEM and VDM, respectively), of which the former originates from kidney tissue under anoxic conditions, whereas the latter has been identified with ferritin (see page 88) and is formed in the liver (Shorr). It has also been demonstrated that patients with advanced cirrhosis of the liver have an abnormal elevation of circulating VDM and, therefore, may be more prone to develop the shock syndrome.

While no proof exists that liver disease can be a cause of renal disease, and vice versa, one must be prepared to treat the patient with hepatic disease who develops renal failure. The renal failure may be due to anoxia or hypotension, such as that taking place after massive bleeding from esophageal varices. It may result from the trauma and tissue damage of surgery or from prolonged anesthesia in such patients. It likewise may result from exposure to toxin equally harmful to the kidney and liver.

With the diminution of urine flow, the blood urea nitrogen may or may not rise, depending upon the status of hepatic function. Perhaps one of the last functions of the liver to be lost is the ability to produce urea from ammonia. If this func-

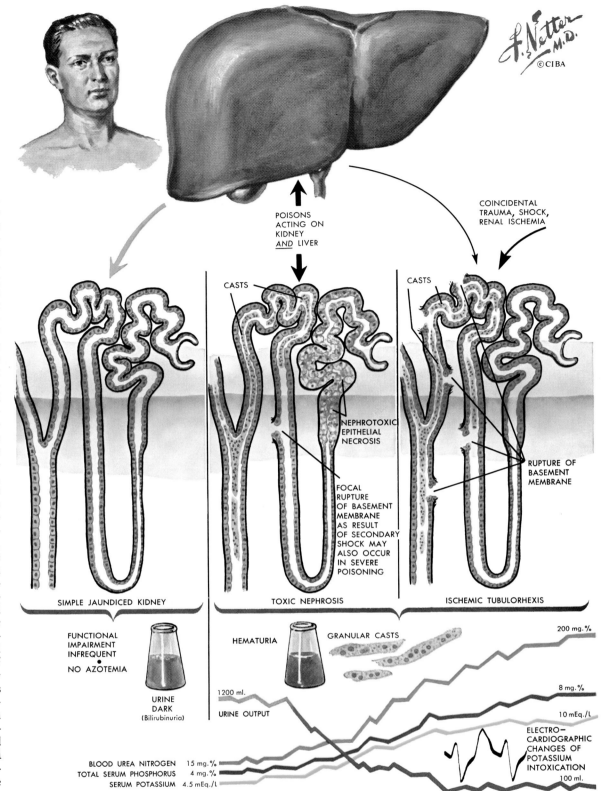

SIMPLE JAUNDICED KIDNEY

FUNCTIONAL IMPAIRMENT INFREQUENT • NO AZOTEMIA

URINE DARK (Bilirubinuria)

BLOOD UREA NITROGEN 15 mg.%
TOTAL SERUM PHOSPHORUS 4 mg.%
SERUM POTASSIUM 4.5 mEq./L

POISONS ACTING ON KIDNEY AND LIVER

CASTS

NEPHROTOXIC EPITHELIAL NECROSIS

FOCAL RUPTURE OF BASEMENT MEMBRANE AS RESULT OF SECONDARY SHOCK MAY ALSO OCCUR IN SEVERE POISONING

TOXIC NEPHROSIS

HEMATURIA   GRANULAR CASTS

1200 ml.
URINE OUTPUT

COINCIDENTAL TRAUMA, SHOCK, RENAL ISCHEMIA

CASTS

RUPTURE OF BASEMENT MEMBRANE

ISCHEMIC TUBULORHEXIS

200 mg.%

8 mg.%

10 mEq./L

ELECTRO-CARDIOGRAPHIC CHANGES OF POTASSIUM INTOXICATION
100 ml.

tion is impaired, the blood urea nitrogen will not rise as high as one might otherwise expect with a comparable degree of anuria. Probably the most important abnormality, and the greatest threat to the patient with a failing renal function, however, is a *rise in the serum potassium level,* leading to potassium intoxication and changes in the myocardium, which are reflected in the *electrocardiogram.* Conduction defects, arrhythmias and cardiac standstill may appear, and death from potassium intoxication alone may result. It should be pointed out, however, that with an adequate urinary output in a patient with chronic liver disease, one might find a lowering of the serum potassium (Artman and Wise). The diminution of serum potassium in chronic liver disease may be due to one factor or a combination of several; namely, a decreased intake of potassium, a greater excretion of potassium because of a negative nitrogen balance and the use of

adrenal steroids and/or intravenous glucose, both of which tend to lower potassium levels.

The development of oliguria or anuria in the patient with a failing liver renders the prognosis extremely grave, and it is a rare person indeed who can overcome such obstacles and survive his illness. Here, as in the case of hepatic coma, close attention to therapeutic detail by the attending physician and nursing staff will result in the greatest success in management. Adequate fluid intake in patients with liver disease, biliary tract disease or similar conditions is of paramount importance in the prevention of this complication.

Most frequently, renal failure in cirrhosis is not associated with recognizable alterations of renal structure; it is considered the result of impaired renal blood flow, which frequently follows abdominal paracentesis or the administration of diuretics.

Nutritional Liver Diseases

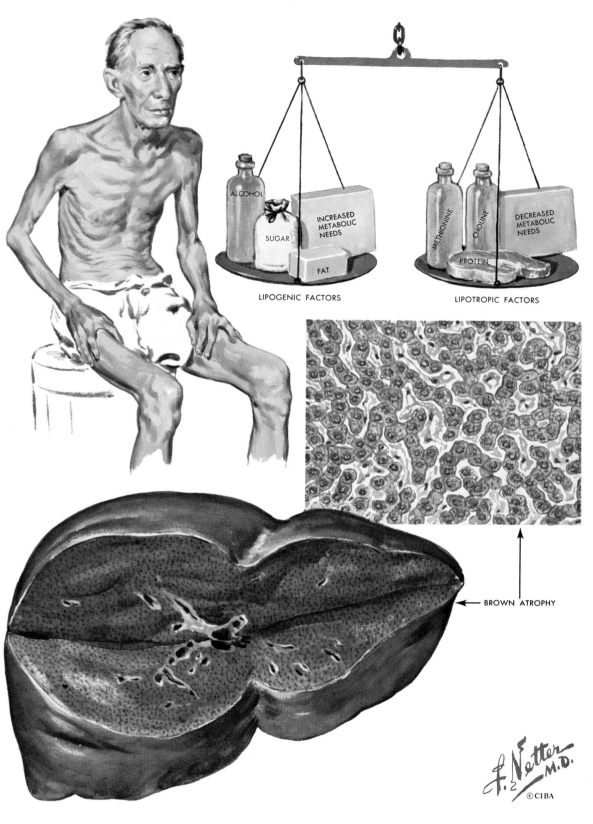

LIPOGENIC FACTORS

LIPOTROPIC FACTORS

BROWN ATROPHY

Starvation, Malnutrition

Hepatic injury can be caused by three kinds of dietary deficiencies: (1) general caloric undernutrition (starvation), (2) lack of one specific dietary component, and (3) imbalanced nutrition. *Starvation, i.e.,* a reduction of the total caloric intake without disturbance of the relation of the different food ingredients, reduces the size of the liver. This shrinkage is a gradual process to which all components contribute. The liver cells become smaller; their cytoplasm contains less proteins, pentose nucleoproteins, glycogen and enzymes, such as cholinesterase. The fat content of the liver is initially diminished, but, at least in some animal species, liver fat in later stages increases. The clinical picture of a balanced caloric undernutrition is seen as a result of famine or in inmates of prisoner-of-war or concentration camps. It is also encountered in debilitating diseases, in senility and in carcinoma of the upper gastro-intestinal tract, especially of the esophagus. Under such circumstances the liver loses more weight than almost any other organ in the body and exhibits the picture of *brown atrophy*. The small organ has very sharp edges and a distinct brown color. On the cut surface, the lobular architecture is preserved or sometimes more marked than normally, because the terminal cardiac failure increases the blood content of the centrolobular zones. The liver cell plates are very slender. The cytoplasm is very dense and, especially around the nuclei, contains granules of brown wear-and-tear pigment which are also found in the Kupffer cells. Quite frequently, hemosiderosis is present. In uncomplicated starvation, fat usually cannot be demonstrated in the liver, but it may be present if complications arise, which happens often because the emaciated body is far more susceptible to a variety of infectious and parasitic afflictions than a normal and well-nourished individual. For the same reason a variety of portal and intralobular inflammatory changes are frequently found in the livers of these undernourished persons. As signs of functional hepatic impairment, the urobilinogen excretion in the urine is increased, the glucose tolerance is altered and serum proteins are decreased. In repatriated prisoners of war, temporary gynecomastia has been observed, which indicates an inability of the liver to inactivate (conjugate) estrogens. In general, however, hepatic insufficiency in starvation is not severe enough to cause death by hepatocellular failure or hepatic coma.

The serious hepatic damage resulting from a deficiency of specific nutritional factors, as observed in recent years in animal experiments, has so far not been established in human pathology. In avitaminosis only little injury to the liver has been recorded. Cystine deficiency in animals produces a hemorrhagic hepatic necrosis, whereas lack of other amino acids and of choline leads to a fatty metamorphosis, which subsequently, and particularly when choline is missing, develops into a hepatic fibrosis and, eventually, into cirrhosis and primary hepatic carcinoma.

On the other hand, examples of injury to the human liver by unbalanced nutrition are very frequent, and the most important imbalance is that between lipogenic and lipotropic factors, the significance of which has been discussed previously (see page 37). The complex interplay of these factors has been symbolized on the accompanying and two following plates by a pair of scales. In a balanced diet, independent of the adequacy of the caloric content, the dishes of the scale, one holding lipogenic and the other lipotropic materials, are in equilibrium. This equilibrium is lost when, *e.g.,* ingestion or absorption

(Continued on page 78)

(Continued from page 77)

of lipotropic factors is reduced absolutely or relatively to the intake of lipogenic factors. Such imbalance, when persistent, leads invariably to metabolic disturbance in the liver and to fat accumulation.

Alcoholism

The most important example of fatty liver in the temperate zone is that seen in *alcoholics,* which constitutes a great proportion of livers with fat content above 12 gm. per cent. It has been claimed in the past that the hepatic effect of alcohol is a "toxic" damage, but it is likely that if a toxic interference plays any rôle at all, it stems from impurities and alcohols other than ethyl alcohol present in beverages. It is far more probable that the harm done the liver is attributable to the nutritional defects resulting indirectly from alcoholism. Alcohol abuse produces gastro-enteritis and pancreatic injury, hindering the absorption of nutrients. Alcoholic intoxication reduces the food intake. Alcohol may, in a manner not yet clearly understood, increase the requirements for choline and, being calorigenic, causes relative deficiency in lipotropic substances. The protein consumption or absorption in chronic alcoholism is usually reduced in spite of excessive caloric intake, which latter is responsible for the characteristic obesity of the alcoholic.

Kwashiorkor

In the tropical zones all over the world, a situation similar to chronic alcoholism is created by a deficiency or inadequacy of dietary protein in the presence of high caloric intake. This tropical or malignant malnutrition, described under various names in Central and South America and the West Indies and also reported from China, Italy, Spain and Hungary, is now usually designated by the African tribal name *Kwashiorkor,* implying "red boy". This name refers to the discoloration of the hair which, together with skin manifestations, is probably caused by accompanying vitamin deficiencies. The principal lesion, however, is a fatty liver, developing in the second or third year of life at the time the child is taken off the mother's breast and receives a high-caloric diet poor in protein. The basic picture of fatty metamorphosis of the liver is modified in various countries, for instance, by association with hemosiderosis, by pancreatic atrophy or by generalized edema. As the child becomes older, the metabolic demands decrease and the fatty liver disappears. Nutritional deficiency in early childhood is frequently coupled with some degree of mental retardation. It may also be related somehow to the high incidence of cirrhosis and of primary hepatic carcinoma observed in young adults in the tropics.

Fatty liver may develop as a complication of any disease in which malnutrition, especially protein deficiency, is present.

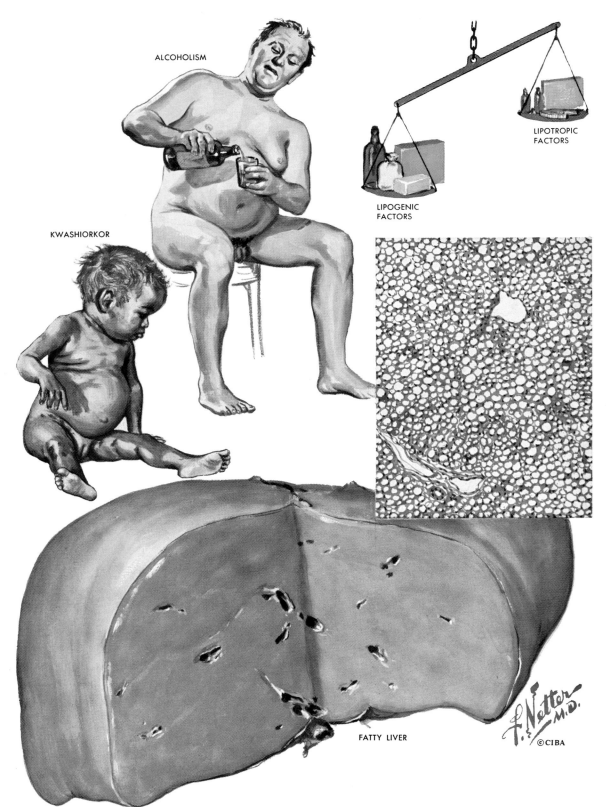

It is seen in gastro-intestinal disorders, such as pancreatitis, ulcerative colitis, enteritis and tuberculous peritonitis, and also in anoxic or toxic conditions. Under such circumstances the underlying diseases essentially dominate the clinical picture, so that nutritional factors produce only a complication in the form of a severe and persistent fatty liver which may assume clinical importance.

Splenomegaly, edema, ascites and spider nevi are not necessarily present in cases with fatty liver. The most frequent functional abnormality is a decreased Bromsulphalein® uptake by the liver. The serum albumin level may be low, the alkaline phosphatase activity is increased and the cephalin flocculation is abnormal in only one third of the cases. Abnormal thymol turbidity is even more rare. Glucose tolerance is more frequently impaired. Only when liver cell degeneration supervenes does jaundice develop, and

the abnormalities of the hepatic test become more significant. Patients with fatty liver seem to be more susceptible to infections; lobular pneumonia especially may take a treacherous course because systemic manifestations, including fever, may be suppressed. Instances of sudden death have been reported and explained by glycogen depletion of the liver or by pulmonary fat embolism as a result of entrance of hepatic fat droplets into the circulation.

At autopsy the liver is found *enlarged,* sometimes to more than 3000 gm. The anterior edges are blunted; the capsule is stretched. The color, depending on the degree of fatty metamorphosis, varies from *light brown to an ochre-yellow.* The consistency is doughy. The lobules may not be seen grossly. In mild degrees the lobular architecture may be accentuated, especially if it is associated with terminal cardiac failure.

(Continued on page 79)

(*Continued from page 78*)

With a fat content of over 20 gm. per 100 gm. of wet tissue, the paraffin sections reveal a *"Swiss cheese" appearance.*

The fat accumulation in early stages is predominantly centrolobular and less often peripheral. Large cysts may result, owing to the fusion of fat drops of several cells. The Kupffer cells are usually fat free. The sinusoids appear narrow, and no perisinusoidal spaces can be found, probably because of the pressure from the expanding fat droplets upon the surrounding tissue. The portal triads may be entirely normal, but small focal necroses and focal accumulations of inflammatory cells are frequently noted.

Fatty Liver with Acute Hepatic Failure (Alcoholic Hepatitis)

Prolonged fatty metamorphosis leads to cirrhosis in rats and other experimental animals. Whether this process takes place in the human being is, however, still an open question. Most observers believe that additional factors, *e.g.,* acute and chronic episodes of hepatic necrosis, are responsible for the transition of the fatty human liver into cirrhosis (see page 66). In the temperate zone such episodes may be provoked by infections elsewhere in the organism, and tropical diseases may play a similar rôle in kwashiorkor (see page 78). A great variety of other factors is apt to influence the course of a nutritional fatty liver disease as, *e.g.,* some toxic components in alcoholic beverages or some toxins in several types of Jamaican "bush teas", which apparently induce an occlusive disease of the hepatic veins. Anemia, as a consequence of hemorrhages from peptic ulcers or esophageal varices, may create hepatic necrosis. Shock or acute or chronic passive congestion may elicit further injurious effects. It is also possible that genetic factors (or some types of body habitus, *e.g.,* a female habitus in a male patient) may play a predisposing rôle.

The understanding of the transition from a fatty liver into cirrhosis is furthered by two stages in the fatty liver-cirrhosis syndrome. One is represented by an *acute hepatic failure* associated with usually *severe jaundice* developing predominantly in patients with a large, fatty liver. This frequently fatal episode eventuates more often than does fatty cirrhosis in younger persons of both sexes. Almost all cases have a history of alcoholism. The duration of symptoms is short; *edema* and *ascites* evolve rapidly. The *liver* is *large,* sometimes weighing over 5000 gm. The capsule is tense; the color varies between yellow and green; the consistency is doughy, owing to the high fat content. On the cut surface the lobular centers appear large and dark green, whereas the peripheral zone is more yellow. In paraffin sections, from which the fat has been removed by solvents, the typical findings are a *"Swiss cheese" appearance,* focal, sometimes

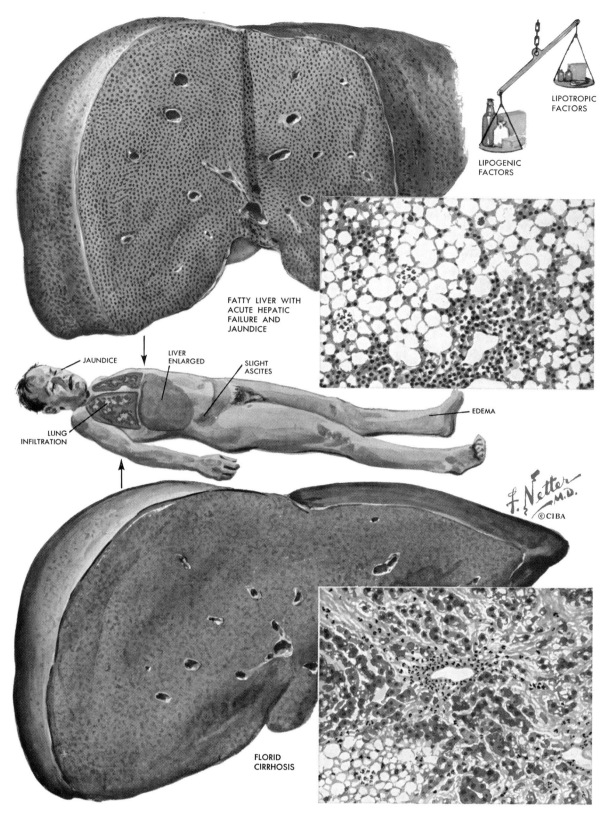

LIPOTROPIC FACTORS

LIPOGENIC FACTORS

FATTY LIVER WITH ACUTE HEPATIC FAILURE AND JAUNDICE

JAUNDICE — LIVER ENLARGED — SLIGHT ASCITES — EDEMA

LUNG INFILTRATION

FLORID CIRRHOSIS

centrolobular necroses, leukocytic infiltration around liver cells with coagulated cytoplasm (hyaline bodies of Mallory) and bile plugs in the bile capillaries. Portal infiltration and bile duct proliferation vary. The portal triads are stellate in shape, but connective tissue septa extend only occasionally into the lobular parenchyma, and the lobular architecture is abolished in only a few places, if at all. The laboratory findings provide evidence of severe hepatic failure, although the cephalin flocculation and thymol turbidity need not be abnormal. The alkaline phosphatase activity is frequently high. Quite evidently, hepatocellular failure is the cause of death, since the circulatory derangement characteristic of cirrhosis (see page 71) is not yet present. Other causes of death in nutritional fatty liver, such as fat embolism into pulmonary arteries or Wernicke's hemorrhagic polio-encephalopathy, are not frequent.

Florid Cirrhosis

Florid cirrhosis, the other, less acute, variety of the same process, has been described under various names such as chronic toxic hepatitis, subacute portal cirrhosis or progressive alcoholic cirrhosis. Although malnutrition is the main etiologic factor for florid cirrhosis, the fat content of the liver is not necessarily high, because it may have disappeared in the course of the disease either as a consequence of starvation or as a result of therapy. The clinical symptoms include weakness, weight loss, gastro-intestinal symptoms, spider nevi and splenomegaly. Jaundice, leukocytosis and azotemia are found in the great majority; ascites occurs in about half of the cases. As in acute hepatic failure of the fatty liver, infections have been held responsible for initiating the acute dete-

(*Continued on page 80*)

(Continued from page 79)

rioration. The brown-to-yellow or green liver is, though not in all instances, enlarged. The surface is, as a rule, smooth but circumscribed; foci of granularity are frequent. The lobular architecture is obscured but is not entirely obliterated and may even appear exaggerated in some areas because of the enlargement of the depressed central zones and the "bridges" connecting them. In one and the same liver, the histologic picture may vary, because hepatocellular degeneration alternates with focal regeneration, or patchy fatty metamorphosis and focal or central necrosis with portal and periportal inflammation. The most distinctive feature is the diffuse *increase of connective tissue* membranes throughout the parenchyma, with some septa transversing the lobule to form portahepatic venous connections. Regenerative nodules, as a rule, still remain scanty. In biopsy specimens of patients surviving the protracted episode, one encounters a similar picture, though usually less severe. The laboratory findings are, again, those of severe hepatocellular degeneration associated with varying degrees of cholestasis, reflected in elevation of serum alkaline phosphatase or total cholesterol.

Fatty Stage of Septal Cirrhosis

The more advanced stage in the course from fatty liver to cirrhosis (see page 66) is *fatty stage of septal cirrhosis,* characterized by a granular or nodular outer and cut surface in an enlarged liver. The growing regenerative nodules have abolished the lobular architecture and are surrounded by a gray-white, firm, connective tissue network. The color of the liver varies between brown and yellow, depending upon the degree of fatty deposition, which is determined essentially by the preceding nutrition. Fatty stage of septal cirrhosis is seen in the temperate zone mainly in alcoholics and, frequently, the term "alcoholic cirrhosis" is applied. But other forms of malnutrition, for instance those caused by intestinal or pancreatic diseases, may lead to the same result. The clinical symptoms, preponderantly in the male, develop most frequently in the fifth or sixth decade. Splenomegaly is present in more than half of the cases. Esophageal varices are found at autopsy in about the same percentage, and in a slightly lower incidence on roentgenologic examination.

Septal (Laennec's) Cirrhosis

As the process, described earlier (see page 68), continues, the fat disappears, the liver becomes smaller and the *Laennec type of septal cirrhosis* results. In this final stage the organ presents the typical "hobnail" appearance. Nodules between 1 and 5 mm. in diameter are surrounded by an evenly spaced, firm, gray-white connective tissue framework. In the

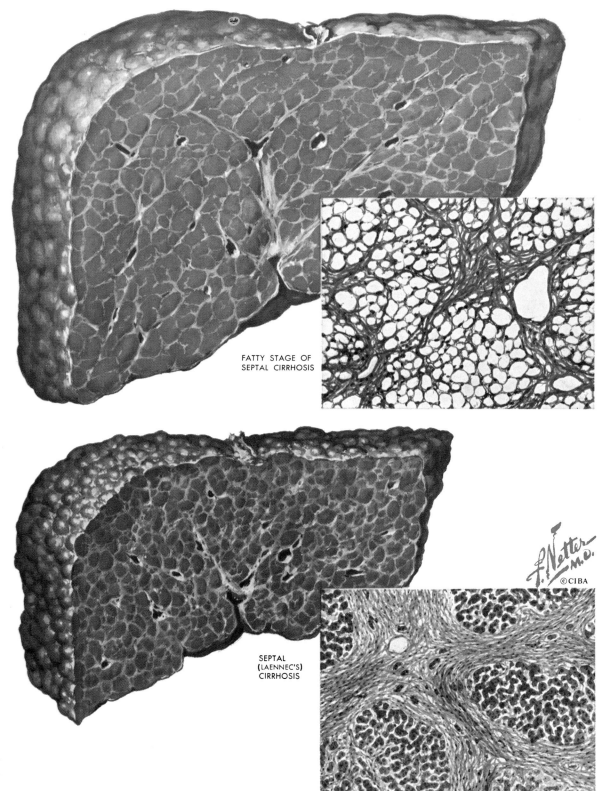

FATTY STAGE OF SEPTAL CIRRHOSIS

SEPTAL (LAENNEC'S) CIRRHOSIS

absence of complicating jaundice, the color is of an ochre-brown which prompted Laennec to coin the name cirrhosis (derived from the Greek word for tawny). Histologically, a round or *elliptic pattern* of the *nodules* dominates the picture. The hepatic veins seem to be compressed. Central veins are not seen. The internodular connective tissue septa are of almost equal widths and merge with the portal triads. Splenomegaly is found almost regularly. Esophageal varices are very frequent on anatomic and roentgenologic examinations, and gastro-intestinal hemorrhage is a common cause of death in almost all types of Laennec's cirrhosis.

The clinical manifestations, the laboratory findings and the microscopic picture depend upon the stage of the disease which has been designated by such terms as "compensated" or "decompensated" cirrhosis. Basically, the course of the disease is controlled by three factors, which are independent of the etiology: (1) degree of liver cell degeneration, (2) the extent of the cirrhotic process and (3) the rate of its progression. These features produce a gamut from the far advanced, actively progressing cirrhosis, with severe liver degeneration, representing a dramatic disease of grave prognosis, to the arrested more or less advanced cirrhosis, with no liver cell damage, which may fail to reveal any clinical or functional manifestations. This latter form, designated as latent cirrhosis, may be encountered as an incidental finding on liver biopsy, which may be the sole device for its recognition.

The etiologic relation of Laennec's cirrhosis with a nutritional disturbance is not always apparent, and the end stage of some forms of viral hepatitis, progressing to postnecrotic cirrhosis (see page 81), and of primary biliary cirrhosis (see page 84) may be indistinguishable from that of nutritional cirrhosis.

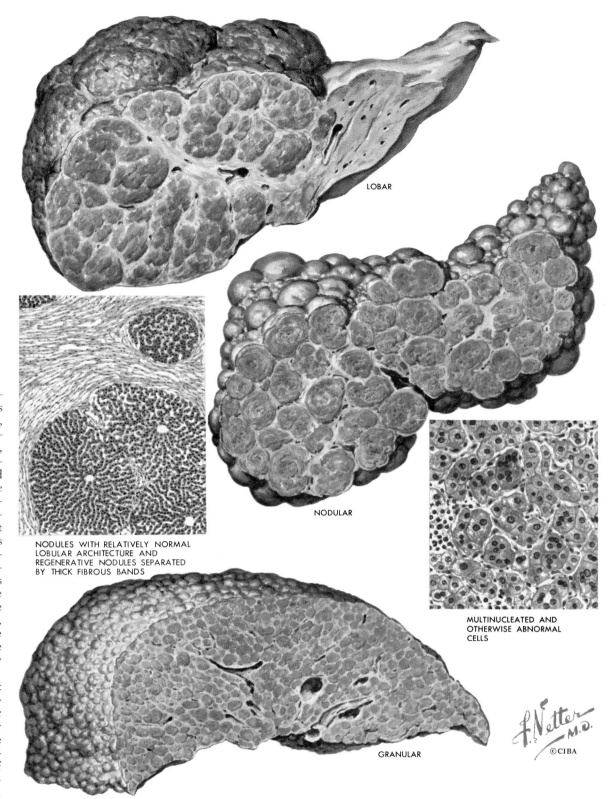

LOBAR

NODULAR

NODULES WITH RELATIVELY NORMAL
LOBULAR ARCHITECTURE AND
REGENERATIVE NODULES SEPARATED
BY THICK FIBROUS BANDS

MULTINUCLEATED AND
OTHERWISE ABNORMAL
CELLS

GRANULAR

POSTNECROTIC CIRRHOSIS

Cirrhosis following massive and submassive collapse has been described as toxic cirrhosis, posthepatitic cirrhosis, postcollapse cirrhosis, coarse nodular cirrhosis, multiple nodular hyperplasia, chronic liver atrophy and under a number of other terms. Although focal and zonal necroses are found in and precede other types of cirrhosis, the term *postnecrotic cirrhosis* appears the most appropriate one from the pathogenetic point of view (see page 67). Massive necrosis in severe viral hepatitis has been established as an etiologic factor, but the incidence of such causal relations seems to vary in different countries. In rare instances a chemical poison and, more frequently, alcoholism or, in the tropics, other nutritional disturbances can be incriminated. In general, however, the etiology remains dubious in the majority of instances.

Postnecrotic cirrhosis is more frequent in women than in men and occurs usually in an earlier age group than do other types of cirrhosis. Clinical symptoms may be severe or may remain latent and be found only incidentally after a long-bygone hepatic insult. The signs of hepatic insufficiency are more conspicuous than those of portal hypertension. Esophageal varices are less frequent than in the nutritional type of cirrhosis, but splenomegaly, spider nevi and, in later stages, ascites are relatively regular findings. Distinct nodules may be palpable, in contrast to the diffuse unevenness in other types.

The results of the hepatic tests depend upon the degree of liver cell damage and the activity of the process. A distinct feature is the very considerable elevation of the serum gamma globulin level, which may reach 4 gm. per 100 ml. and more, whereas in other types of cirrhosis elevations above 3 gm. per 100 ml. are unusual. In keeping with such gamma globulin elevation, as a rule, a high thymol turbidity is obtained.

A coarse *nodular liver* is the most frequent picture encountered at autopsy.

Its characteristic features are an uneven distribution of nodules varying from 1 to 20 mm. in size and an irregular arrangement of intervening connective tissue forming, in many places, broad white bands, containing many vessels. The small nodules are devoid of a central vein and are composed of newly formed parenchyma. Other *nodules* represent the *pre-existing lobular parenchyma* and contain fairly *normal-appearing portal triads* and central fields, the presence of which in an otherwise severely cirrhotic liver is the most reliable diagnostic criterion of postnecrotic cirrhosis. Biopsy specimens taken from such areas may present a perfectly normal hepatic architecture, and the cirrhosis may thus be overlooked. The lobular as well as the nodular parenchyma sometimes assumes bizarre expressions of regeneration. The *cells* are *multinucleated* or have large nuclei, and the cell plates are thick. In active cases the liver parenchyma shows focal or zonal necrosis, and the cellular infiltration in the septa is dense. The gross anatomic appearance is subject to a great deal of variation, in so far as large areas may have become necrotic and collapsed. The *left lobe,* especially, may form a small *shrunken* appendix to the liver, whereas the right lobe becomes hypertrophic and irregularly deformed. Such a *"lobar"* type is bound to cause most confusing palpatory findings.

Another extreme is the *granular type* of uniform size and distribution of the nodules, with only sparsely allotted broad bands between them. The gross and microscopic pictures and the palpatory findings resemble greatly those of Laennec's cirrhosis (see page 80). In some instances the appearance becomes indistinguishable from the latter, and only the history of a pre-existing severe hepatic necrosis suggests that the case be designated as postnecrotic cirrhosis.

COMPLETE OBSTRUCTION   INCOMPLETE OBSTRUCTION

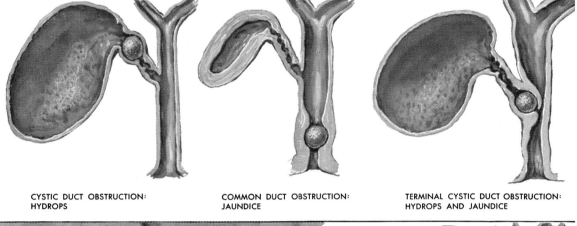

EXTRINSIC CANCER FIXING AND COMPRESSING DUCT

INTRINSIC CANCER

IMPACTED STONE WITH EDEMA

BALL–VALVE STONE

STRICTURE

Extrahepatic Biliary Obstruction I

Mechanism

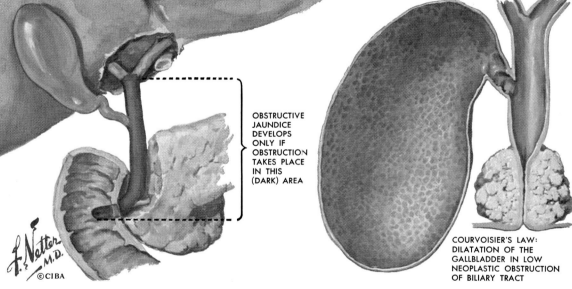

CYSTIC DUCT OBSTRUCTION: HYDROPS

COMMON DUCT OBSTRUCTION: JAUNDICE

TERMINAL CYSTIC DUCT OBSTRUCTION: HYDROPS AND JAUNDICE

Extrahepatic biliary obstruction causes jaundice only if it is located between the site of confluence of the right and left hepatic ducts and the tip of the papilla of Vater. Obstruction of a single branch of the main hepatic duct does not produce jaundice, because the nonobstructed part of the liver takes over in a compensating fashion. The excretion of bile components other than the bile pigments, however, may not be as readily compensated, and serum alkaline phosphatase or total serum cholesterol may be elevated in the absence of jaundice. The *obstruction* may be *complete* or *incomplete* and, in the latter case, it is often intermittent.

Complete obstruction is most frequently caused by tumors, which initially produce an incomplete and, subsequently, a permanent complete occlusion. Occasionally, regressive changes or hemorrhage into a tumor may result in sloughing off of obstructive tissue, with temporary relief of a complete obstruction. Such a happening is usually associated with at least chemical evidence of melena. *Intrinsic obstructive tumors* are usually malignant, represented by either cancer of the biliary ducts or cancer of the papilla of Vater. Carcinoma of the pancreas (see page 148), which may compress or kink the ducts, extension of carcinoma of the gallbladder (see page 149), carcinomatous metastases to the hepatic lymph nodes and metastatic carcinoma to the areolar tissue on the hepatic hilus, in other words, *extrinsic carcinoma*, must invade the wall of the bile duct to produce obstruction. A tumor not fixed to the duct remains movable and cannot cause complete obstruction. For this reason even large metastases to the hepatic lymph nodes, such as occur in Hodgkin's disease or leukemia or reticulum cell sarcoma, only seldom produce obstructive jaundice. Jaundice, if appearing in such conditions with inflammatory swelling of the hepatic lymph nodes, is almost always due to intrahepatic causes.

Gallstones (see pages 125 and 126),

OBSTRUCTIVE JAUNDICE DEVELOPS ONLY IF OBSTRUCTION TAKES PLACE IN THIS (DARK) AREA

COURVOISIER'S LAW: DILATATION OF THE GALLBLADDER IN LOW NEOPLASTIC OBSTRUCTION OF BILIARY TRACT

entering the biliary ducts and becoming impacted there, cause initially spasm and edema and, therewith, complete obstruction which is usually transient, since spasm and/or edema as a rule quickly subside. If the stone is not expelled from the duct, incomplete obstruction persists. If a stone moves or acts like a ball valve, the obstruction may become intermittent. In calculous obstruction a variable, usually short, period of complete obstruction is followed generally by intermittent obstruction reflected in spiking urinary urobilinogen excretion.

Strictures, whatever their cause may be (see page 133), whether produced by surgical injury to the biliary ducts or resulting from inflammatory lesions, cause incomplete or intermittent obstruction. Rarer causes of biliary obstruction are congenital atresia (see pages 118 and 119), inflammatory processes in neighboring organs (peptic ulcers, pancreatitis),

duodenal diverticula, foreign bodies or parasites.

Mechanical obstruction leads rapidly to dilatation of the biliary system above the site of obstruction. *Obstruction of the cystic duct* leads to dilatation of the gallbladder and to phenomena described elsewhere (see page 127). If the *obstruction* involves the *terminal portion of the cystic duct,* the stone may bulge into the lumen of the common duct and produce jaundice together with hydrops of the gallbladder. *Obstruction of the common duct* by stone (see page 126) is usually associated with inflammation of the gallbladder which is fibrotic and does not dilate significantly. Obstruction of the duct by a tumor, located usually near the major papilla (see page 137), is mostly associated with a normally expanding gallbladder that readily dilates and which may be palpated as a thin-walled large cyst (Courvoisier's law).

EXTRAHEPATIC BILIARY OBSTRUCTION II
Stages

CUT SURFACE OF LIVER IN BILIARY OBSTRUCTION

3. → MICROCALCULI IN DILATED BILE DUCTULES

← 1. CENTRILOBULAR BILE CASTS AND FEATHERY DEGENERATION OF LIVER CELLS

4. → EXTRAVASATION OF BILE

← 2. PORTAL FIBROSIS AND INFLAMMATION

5. → BILE INFARCT

The effects of biliary obstruction upon the liver itself, best observed in biopsy specimens, develop more rapidly in complete than in incomplete obstruction. The change first to appear is the *accumulation of bile pigment* in the liver cells and Kupffer cells in the *central zone* of the lobule. Simultaneously, bile may amass in the form of ramified bile plugs in the dilated bile capillaries. The cytoplasm of some liver cells adjacent to the bile capillaries is rarefied and pyknosis (*"feathery degeneration"*) may be seen, whereas the liver cells of the intermediate and peripheral zones still appear normal. At this stage hyperbilirubinemia and bilirubinuria appear, the activity of serum alkaline phosphatase is elevated and the urinary urobilinogen excretion is reduced.

Subsequently, *cellular infiltration* of the portal triads takes place, with some proliferation of perilobular cholangioles and periportal ducts. An *inflammatory reaction* ensues, without bacterial infection, probably as a result of a reaction to the bile stasis. As a rule, in this stage the alkaline phosphatase elevation is more marked and, in addition, the total serum cholesterol has risen. The cholesterol ester ratio may or may not be normal. The flocculation tests and other serum protein reactions are still normal; the serum γ-globulin is sometimes slightly elevated.

With prolonged obstruction the proliferation of the cholangioles becomes more marked, and bile casts form even in peripheral bile capillaries. The *dilated cholangioles* contain thick bile plugs, *microcalculi,* especially on the border between the lobular parenchyma and the connective-tissue-enlarged portal triads.

These alterations described so far may be found in intra- and extrahepatic cholestasis, whereas two features, the *extravasation of bile* and *bile infarcts,* are diagnostic criteria for extrahepatic obstruction, though their absence does not exclude it. Both, incited by marked dilatation of the intrahepatic bile ducts (hydrohepatosis), appear only after very prolonged obstruction and when the obstruction is complete. Necroses of the epithelial lining of the interlobular bile ducts permit escape of bile into their walls, and granulation tissue appears around the golden-yellow bile in the portal triad. In circumscribed foci the cytoplasm of liver cells is rarefied but bile pigmented, whereas their nuclei remain unstained. Compression of supporting blood vessels by the markedly dilated neighboring bile ducts has been thought to explain the formation of these bile infarcts. Infarcts near the portal triads are found only in extrahepatic obstruction. Very small infarcts, apparently caused by compression of intralobular arterioles, develop within the parenchyma in severe nonobstructive hepatic disorders.

In the late stages of obstruction, secondary hepatocellular damage may be severe and reflected in abnormalities of the tests indicative of liver cell degeneration. However, only late and very exceptionally do the serum protein reactions (cephalin flocculation and thymol turbidity) become abnormal, except in the presence of a complicating bacterial infection.

The *liver in the late stages of biliary obstruction* is enlarged, and of a dark-green color, accentuated in the lobular centers. On the cut surface the bile ducts appear greatly dilated. Eventually, formation of connective tissue membranes and fibers and of some regenerative nodules marks the beginning of cirrhosis.

BILIARY CIRRHOSIS

The term *"biliary cirrhosis"* is applied to several etiologically and also morphologically different types of cirrhosis, all of which have in common a long history of extra- or intrahepatic cholestasis and, morphologically, an enlarged, finely granular and firm liver with a green hue, the shade of which parallels the degree of jaundice. The lobular architecture is obscured by a *network of fine connective tissue* and fibrosed septa, which, on microscopic examination, are found to connect the enlarged portal triads. Connective tissue septa extending into the lobular parenchyma are sparse. The bile capillaries and ductules contain bile plugs and the liver cells frequently a green pigment. Regenerative nodules are rarer, compression of hepatic vein branches is less significant, and anastomoses between hepatic artery and venous branches are less developed than in other types of cirrhosis and, consequently, portal hypertension, ascites and bleeding from esophageal varices are also less eminent clinical features. The described stage of biliary cirrhosis is surprisingly well tolerated. But this situation, actually representing a "pseudocirrhosis", may eventually progress to real cirrhosis, which then is clinically and pathologically indistinguishable from Laennec's cirrhosis.

A classification of the various etiologic types of biliary cirrhosis has been proposed by MacMahon:

1. Obstructive biliary cirrhosis or cholestatic cirrhosis is the result of very prolonged intrahepatic biliary obstruction without bacterial infection. Adults, however, do not survive complete biliary obstruction long enough, or they succumb to its underlying cause (usually cancer) before cirrhotic transformation has become significant. In contrast, children with congenital biliary atresia (see pages 118 and 119) tolerate complete biliary obstruction for a considerable time.

2. *Cholangitic biliary cirrhosis,* or secondary biliary cirrhosis, or infectious cirrhosis of Mallory, results from biliary obstruction complicated by bacterial infection, which develops from prolonged obstruction by calculi or from strictures of the extrahepatic ducts (see page 133). This type of obstruction is mostly incomplete and frequently intermittent and, therefore, the degree of jaundice need not be very pronounced. The clinical picture is dominated by the infectious mani-

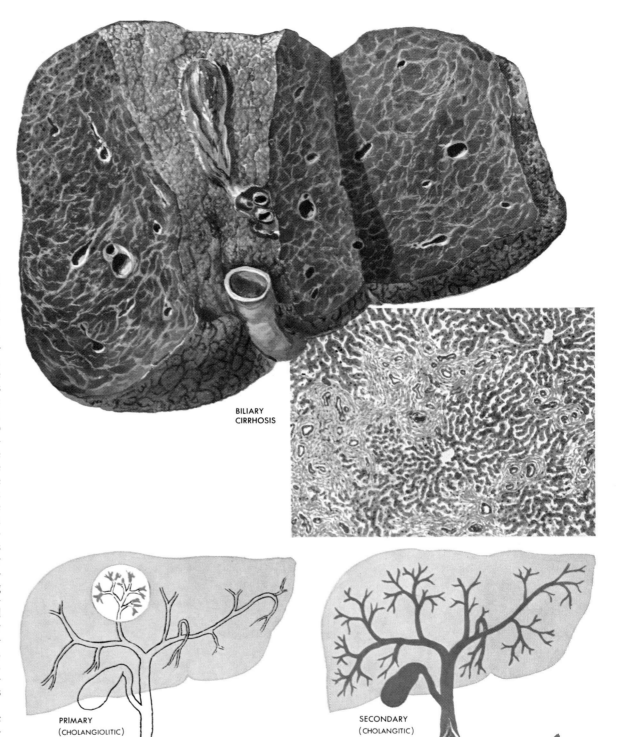

BILIARY
CIRRHOSIS

PRIMARY
(CHOLANGIOLITIC)

SECONDARY
(CHOLANGITIC)

PUS

festations (intermittent Charcot type of fever). The liver is large and tender, the spleen usually enlarged. Chronic biliary infection causes significant γ-globulin elevation; cephalin flocculation and thymol turbidity are usually abnormal. The manifestations of bile stasis are severe. The perilobular cholangioles and smallest bile ducts are dilated and contain inspissated bile in concrement form. Scarring of the portal triads and sometimes a gray-white network of the thickened portal fields, justifying the term "pipe stem cirrhosis", obscure the lobular architecture. Liver abscesses may complicate the picture and are frequently the cause of death. The spleen is usually enlarged and portal hypertension is present, both the result of the chronic biliary infection.

3. *Cholangiolitic cirrhosis,* also known as primary biliary cirrhosis or hypertrophic cirrhosis of Hanot, probably results from intrahepatic bile duct disease

(see page 97). In this disease the extrahepatic biliary tract is not involved. The lesions are primarily located in the smallest intrahepatic cholangioles. Jaundice is present, and ascites absent. Itching is the most significant clinical symptom, and the condition is tolerated relatively well for a considerable period of time. Severe liver cell damage and portal hypertension endanger the life of the patient only when the typical cirrhotic transformation (vascular anastomoses, regenerative nodules) is accelerated.

4. Acholangic biliary cirrhosis is a rare congenital defect of the intrahepatic bile duct system (see pages 118 and 119).

5. Fibroxanthomatous biliary cirrhosis is an extremely rare congenital lesion in children (MacMahon). It represents the rare example of a systemic disease, causing abnormal lipid deposition in portal histocytes.

METABOLIC INJURIES I

Amyloidosis

Amyloid is a protein (probably corresponding to α-globulin) attached to a polysaccharide (probably chondroitin sulfate). Why it is deposited in organs, selectively around and within the walls of blood vessels, is unknown. Experimentally, amyloidosis has been produced by feeding large amounts of protein, especially cheese or casein, and it has been claimed that the disease is rare in countries with little milk or cheese consumption, whereas it is a frequent finding in animals, *e.g.*, horses, which have been immunized over long periods of time against diphtheria or tetanus. Amyloid deposit gives the liver a dry, waxy appearance. After treatment with Lugol's solution, a brown color appears which changes to blue with the addition of diluted sulfuric acid. This color reaction, resembling that of starch (amylum), explains the classic connotation of the material as amyloid. Another staining reaction used histologically rests upon the elective affinity of amyloid to Congo red, which is also utilized in the clinical diagnosis of amyloidosis. Methyl violet staining amyloid red is also used histologically.

Two types of human amyloidosis, though considerably overlapping, are differentiated according to their distribution tendencies. Systemic amyloidosis, usually designated as *secondary amyloidosis*, develops in diseases with prolonged tissue breakdown and suppuration, as in *pulmonary tuberculosis,* other chronic pulmonary or pleuropulmonary suppurations, chronic *osteomyelitis,* protracted rheumatoid arthritis, trichinosis, neoplastic diseases, and especially Hodgkin's disease and ulcerative colitis. In this secondary amyloidosis, the liver is supposedly involved in 80 per cent of the cases. (For discussion re involvement of various organs see other CIBA COLLECTION volumes.)

The sometimes markedly and uniformly enlarged liver has a smooth surface and rounded edges. The *color is brown* to pale yellow, depending on the degree of anemia. The lobular architecture is indistinct, the consistency very firm and usually described as "rubbery". Amyloid, as seen histologically, is deposited in the interstitial spaces in the form of an eosinophilic homogeneous, amorphous material. The liver cell plates, which are free

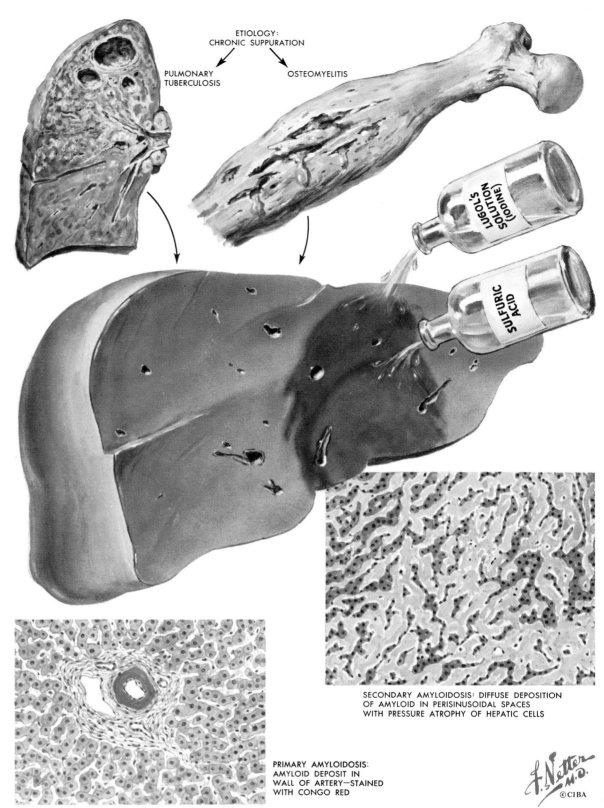

SECONDARY AMYLOIDOSIS: DIFFUSE DEPOSITION
OF AMYLOID IN PERISINUSOIDAL SPACES
WITH PRESSURE ATROPHY OF HEPATIC CELLS

PRIMARY AMYLOIDOSIS:
AMYLOID DEPOSIT IN
WALL OF ARTERY—STAINED
WITH CONGO RED

of amyloid, become initially more and more basophilic and then compressed by the progressing amyloid deposition until they disappear, clearing the way for large masses of eosinophilic material. The sinusoids also suffer from compression. The walls of the vessels are involved only in the minority of cases. The bile ducts are always free. The clinical and laboratory manifestations of even severe hepatic amyloidosis are few, except for hepatomegaly. Jaundice is rare and accompanied by a mild hyperbilirubinemia. Far more significant are the renal manifestations, which are responsible for the low serum albumin level. For the diagnosis of amyloidosis, liver biopsy has recently become very popular. Hepatic amyloidosis is strongly suggested if more than 60 per cent of intravenously injected Congo red is removed from the blood stream within 30 minutes.

The relatively rare *primary amyloidosis* is not asso-

ciated with inflammatory conditions in other organs. Though no apparent cause can be detected in many instances, further studies might prove that the abnormal globulin is formed by plasma cells, because in an appreciable number of cases it is associated with multiple plasma cellular myeloma or diffuse plasmacytosis of the bone marrow. Typical primary amyloidosis involves mesodermal organs (heart muscle, skeleton muscle, tongue, cutis, kidney or spleen), including the liver, where it is typically deposited in the wall of the hepatic arteries and arterioles, without narrowing their lumen. The tissue spaces are usually but not necessarily free. In primary amyloidosis the deposits give less convincingly the staining reactions, so that the term para-amyloidosis has been coined. The hepatic involvement in primary amyloidosis produces no gross changes of the liver and, as a rule, has no functional significance.

METABOLIC INJURIES II

Gierke's Disease, Galactosemia, Niemann-Pick's Disease

In *glycogen storage* or *Gierke's disease*, an inborn error of the metabolism, excessive quantities of glycogen accumulate in the liver cells, which become enlarged and exhibit a finely vacuolized or granulated cytoplasm with a central nucleus. The distended liver is smooth, glassy and pink-brown. The fat content is usually higher than normal. Excessive glycogen deposition may occur also in other organs, especially kidneys and heart. The pathogenesis of the glycogen deposition and its unusually long persistence after death appear to be explained by the deficiency of one of several enzymes of carbohydrate metabolism. In typical Gierke's disease, glucose-6-phosphatase, essential for conversion of glycogen to glucose, is absent. In another form, the enzyme which debranches glycogen, amylo-1,6-glucosidase, is missing, resulting in an altered glycogen structure. Deficiency of the branching enzyme is rare. In still another form, with normal glycogen structure (Hers' disease), liver phosphorylase is absent. The glucose release from the liver being reduced and its carbohydrate uptake by the liver therefore impaired, the blood sugar level is unstable. Occurring in early childhood, the disease leads to retardation of development and growth, marked hepatomegaly (without jaundice) and splenomegaly. The children succumb easily to infections. Only few have lived into adolescence. Glucose-tolerance curves show a diabetic tendency, and glycosuria may be present. Ketosis develops if food is withheld. The hepatic tests are not necessarily abnormal, but liver biopsy reveals characteristic changes.

Galactosemia, another rare, inborn disturbance of the carbohydrate metabolism, is presumably caused by a defect of a hepatic enzyme required for the transformation of galactose-1-phosphate to glucose-1-phosphate. Excess galactose, not being converted to glucose and/or glycogen, accumulates in the body, injures the lens, and probably also brain and kidney, causing cataracts, mental retardation or amino-aciduria, respectively. Though no evidence indicates that galactose is hepatotoxic, the liver suffers, owing to reduced blood glucose, from endogenous malnutrition, which leads to fatty liver and subsequently fatty cirrhosis and splenomegaly from portal hypertension. The diagnosis is substantiated by high blood galactose and depressed glucose levels and by liver biopsies which reveal fatty metamorphosis, focal necroses and fibrotic changes. With milk losing its dietary importance at the age of about 5 years, the clinical manifestations of the survivors subside, though the damage inflicted persists through life.

Niemann-Pick's disease, again a rare

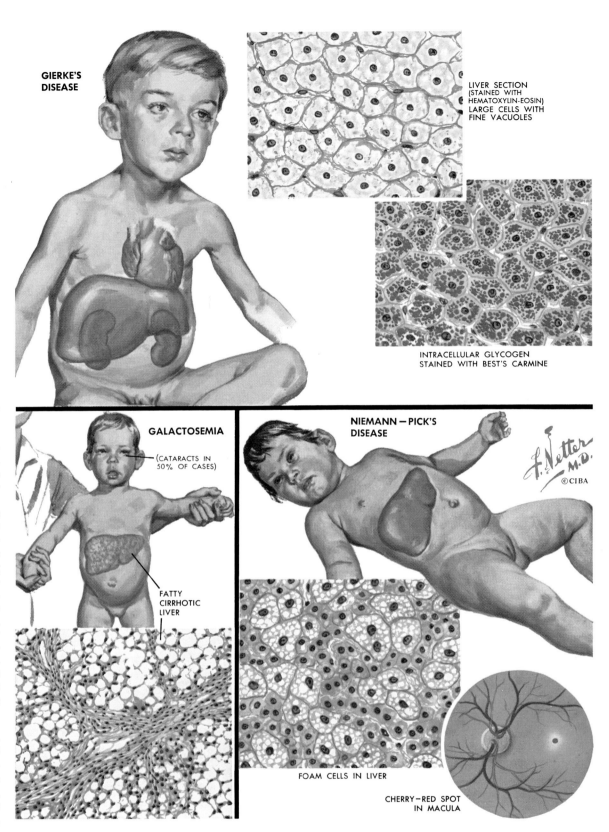

GIERKE'S DISEASE

LIVER SECTION (STAINED WITH HEMATOXYLIN-EOSIN) LARGE CELLS WITH FINE VACUOLES

INTRACELLULAR GLYCOGEN STAINED WITH BEST'S CARMINE

GALACTOSEMIA

(CATARACTS IN 50% OF CASES)

FATTY CIRRHOTIC LIVER

NIEMANN—PICK'S DISEASE

FOAM CELLS IN LIVER

CHERRY—RED SPOT IN MACULA

hereditary condition found almost only in Jewish children, is a disorder of lipid metabolism. Phosphatides, particularly sphingomyelin, are excessively stored in the reticulo-endothelial cells of the liver and spleen, but also of other tissues. The Kupffer cells are greatly enlarged, have increased in number and frequently have changed into foam cells with central nuclei. Occasionally, two nuclei are found in the enlarged cells. The excessive proliferation and enlargement of the Kupffer cells distort the hepatic architecture but cause no fibrosis, and no evidence for hepatic insufficiency exists. The clinical manifestations, which start within the first 3 months of life, are dominated by anemia, cachexia and mental retardation. The children are blind and deaf and hardly ever survive the second year. Cherry-red spots in the macula of the eye fundus are characteristic but are found also in Tay-Sachs disease which is associated with idiocy

and never involves the liver.

In cerebroside lipidosis, or Gaucher's disease, characterized by an accumulation of kerasin in the reticulo-endothelial system, the liver is moderately enlarged. Its lobular architecture is but slightly distorted by the "Gaucher cells", large polygonal cells, with small eccentric nucleus and an opaque homogeneous cytoplasm, or sometimes multinucleated giant cells. Only in an acute infantile form is this familial disease life-threatening, while the enormously enlarged spleen, the spontaneous bone fractures and hematologic manifestations of the chronic adult form do not severely interfere with life expectancy.

In primary essential xanthomatosis with cholesterol storage, the liver is not involved. A very rare exception is fibroxanthomatous biliary cirrhosis (see page 84). The xanthomatosis in cholangiolitis is a secondary sign of a primary liver disease (see page 97).

METABOLIC INJURIES III

Wilson's Disease

Originally, *Wilson's disease,* or hepatolenticular degeneration, was considered to be a congenital disorder mainly seen in children and young adults. It is characterized by a triad consisting of *symmetric basal ganglia degeneration, cirrhosis of the liver* and a greenish-brown pigmented ring on the margin of the cornea (*Kayser-Fleischer ring*). This condition now has been identified as a disturbance of copper metabolism, on a genetic basis, with many gradations from asymptomatic siblings to patients with the fully developed disorder. Since treatment with copper-chelating agents prevents progression, recognition of oligosymptomatic forms becomes important. Although considerable argument still exists about the underlying mechanism, affected patients appear to be homozygous for an autosomal recessive gene which is responsible for transmission of the inability to form a normal quantity of protein containing copper. This results in a reduced or altered amount of a blue serum protein with oxidase activity, containing copper, called ceruloplasmin. It travels electrophoretically with α-globulin and is probably formed in the liver. The defect results in an increased copper absorption from the diet; more important, nonceruloplasmin copper is increased in the plasma. This is associated with increased copper deposition in various organs, particularly in the liver, brain, kidney and Descemet's membrane of the cornea. The excess deposition in tissue is considered injurious and probably is responsible for the tissue changes. Deficiency of ceruloplasmin deprives the body of an important regulatory mechanism in copper metabolism. However, the possibility exists also that copper binding to ceruloplasmin or transfer to the liver may be defective, since the ceruloplasmin level does not necessarily reflect the severity of Wilson's disease. Also, excess copper is excreted in the urine in the form of copper-amino acid and peptide complexes. It has been claimed that the loss of amino acids, even with no change in blood levels, causes the hepatic alteration, but it probably is not sufficient to do this.

The hepatic alterations are extremely variable. In asymptomatic siblings, the only significant change may be ballooning of the nuclei in the periportal zone, due to deposition of glycogen associated with an accumulation of cytoplasmic lipofuscin pigment and varying degrees of fatty metamorphosis. In early symptomatic cases the fatty metamorphosis is usually more advanced, and some portal fibrosis is noted. In more advanced cases all the manifestations of *postnecrotic cirrhosis* are found, frequently associated with many liver cells with glycogen-containing ballooned nuclei. Histochemically, acid phosphatase may be reduced in liver cells, but increased in Kupffer cells. Some patients show acute necro-

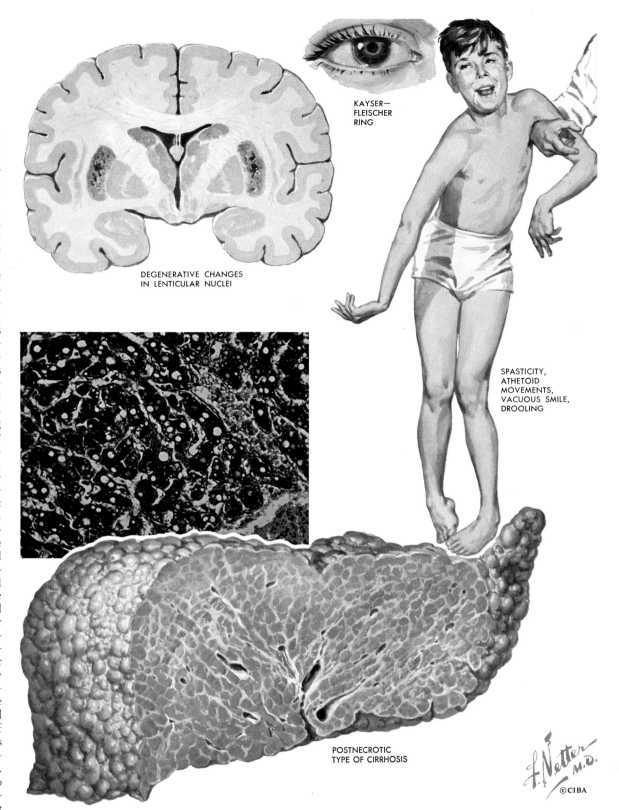

KAYSER—FLEISCHER RING

DEGENERATIVE CHANGES IN LENTICULAR NUCLEI

SPASTICITY, ATHETOID MOVEMENTS, VACUOUS SMILE, DROOLING

POSTNECROTIC TYPE OF CIRRHOSIS

sis of liver cells, usually associated with vacuolization and much pigmentation of these cells which is explained, in part, by excess copper. In general, the gross and microscopic changes of the fully developed stage of postnecrotic cirrhosis are not necessarily characteristic, and any case of juvenile cirrhosis should be suspected of being Wilson's disease. A low ceruloplasmin level has been considered diagnostic, but Wilson's disease with normal ceruloplasmin levels has been reported also, as have cases of liver diseases with low ceruloplasmin levels without other indications of this illness. A family history and the demonstration of some morphologic changes may assist in establishing the diagnosis.

The neurologic manifestations: tremor with *athetoid movements, rigidity,* a fixed *smiling* expression, *drooling,* and eventually mental deterioration result from *degeneration of ganglion cells* in the *lenticular nuclei,* especially in the putamen, in the internal capsule or in the frontal lobe. The site of degeneration is grayish-brown, and, microscopically, many minute cysts and a distinct glial proliferation are visible.

The course of Wilson's disease is variable. Revealing itself in preadolescence and adolescence, it may be a rapidly progressing illness, but it may also stretch over years or even decades. In a more chronic form in young adults (pseudosclerosis of Westphal-Strümpell), hepatic manifestations may be virtually absent. Conversely, in the abdominal form, the metabolic changes and Kayser-Fleischer rings are present. Idiopathic juvenile amino-aciduria, with normal liver function but without Kayser-Fleischer rings and clinical symptoms, has also been described. Therapy with penicillamine or other chelating agents is usually effective against the neurologic manifestations but is of only limited efficacy in the liver disease.

HEMOSIDEROSIS, HEMOCHROMATOSIS

Normal Iron Metabolism

Iron is taken up with food, mainly in a trivalent *ferric form*. The hydrochloric acid of the stomach reduces the ferric to the ferrous form, which passes through the intestinal mucosa. There it is reoxidized, and the ferric iron is bound to a protein, *apoferritin*. The iron-protein complex, *ferritin,* is the main organic storage form of iron but before iron is released to the blood, ferritin is split into apoferritin and ferric iron. The latter enters the blood stream in the ferrous form, where it is bound to a β-globulin after undergoing another oxidation to trivalent iron. The globulin-iron complex, *transferrin (siderophilin),* is the transport form of iron in the body. Ferrous iron, liberated by the breakdown of hemoglobin, myoglobin or of cytochrome enzymes, is similarly taken up by transferrin.

Transferrin carries iron to the tissues, where it is utilized in the ferrous form for the formation of hemoglobin and respiratory enzymes. It also delivers iron to the liver, which stores it as ferritin. The iron can be released according to need, can be taken up from the *blood* or can be excreted in the *bile*. Ferritin has an iron content up to 25 per cent. Under electron microscopy, it has a characteristic appearance. Ferritin accumulates in *Kupffer cells* and hepatocytes in circumscribed membrane-enclosed structures corresponding to lysosomes and frequently called siderosomes. These bodies or their aggregates are the *brown-pigmented granules* giving an iron reaction on conventional microscopy. They are frequently designated as *hemosiderin,* though some reserve this term for nonferritin iron accumulation. While some iron in liver tissue, recognized chemically and by the electron microscope is normal, a positive iron reaction with the Prussian blue technique on conventional microscopy is excessive, except for a few granules in Kupffer cells. Excess iron accumulates around local hemorrhage. After liver cell breakdown, Kupffer cells usually show accentuated iron reactions focally. Diffuse and conspicuous histologic iron, mainly in Kupffer cells, indicates either widespread alteration of liver cells (for example, in malnutrition) or, more often, an excess supply of iron, mostly in forms other than transferrin. This includes intravascular hemolysis either spontaneously or after blood transfusions, and therefore it accompanies most hematologic disorders. It also results from intravenous iron therapy or oral administration, if very prolonged, or accompanied by increased intestinal iron absorption as in malnutrition. When iron in Kupffer cells is extensive, the liver cells also contain some in conditions designated as

hemosiderosis. Reticulo-endothelial storage is prominent, involving the *spleen, lymph nodes* and, to some extent, *bone marrow* in addition to the *liver*. These organs all appear *rusty-brown*.

Reticulo-endothelial hemosiderosis induced by excess iron is supposedly differentiated from *hemochromatosis* in which parenchymal iron storage is presumably the result of disturbed iron metabolism or of increased avidity of cells for iron. Some insist that the difference between hemosiderosis and hemochromatosis is only one of degree and, especially, of duration. In hemochromatosis melanin and iron are found in the *skin,* but iron alone in most glands, smooth muscles and the *myocardium*. The *pituitary* and *adrenal glands,* the *testes* and the *pancreas* are deeply pigmented by iron deposits in hemochromatosis. *Testicular atrophy,* with *azoospermia,* loss of libido and regression of secondary sex characteristics, is probably the

result of pituitary insufficiency. The *gastric mucosa* contains excess iron. Myocardial iron deposition can result in heart failure. Degeneration of iron-laden epithelial cells may lead to *fibrosis* as in the pancreas and the liver. In the former the islands of Langerhans may be involved, so that diabetes is a frequent manifestation of hemochromatosis ("bronze diabetes"). The liver is the main storage site, its iron content reaching more than 25 gm. Characteristically, in early stages iron is found in epithelial cells on the lobular periphery, whereas Kupffer cells contain relatively little except where liver cells disintegrate. With increasing iron deposition, the bile duct epithelium becomes involved, and eventually much extracellular iron is found in portal tracts. Fibrous septa form, and ultimately cirrhosis develops (see page 68). Since diabetes can now be controlled, hepatic coma, often

(Continued on page 89)

(Continued from page 88)

precipitated by bleeding esophageal varices, is the leading cause of death in older patients, while cardiac failure predominates in the rare cases of fatality from hemochromatosis before the age of 45. The spleen may be enlarged from portal hypertension and contains little iron; nor do the bone marrow and lymph nodes except those draining the liver.

The classification and pathogenesis of hemochromatosis are much debated. The existence of primary hemochromatosis is accepted as a familial inborn error of metabolism. Healthy siblings have either excess lipofuscin in the centrolobular zone or excess iron in the peripheral zone in an otherwise normal liver. A fundamental defect, possibly a faulty mechanism regulating iron absorption, is thought to produce a minimal daily increment of iron, with excessive accumulation eventually producing symptoms. This condition occurs overwhelmingly in men. Repeated bleedings or the use of iron-chelating agents are therapeutically efficacious.

In contrast to this probably rare primary congenital form is hemochromatosis secondary to hepatic or hematologic disorders. In cirrhosis, particularly from alcoholism, secondary parenchymal iron accumulation may develop and cause clinical symptoms of hemochromatosis. Since this happens following portacaval shunts, spontaneous intrahepatic shunts (see page 68) may also be responsible for hemochromatosis. Separation of primary hemochromatosis and that secondary to liver disease is difficult in individual cases. This secondary form is widespread.

Hemochromatosis secondary to hematologic diseases is of practical importance. The fully developed picture with cirrhosis is rare except in thalassemia or pyridoxine-responsive anemia. In other types of anemias, the manifestations are few. This condition has been seen with increasing frequency since blood transfusions have been used. Because of the many transfusions used, hemochromatosis has been considered secondary to the blood administration. However, transfusion siderosis or secondary exogenous hemochromatosis, as it has been called, also develops in patients who have received few or no blood transfusions. Prolonged anemia probably leads to increased uptake of dietary iron. If utilization in erythrocyte formation is impaired, the parenchymal organs become overloaded. Blood transfusion seems to aggravate this. The iron distribution shows the characteristics of both hemochromatosis and simple hemosiderosis influenced only by the underlying disease.

The diagnosis of hemochromatosis often rests upon the demonstration, by biopsy, of iron excess in the skin, liver or gastric mucosa. The presence of the classical triad (brown and atrophic skin, diabetes and an enlarged and firm cirrhotic liver) leaves no doubt as to the diagnosis. Frequently, however, all features are not present. Serum iron is elevated, with a high degree of saturation of the iron-binding serum protein which is also increased.

HEMOSIDEROSIS

LIVER BROWN BUT OTHERWISE NORMAL

IRON DEPOSITS CHIEFLY IN KUPFFER CELLS, LESS IN LIVER CELLS

SKIN NORMAL

SPLEEN VARIABLE AND DARK BROWN

BONE MARROW PIGMENTED

HEART NORMAL

LYMPH NODES PIGMENTED

ADRENAL CORTEX NORMAL

PANCREAS NORMAL, NO URINARY SUGAR

PITUITARY NORMAL

GASTRIC MUCOSA NORMAL

GONADS NORMAL

HEMOCHROMATOSIS

LIVER CIRRHOTIC AND BROWN

IRON DEPOSITS CHIEFLY IN LIVER CELLS, BILE DUCT EPITHELIUM AND FIBROUS BANDS, LESS IN KUPFFER CELLS

SKIN PIGMENTED

SPLEEN ENLARGED, SLIGHTLY BROWN

BONE MARROW RELATIVELY NORMAL

HEART PIGMENTED

LYMPH NODES RELATIVELY NORMAL

ADRENAL CORTEX PIGMENTED

PANCREAS PIGMENTED AND FIBROTIC, URINARY SUGAR ++++

PITUITARY PIGMENTED

GASTRIC MUCOSA PIGMENTED

TESTIS PIGMENTED AND ATROPHIC (AZOOSPERMIA)

F. Netter M.D. ©CIBA

SECONDARY HEMOCHROMATOSIS ASSOCIATED WITH ANEMIA (TRANSFUSION SIDEROSIS)

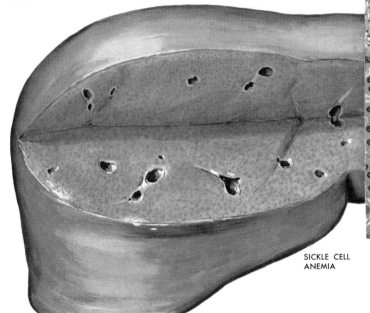

SHOCK LIVER

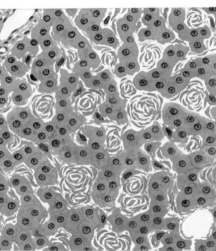

SICKLE CELL ANEMIA

HYPOXIC CONDITIONS

Shock, Sickle Cell Anemia, Erythroblastosis

Profound alterations of the liver may be induced when the hepatic blood flow or oxygen supply suffers secondarily to disturbances elsewhere in the organism. A typical example is *shock,* which might induce hepatic hyperemia with focal extravasation of blood into the tissue spaces and focal necrosis. If shock is more severe, central necrosis develops with or without disappearance of the liver cells, which are usually replaced by segmented leukocytes. Diverse factors can be responsible for such changes: (1) general circulatory failure associated with a reduced volume of circulating blood; (2) oxygen lack, especially in hemorrhagic shock; (3) impeded hepatic circulation, essentially by a throttle mechanism of the hepatic veins, leading to centrolobular stasis because of reduced outflow of blood; (4) increased permeability of the sinusoids, prompting edema and increased lymph flow; (5) release of vasodilating ferritin (see page 88) (V.D.M. of Shorr) by the anoxic liver. The significance of the hepatic injury upon the prognosis in shock is not established. Some consider it of crucial importance in irreversible shock.

Owing to hereditary anomaly in the formation of hemoglobin, restricted to the Negro race, the red blood corpuscles in *sickle cell anemia* contain hemoglobin S which differs from normal hemoglobin A and crystallizes readily, in contrast to the latter, under reduced oxygen tension. This characteristic of hemoglobin S alters the erythrocytes, which become sickle-shaped, exceedingly fragile, easily agglutinable and short-lived. As a result, thrombi form, vascular occlusion occurs, and the typical picture of a hemolytic anemia evolves. The dominant feature for the liver is the vascular obstruction. The organ is enlarged and has a tense capsule and a purplish cyanotic hue. The lobular architecture is almost lost because of distention of all sinusoids by packed, crescent-shaped, red cells. The liver cell plates are compressed and frequently broken, and exhibit focal degenerative and necrotic changes. The Kupffer cells are enlarged and contain iron pigment and engulfed erythrocytes.

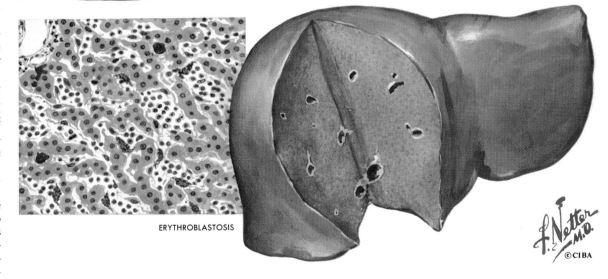

ERYTHROBLASTOSIS

Most of these alterations develop shortly before death. Jaundice is found in half of the patients during the crises, when elevated prompt-reacting bilirubin indicates functional hepatic injury. When, exceptionally, jaundice becomes severe, the question of a complicating hepatic disease, such as serum hepatitis from blood transfusion, arises.

In an individual who has inherited the ability to form normal adult hemoglobin, as well as hemoglobin S, the liver alterations are of minor importance in accordance with the milder course of this condition, called "sickle cell trait".

Blood group incompatibility between fetus and mother induces hemolysis, which is associated with a severe hematopoietic reaction, which gave rise to the name *"erythroblastosis fetalis"* (see also pages 118 and 119 and THE CIBA COLLECTION, Volume 2, page 233). The functional insult produced by the

anemia and the hemolysis is aggravated by the liver's immaturity, which prevents bilirubin excretion. The liver is enlarged, smooth, green and, as is usual for the neonatal organ, has few signs of lobular delineation. Excessive erythropoiesis is reflected in irregularly distributed cellular nodules mainly within the sinusoids. In the portal triads erythropoietic cells are mixed with myelopoietic cells. All cells are filled with bile pigment and the bile capillaries with bile plugs, in line with the severe jaundice. The liver cell plates appear frequently disorganized. Focal and midzonal necroses develop because of anoxia. These lead later to collapse and fibrosis. Cirrhosis in infants has been associated with erythroblastosis fetalis. Liver function appears to be not severely impaired, except for Bromsulphalein® retention. Jaundice develops rapidly, with serum bilirubin exceeding 10 mg. per 100 ml. within the first days.

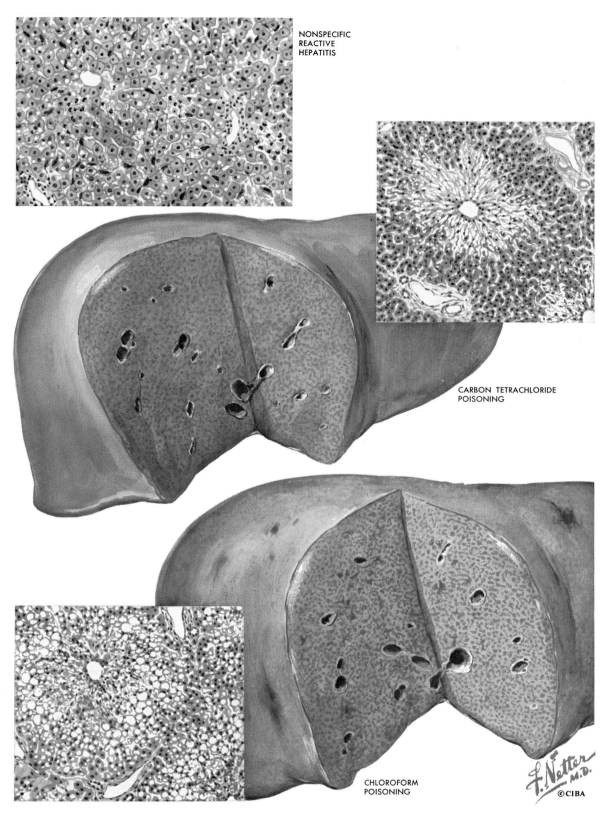

NONSPECIFIC
REACTIVE
HEPATITIS

CARBON TETRACHLORIDE
POISONING

CHLOROFORM
POISONING

Toxic Injuries

A great variety of clinical manifestations may result from liver injury by toxic substances which may belong to some not-well-defined endogenous factors (breakdown products of tissue and blood), or to hormones (thyrotoxicosis, eclampsia [?]), or to drugs and poisons, or to bacterial toxins. Exogenous factors may be classified into: (1) agents such as phosphorus, organic solvents or plant poisons (muscarine, amanita toxin), which regularly produce liver injury when absorbed in sufficient amounts; (2) agents such as anesthetics, which damage the liver in the presence of other contributing factors (infectious diseases, malnutrition); (3) agents such as sulfonamides, antibiotics, thiouracils, methyltestosterone and other drugs to which a few individuals are sensitive while the vast majority tolerate them; (4) agents which primarily impair other organs and affect the liver only secondarily as a result of anoxia, anemia, shock or tissue breakdown. The frequent hepatic changes in alcoholics seem to be primarily the result of malnutrition (see page 78).

The liver may respond to toxic agents of any kind with more or less localized degeneration of liver cell, such as described on page 62 (cloudy swelling, fatty degeneration) or on page 97 ("allergic" cholangiolitis). With more severe injuries, necroses of liver cells develop, presenting the picture of a nonspecific reactive hepatitis and zonal necrosis, mainly centrolobular, which rarely progress to massive necrosis (see pages 64 and 65). *Nonspecific reactive hepatitis* is the most frequent alteration encountered in biopsy specimens taken from a great variety of cases. It is characterized by slight but diffuse liver cell damage, small focal necroses with accumulation of segmented leukocytes, mobilization of Kupffer cells and accumulation of inflammatory cells in the portal triads and sometimes around proliferated cholangioles. All features can vary greatly in extent and distribution. They are found in gallbladder disease, peptic ulcer, ulcerative colitis and gastro-intestinal carcinoma, in diffuse systemic disorders, subacute bacterial endo-

carditis, in septicemias, pneumonia and Rickettsial and viral diseases. These changes are also prominent and only modified by pigment deposits in malaria. The nonspecific character of the lesion excludes an etiologic diagnosis, and sometimes even the differentiation from a subsiding viral hepatitis is difficult. Nonspecific reactive hepatitis probably represents the anatomic substrate for the abnormalities in hepatic tests frequently found in conditions such as mentioned. However, the correlation between the functional aberration indicated by the tests and the histologic changes is poor, probably because the morphologic aspect reflects only inadequately the degree of diffuse liver cell damage.

In *carbon tetrachloride poisoning*, now frequently observed as a result of exposure to cleaning fluids, the liver is enlarged, usually yellow, and the lobular architecture is frequently exaggerated because the

central necrosis produces central hyperemia and even hemorrhage. Histologically, the liver cells are missing in the central zone. The framework has collapsed, while the peripheral zone and the portal triads usually remain normal and the intermediate zone is filled with fat droplets. Portal inflammation develops in persons surviving the first week, during which period of time renal failure with anuria is more often fatal than is hepatic insufficiency.

Chloroform poisoning following anesthesia, more familiar to a previous generation than to ours, produces a picture similar to carbon tetrachloride poisoning, except that the fatty metamorphosis in the liver is usually far more severe and hemorrhages are more conspicuous. Phosphorus poisoning, also more frequent in previous years, produces similarly fatty liver with a severe necrosis, the localization of which is mainly peripheral.

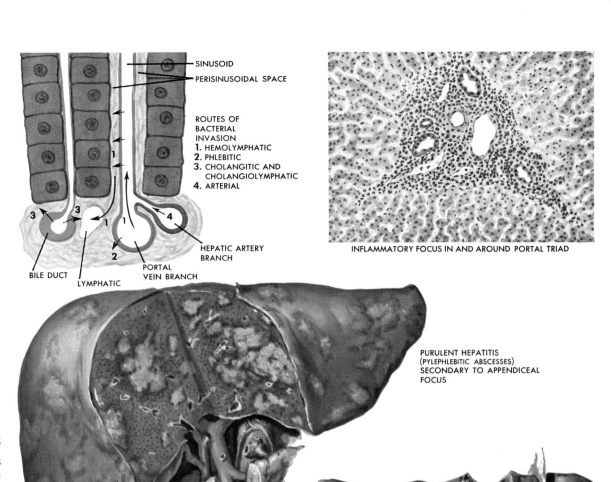

ROUTES OF
BACTERIAL
INVASION
1. HEMOLYMPHATIC
2. PHLEBITIC
3. CHOLANGITIC AND
   CHOLANGIOLYMPHATIC
4. ARTERIAL

INFLAMMATORY FOCUS IN AND AROUND PORTAL TRIAD

PURULENT HEPATITIS
(PYLEPHLEBITIC ABSCESSES)
SECONDARY TO APPENDICEAL
FOCUS

CHOLANGITIC
ABSCESSES:
(STONE IN COMMON
DUCT)

Bacterial Hepatitis

Minor lesions of the intestinal wall may be responsible for the permeation of bacteria, so that the *portal vein* becomes the most important and frequent route by which a *bacterial invasion* of the liver comes to pass. In some animals, such as the dog, intestinal bacteria are always present in the liver, but in the human this happens only under abnormal circumstances, *suppurative appendicitis* being the most prevailing. It is followed in incidence by inflammatory lesions of gallbladder and bile ducts, pancreas, spleen, diverticula and other alterations of the large and small intestine, and in newborn children by omphalic infections (see page 118). But even before the availability of chemotherapeutics, bacteria entering through the portal vein led only exceptionally to pylephlebitis (see also page 108). If the microorganisms reach the sinusoids, they are either taken up and destroyed by the Kupffer cells or they pass into the tissue spaces, whence they are drained to the lymphatics in the portal triads to set up an *inflammation within and around the lymphatics*. Polymorphonuclear leukocytes predominate around the dilated lymphatics, and in acute infections the cellular exudate extends in strand form into the lobular parenchyma.

Another *route of infection,* which, contrary to a frequently encountered belief, is relatively rare, follows the *bile duct system* and occurs mainly when bile stagnates owing to incomplete and, less frequently, to complete biliary obstruction. Under these circumstances, bacteria pass through the wall of the larger and smaller bile ducts and produce inflammation in the tissue of the portal triads, especially around the lymphatics. More often than by any other mode of *transmission,* bacteria reach the portal triads by way of the *lymphatics* and *arterial blood,* when the primary infection spreads from elsewhere in the organism (pyemia, osteomyelitis, endocarditis, etc.).

Infection in the portal triads may progress to abscess formation (*purulent*

hepatitis), which may involve the portal vein branches to produce *pylephlebitic abscesses,* with further thrombotic extension along the portal vein tree. But the pylephlebitic abscesses may develop from purulent infections anywhere in the portal system and subsequent multiple embolisms in the intrahepatic portal vein branches. Inflammation of the bile ducts can lead to *cholangitic abscesses,* almost always associated with *biliary obstruction* and mostly with jaundice. They are characterized, even in histologic sections, by the gold-green color of the pus and of their pyogenic membrane. In most cases they are a complication of a biliary fistula or of strictures of the common duct.

The clinical signs of hepatic abscesses are pain in the right upper quadrant, chills and fever of a spike (picket-fence) type. The enlarged liver is tender. Leukocytosis is conspicuous. Roentgenologically, the diaphragm is elevated and fixed. Of diagnostic impor-

tance is that the liver function tests in infected biliary obstruction will yield abnormal findings which are otherwise characteristic of primary hepatitis or cirrhosis. The serum protein reactions, normal in noncomplicated extrahepatic biliary obstruction, become abnormal in infected biliary obstruction, and the cholesterol ester ratio is usually markedly depressed. The essential point is that the clinical signs of bacterial infection, such as fever, chills and leukocytosis, supported by the laboratory findings of a primary hepatic (medical) jaundice, do not exclude an extrahepatic biliary obstruction (see also page 51). The significance of the liver injury, induced by infections, depends more upon the degree, site and extent of the infection, whereas in the case of extrahepatic biliary obstruction it is the duration and the completeness of the bile flow impairment that determine the grade of hepatic damage.

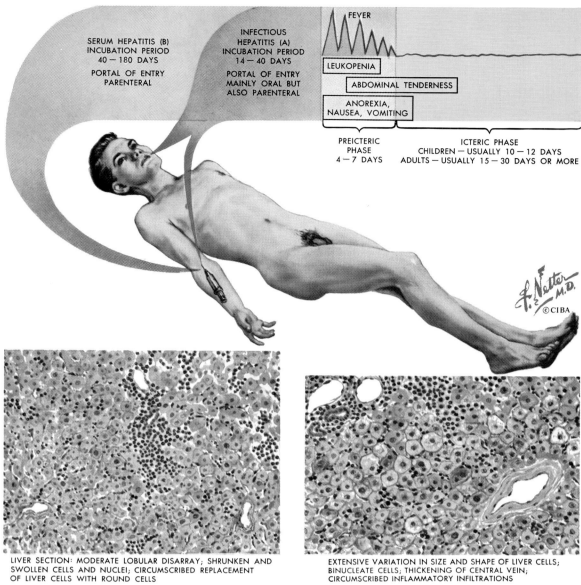

| | | | FEVER |
| SERUM HEPATITIS (B) INCUBATION PERIOD 40 — 180 DAYS PORTAL OF ENTRY PARENTERAL | INFECTIOUS HEPATITIS (A) INCUBATION PERIOD 14 — 40 DAYS PORTAL OF ENTRY MAINLY ORAL BUT ALSO PARENTERAL | | |

LEUKOPENIA

ABDOMINAL TENDERNESS

ANOREXIA, NAUSEA, VOMITING

PREICTERIC PHASE 4 — 7 DAYS

ICTERIC PHASE
CHILDREN — USUALLY 10 — 12 DAYS
ADULTS — USUALLY 15 — 30 DAYS OR MORE

Viral Hepatitis I

Acute Form

Catarrhal jaundice and acute yellow atrophy of the liver, formerly thought to be two different entities, are now recognized, mainly through the knowledge acquired in the First World War, as different stages of one primary hepatic disease. The available evidence, corroborated by epidemiologic experience and by transmission to human volunteers, has established the viral origin of this disease and has justified the designation of *viral hepatitis*, although neither culture nor animal transmission has yet been possible. At least two types of virus play the pathogenetic rôle:

1. Virus A or IH produces *"infectious hepatitis"*. It is transmitted mainly by the oral route and is, therefore, a food-borne or water-borne infection, although the parenteral route is not excluded. The incubation period is relatively short, not exceeding 40 days with any mode of transmission. The virus is excreted in the feces, sometimes over very long periods. Gamma globulin administration provides protection. The disease occurs usually in persons under 30 years of age.

2. Virus B or SH (*"homologous serum hepatitis"*) is transmitted only by the parenteral route and mostly by healthy-appearing carriers who give blood for transfusion. Small amounts of the blood of such carriers are infective, so that syringes, needles or lancets which are not steam-sterilized may transmit the relatively heat-resistant virus. The incubation period of homologous serum hepatitis may be very long, usually more than 40 days. The virus appears in the feces. Gamma globulin provides no protection. The serum hepatitis has no preference for age periods.

The clinical manifestations of both types of viral hepatitis are identical, except that the onset in the infectious form is perhaps more abrupt, with the constitutional symptoms more prominent. In the few days of the preicteric prodromal period, gastro-intestinal or influenzalike symptoms (fever and chills) appear, and leukopenia and tenderness of the liver or right costovertebral angle may be present. When jaundice becomes conspicuous, the

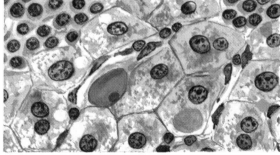

LIVER SECTION: MODERATE LOBULAR DISARRAY; SHRUNKEN AND SWOLLEN CELLS AND NUCLEI; CIRCUMSCRIBED REPLACEMENT OF LIVER CELLS WITH ROUND CELLS

EXTENSIVE VARIATION IN SIZE AND SHAPE OF LIVER CELLS; BINUCLEATE CELLS; THICKENING OF CENTRAL VEIN; CIRCUMSCRIBED INFLAMMATORY INFILTRATIONS

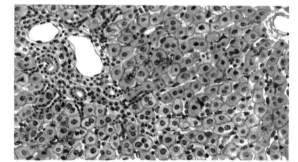

VERY HIGH POWER: CHANGES IN LIVER CELLS; BINUCLEATE CELLS, INFILTRATION, COUNCILMANLIKE BODY

RECOVERY STAGE: LIPOFUSCIN DEPOSITS IN KUPFFER CELLS; BILE CASTS IN CAPILLARIES; INCREASE IN BINUCLEATE CELLS; OCCASIONAL TRINUCLEATE CELLS

picture gradually changes. The fever subsides; anorexia and vomiting are aggravated but gradually subside, while the jaundice increases. In this early icteric period a great variety of manifestations, including arthropathy and urticaria, may confuse the picture. The spleen is seldom palpable. The entire icteric phase lasts in children usually not longer than 10 days and in adults not more than 4 weeks. Almost the same clinical picture unfolds without any jaundice, and these anicteric forms present the greatest diagnostic difficulties. The laboratory findings are in line with those of a diffuse hepatocellular degeneration. The thymol turbidity is very regularly elevated. Evidence of cholestasis is reflected in moderate elevation of the activity of the serum alkaline phosphatase.

The pathologic picture of the noncomplicated, self-limited form of viral hepatitis has been established almost entirely on the basis of liver-biopsy specimens.

The principal lesion, in the icteric and anicteric forms alike, is a diffuse degeneration of the liver cells throughout the lobule with *disorganized liver cell plates*. Isolated cells become necrotic, disappear and are replaced by mononuclear exudate cells which accumulate in small foci within which also the Kupffer cells markedly proliferate. With a sprinkling of eosinophilic infiltrates in the portal triads, in general the full picture of an eosinophilic degeneration with Mallory- and *Councilmanlike bodies* (see page 62) presents itself. An extensive regenerative tendency is evidenced by numerous *binucleate cells*. Golden-brown wear-and-tear *pigment of lipochrome character* accumulates in the Kupffer cells and in the portal triads. Later, in the recovery stage the regeneration dominates the picture, and quite often *bile plugs* may be found in the bile capillaries, indicating functional restoration of bile secretion.

GROSS APPEARANCE OF LIVER

CUT SURFACE: ACUTELY CONGESTED, "SPLEENLIKE"

CUT SURFACE: MORE COMMON "NUTMEG" LIVER

HIGH MAGNIFICATION: CELLULAR EXUDATE CONSISTS CHIEFLY OF MONONUCLEAR CELLS AND PLASMA CELLS; COMPLETE LOSS OF PARENCHYMAL CELLS

LOW MAGNIFICATION: MASSIVE NECROSIS, INFILTRATION OF LOBULES AND PORTAL AREAS, BILE DUCT PROLIFERATION

RETICULUM STAIN: RETICULAR NETWORK INTACT

VIRAL HEPATITIS II

Fulminant Form
(Acute Massive Necrosis)

It is now believed, on epidemiologic evidence, that almost all cases of "acute yellow atrophy" or massive necrosis, at least as seen in Western Europe and North America, are the result of the most severe phase of viral hepatitis, for which the term "fulminant hepatitis" has been recommended. It is mostly the homologous serum hepatitis (see page 93) which appears in this fulminant form in civilians (including children), as well as in military personnel. But it should not be concluded that this indicates a greater virulence of serum hepatitis, as compared to infectious hepatitis, because it is more probable that the disease which prompted the administration of plasma, blood and the like plays the rôle of an aggravating factor.

The disease is ushered in either by symptoms and signs of an infection such as high fever and malaise or by gastrointestinal manifestations, much the same as in the acute, nonfatal form (see page 93), but within 10 days after the onset neurologic changes (restlessness, lethargy or excitation) dominate the picture until the rapidly approaching end in coma (see page 75). The fever may temporarily drop when jaundice appears but rises before death. Ascites and severe hemorrhages are frequent. The liver shrinks during the short course of the disease, disappearing behind the costal arch. All hepatic tests indicate severe liver cell damage, though sometimes the serum protein tests may appear normal, because within a period of a few days the serum does not yet reflect the metabolic disturbance. Hepatogenic hypoglycemia also may not necessarily develop.

At autopsy the liver is small, weighing in adults as little as 700 gm. Its *surface* is smooth or wrinkled, and the anterior edge is sharp. Placed on a table, the liver flattens completely; its consistency permits bending it in any direction. On the cut surface the lobular architecture may be exaggerated, with dark-red depressed and enlarged lobular centers and a brown-to-gray peripheral zone (*nutmeg* appearance). In other areas the lobular architecture is entirely missing, so that the dark-red congested surface resembles the cut *surface of a spleen. Microscopically,* all or almost all liver cells have disappeared, and small, hardly recognizable breakdown products can be seen, some of them engulfed by Kupffer cells, some by *mononuclear scavenger cells. Plasma cells* and, occasionally, eosinophilic leukocytes are present. These exudate cells entirely replace the liver cells and infiltrate the portal triads. When the exudate cells gradually disappear, red cells will predominate, and then the lobular markings are best recognized by the proliferating cholangioles. At still later stages complete collapse (see pages 64 and 65) of the denudated framework is seen. Wherever the *massive necrosis* develops, the *reticulum framework* of the liver appears intact and hardly varies from that in normal livers, even if specific histologic staining techniques are applied.

The pathologic findings of acute massive necrosis, however, are not restricted to the fulminant type of viral hepatitis. Chemical poisons (trinitrotoluene, carbon tetrachloride) or even drugs (cinchophen, gold preparations, etc.) can produce massive necrosis. Though the presence of fat in many of these toxic injuries permits, sometimes, a differentiation, it is notoriously difficult to establish the responsible agent in many instances of hepatitis following therapeutic administration of drugs, and infection by serum hepatitis virus cannot usually be excluded. The SH or B virus seems to account for most cases of fulminant hepatitis following antisyphilitic treatment by arsenicals or bismuth. The long incubation period of serum hepatitis complicates the recognition of the etiologic factor.

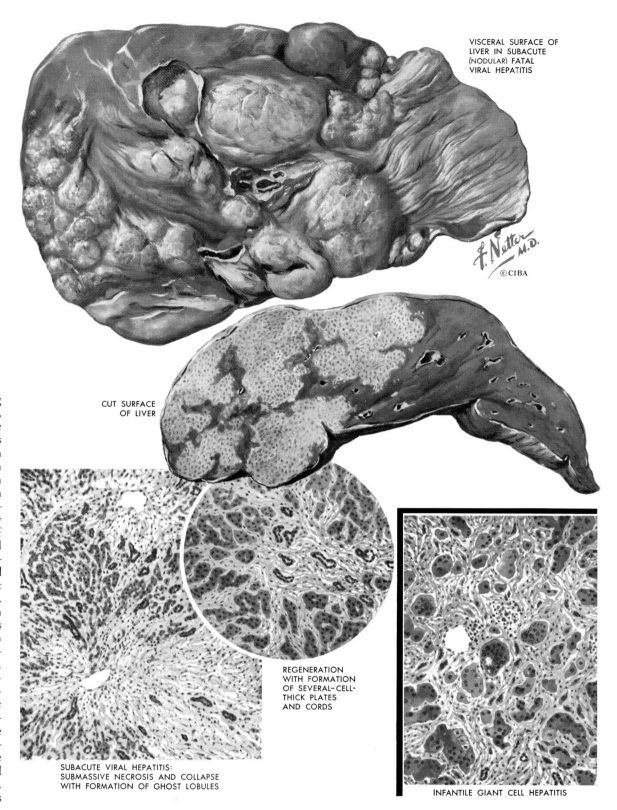

VISCERAL SURFACE OF
LIVER IN SUBACUTE
(NODULAR) FATAL
VIRAL HEPATITIS

CUT SURFACE
OF LIVER

REGENERATION
WITH FORMATION
OF SEVERAL-CELL-
THICK PLATES
AND CORDS

SUBACUTE VIRAL HEPATITIS:
SUBMASSIVE NECROSIS AND COLLAPSE
WITH FORMATION OF GHOST LOBULES

INFANTILE GIANT CELL HEPATITIS

Viral Hepatitis III

Subacute Fatal Form

If massive necrosis, instead of seizing more or less simultaneously all lobules, as in acute fulminant hepatitis (see page 94), is restricted to only some lobules at one time but proceeds at intervals from one part of the liver to another, death may result from *subacute hepatitis,* when eventually sufficient liver tissue has been destroyed. The duration of such a process varies from several weeks to many months, depending upon the speed of necrosis and the acuity of the individual bouts. Similarly as with fulminant hepatitis, the etiology of the subacute fatal hepatitis is not definitely established, but it apparently is caused by hepatitis virus, since it occurs in epidemics, especially in some European countries, where it seems to involve primarily women beyond 30 years of age, in whom it produces a protracted course of up to 1 year's duration. A short preicteric period is usually followed by a long icteric phase and a terminal period of acute severe hepatic insufficiency, dominated by central nervous system manifestations and severe hemorrhages. Sometimes only the terminal period is associated with severe jaundice. The laboratory findings depend greatly upon the stage of the disease. Evidence of liver cell degeneration is reflected in abnormal cephalin flocculation and thymol turbidity, the latter being, as a rule, exceedingly high. Increased activity of serum alkaline phosphatase is noted in some instances when severe jaundice heralds in the terminal stage. Serum albumin is usually low, whereas the serum γ-globulin may reach levels up to 4 gm. per ml. Except for a sudden drop in the cholesterol ester ratio and the appearance of amino-aciduria in a period of abrupt increase of jaundice, the clinician can get little if any help from the laboratory that would permit him to recognize the dangerous transition of a benign "spotty necrotic" type of hepatitis to the massive necrotic form.

The pathologic findings also vary greatly, depending upon the degree of necrosis, collapse and regeneration. As a

rule, the lesion is more severe or older in the left lobe. Shrunken, atrophic and nodular regenerative areas alternate with irregularly demarcated green or yellow areas, in which the lobular architecture is not only preserved but exaggerated. Recent massive necrosis in previously apparently intact areas accounts for the acute hepatic failure. In these grossly preserved areas one may find, microscopically, all graduations from "spotty necrotic" acute hepatitis, with loss of only individual cells and focal accumulation of mononuclear cells, to submassive and massive necrosis. Only *"ghost" lobules* remaining after complete disappearance of the hepatic cells can be recognized in the collapsed areas. The borders of the lobules are marked by the persisting and proliferating perilobular cholangioles. Where submassive necrosis has left part of the lobules intact, intensive *regeneration* results in the formation of nodules of various sizes, up

to several centimeters in diameter. The degree of regeneration depends upon the acuity of necrosis, but numerous *several-cell-thick liver cell plates* are dispersed throughout the liver.

A hepatitis with specific morphologic features occurs in childhood and particularly in infancy (see pages 118 and 120). It is characterized by *epithelial giant cells* with multiple nuclei, usually containing pigmented or vascular inclusions. The lesion is probably an expression of the excessive regenerative ability of the infantile liver in a hepatitis induced by various agents, including virus. Clinical and laboratory evidence of severe cholestasis is frequent, and this raises a problem of differential diagnosis from extrahepatic biliary obstruction. Though the liver shows sometimes only milder changes, the sequelae are serious because cirrhosis develops, which is often discovered only in a far-advanced stage.

SEQUELAE OF VIRAL HEPATITIS
(CHRONIC NONFATAL HEPATITIS)

NORMAL HEALING — CHOLANGIOLITIS — RECURRENT — GRANULOMA FORMATION — FIBROSIS — NONSPECIFIC CHANGES — NODULE FORMATION

Viral Hepatitis IV

Sequelae of Hepatitis
(Chronic Nonfatal Hepatitis)

The military experiences during and following World War II have alerted us to the relatively high incidence of the sequelae of benign, apparently self-limited, viral hepatitis. In children the disease completely heals shortly after the disappearance of jaundice, whereas in adults clinical, laboratory or anatomic residual alterations frequently persist with no, little or conspicuous jaundice. In most cases these residual changes are relatively mild and may disappear within 1 year. The incidence of permanent disease seems to be rather small. The picture in some patients is confusing, because clinical and laboratory findings and histologic alterations as recognized by liver biopsy do not match. Quite frequently, only one of the three factors may point to a persisting pathologic process. In this condition liver biopsy is of special diagnostic help. In view of the vagueness of the clinical complaints and of the difficulty in interpreting abnormal laboratory findings, the final decision as to complete recovery from viral hepatitis may depend upon biopsy interpretation.

After subsidence of the acute stage of hepatitis, complete healing may set in or a picture of a persistent intrahepatic cholestasis ("cholangiolitis") may develop (see page 97), with all its clinical, laboratory and morphologic characteristics. Before recovery is complete, an acute hepatitis may exacerbate. Such a relapse may sometimes be very severe and even proceed to massive necrosis. In other patients, after a period of apparent recovery, acute *hepatitis recurs,* and the possibility exists that infection by a different virus (for instance the SH or B virus with much longer incubation period) may have been superimposed upon the first attack. At any rate, the histologic, clinical and laboratory picture does not differ from that of acute viral hepatitis.

In some patients with apparent clinical recovery, mononuclear cells, including plasma cells, accumulate in nodular form (*granuloma formation*) within the lobular parenchyma and sometimes in the portal triads. In these cases serum γ-globulin is quite often elevated without other significant laboratory changes. In other patients biopsies following apparent recovery reveal increased connective tissue of the portal triads which assume a stellate appearance. Connective tissue membranes (*perilobular fibrosis*) may stretch from one triad to the other. It seems that eventually this fibrosis disappears again. In other instances dissection of the lobule has set in, and more or less actively *regenerating nodules* are noted. They sometimes result from focal massive necrosis and sometimes apparently from progression of the just-mentioned perilobular fibrosis. A postnecrotic cirrhosis can develop, as described on pages 67, 68 and 81. Quite frequently, however, the changes in the liver are those of a *nonspecific reactive hepatitis,* with small focal necroses, diffuse slight liver cell degeneration, cholangiolar proliferation, Kupffer cell mobilization and portal inflammatory infiltration. The histologic appearance usually does not permit the diagnosis of viral hepatitis.

The clinical manifestations may be referable to the cholangiolitis or may be characteristic of a relapse or of a recurrence, but they may also be restricted to neurasthenic or vague gastro-enterologic symptoms with fat intolerance. Sometimes a mild hyperbilirubinemia persists, caused either by altered bilirubin uptake by the liver or by hemolysis. The laboratory may report Bromsulphalein® retention, increased urinary urobilinogen excretion or abnormal cephalin flocculation and, especially, abnormal thymol turbidity which may persist for long periods. These findings need not be correlated with clinical or morphologic manifestations; sometimes they may even not match each other.

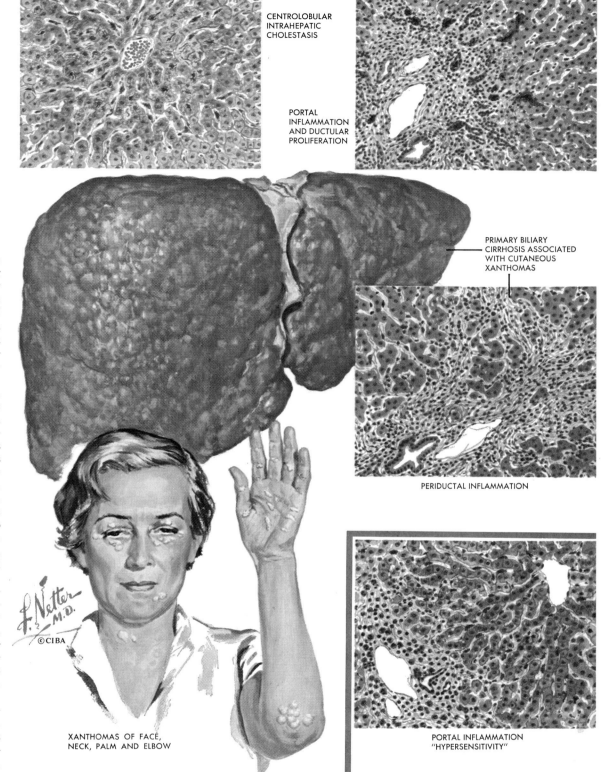

CENTROLOBULAR
INTRAHEPATIC
CHOLESTASIS

PORTAL
INFLAMMATION
AND DUCTULAR
PROLIFERATION

PRIMARY BILIARY
CIRRHOSIS ASSOCIATED
WITH CUTANEOUS
XANTHOMAS

PERIDUCTAL INFLAMMATION

XANTHOMAS OF FACE,
NECK, PALM AND ELBOW

PORTAL INFLAMMATION
"HYPERSENSITIVITY"

INTRAHEPATIC CHOLESTASIS

Clinical and laboratory manifestations of cholestasis, in the absence of "liver cell damage", present a major difficulty in the differential diagnosis of jaundice if the extrahepatic bile ducts are free of obstruction. This condition has been designated *intrahepatic cholestasis*. In some instances of viral hepatitis, alcoholic hepatitis, or *cirrhosis,* the morphologic liver cell injury can be detected by liver biopsy, although the biochemical alterations resemble those of extrahepatic biliary obstruction. There are, however, occasional instances in which, histologically, no significant liver cell injury is noted, and only cholestasis is seen. This condition previously was called "cholangiolitis", more for lack of a better term than on histologic evidence. However, recent electron microscopic investigations have confirmed the opinion of those who localized the lesion in the liver cells (see page 177), and the term "cholangiolitis", though still widely used, is being replaced by *intrahepatic cholestasis*.

The etiology of pure, acute intrahepatic cholestasis is frequently not established. Now and then, the past history points to viral hepatitis. In some instances, hepatocellular damage may have subsided, whereas manifestations of cholestasis persist. In other cases, cholestasis is associated with drug administration (see page 181). It is also found in toxic injuries or in infections such as pneumonia, and occasionally after operations.

This acute *centrolobular cholestasis* is frequently accompanied by *portal inflammation* and *proliferation of bile ductules,* particularly if the lesion lasts long. In drug-induced hepatic injuries, transient portal inflammation, edema and the accumulation of eosinophils are often noted, but these may disappear even if the process progresses. The old assumption that this portal inflammation mechanically produces the cholestasis can therefore no longer be entertained. However, the portal inflammatory reaction, at least in some instances, possibly represents a *hypersensitivity* reaction triggering the cholestasis.

Previously, primary biliary cirrhosis was considered to be chronic cholestasis, developing from acute centrolobular cholestasis, just described. This disease occurs somewhat more frequently in females and usually in the later reproductive period. An insidious onset of itching usually precedes the occurrence of jaundice, which is characterized by high activity of serum alkaline phosphatase and much retention of Bromsulphalein®. Serum γ-globulin levels are high and variable. In early stages, inflammation around the intrahepatic bile ducts is noted, but centrolobular cholestasis may be absent, suggesting that regurgitation of biliary substances through the ducts explains the jaundice and pruritus. Later, proliferation of the ductules, with *periductal inflammation* and fibrosis, sets in and is associated with central and peripheral cholestasis. In some patients the serum cholesterol level rises to extreme heights, although otherwise these individuals do not differ morphologically, clinically or in their laboratory findings from the majority of cases. The phospholipids usually parallel the cholesterol elevation. If the total lipid level exceeds 1800 mg. per 100 ml. serum, cholesterol is deposited in the skin in the form of yellow plaques (flat or eruptive *xanthomas*) which appear on the *palms, neck* and chest, or as more elevated tuberous xanthomas on the wrists, *elbows* and ankles. Such cholesterol infiltrations may develop in the *eyelids,* as xanthelasmas, at considerably lower cholesterol levels. The consensus now is that the serum cholesterol increases, and the skin phenomena are the results of primary liver disease. The term "xanthomatous biliary cirrhosis", introduced under the assumption that xanthomas in the bile ducts account for the biliary obstruction, should be abandoned. Eventually, fibrosis obscures the lobular architecture but initially does not destroy it. Only after many years, typical cirrhosis, with all its manifestations (see page 84), develops. While the cirrhosis progresses and liver cell damage becomes more evident, the xanthomas may disappear as the serum cholesterol drops.

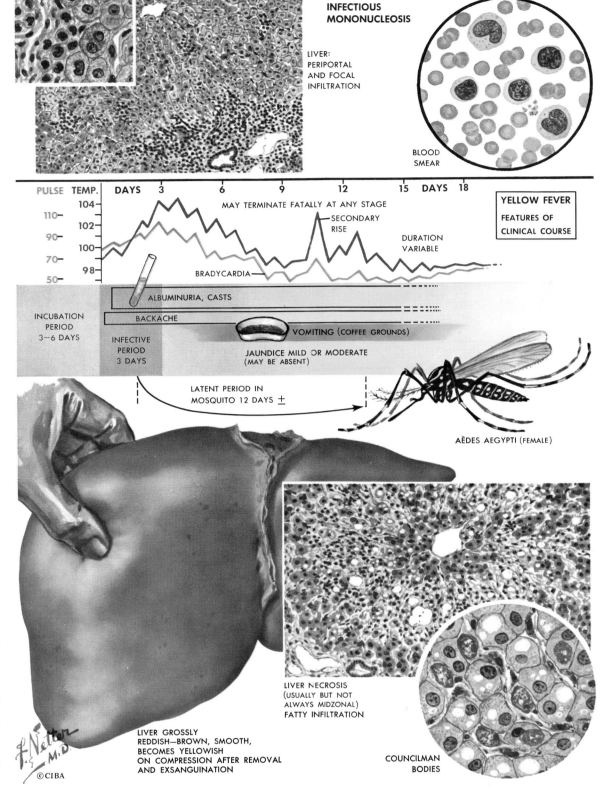

INFECTIOUS
MONONUCLEOSIS

LIVER:
PERIPORTAL
AND FOCAL
INFILTRATION

BLOOD
SMEAR

MAY TERMINATE FATALLY AT ANY STAGE

SECONDARY
RISE

DURATION
VARIABLE

BRADYCARDIA

YELLOW FEVER
FEATURES OF
CLINICAL COURSE

INCUBATION
PERIOD
3—6 DAYS

ALBUMINURIA, CASTS

BACKACHE

INFECTIVE
PERIOD
3 DAYS

VOMITING (COFFEE GROUNDS)

JAUNDICE MILD OR MODERATE
(MAY BE ABSENT)

LATENT PERIOD IN
MOSQUITO 12 DAYS ±

AËDES AEGYPTI (FEMALE)

LIVER NECROSIS
(USUALLY BUT NOT
ALWAYS MIDZONAL)
FATTY INFILTRATION

LIVER GROSSLY
REDDISH—BROWN, SMOOTH,
BECOMES YELLOWISH
ON COMPRESSION AFTER REMOVAL
AND EXSANGUINATION

COUNCILMAN
BODIES

©CIBA

INFECTIOUS MONONUCLEOSIS, YELLOW FEVER

Infectious mononucleosis is a febrile disease, presumably viral in origin. Infiltration of spleen, lymph nodes and bone marrow by mononuclear cells, resembling immature lymphocytes, is its main feature. The spleen and lymph nodes (glandular fever) are enlarged and tender. Moderate leukocytosis and atypical lymphocytes with somewhat foamy cytoplasm and indented nuclei are found in the peripheral blood. The serum contains heterophil antibodies agglutinating sheep cells. Jaundice, known for many years to be associated with infectious mononucleosis, is not caused by enlarged lymph nodes obstructing the extrahepatic biliary ducts but by a hepatitis. Therefore, a problem of differential diagnosis from viral hepatitis may sometimes arise, to be solved by serologic and hematologic examinations, though even in viral hepatitis a few atypical lymphocytes may be detected, and the heterophil antibody reaction may become positive only late in infectious mononucleosis. Nonspecific hepatic alterations, particularly extensive infiltrations with lymphoid cells, have been the findings at autopsy of patients who have died from complications of the disease, such as rupture of the spleen. Recent biopsy studies revealed, in the acute stages with jaundice, changes resembling those in nonfatal viral hepatitis. The liver cell plates are irregular, focal necroses are present and even acidophilic round bodies may be seen. Most characteristic is the *portal and intralobular infiltration* with round cells, some of which have indented nuclei. These changes may be present in cases with or without jaundice. In absence of jaundice, abnormal flocculation reactions and increased Bromsulphalein® retention may be detected. In

jaundiced patients, alkaline phosphatase is elevated.

Yellow fever is produced by a virus present in the blood in the first 3 days of the disease. The urban form is transmitted from man to man by the female of the mosquito *Aëdes aegypti,* while in the jungles white monkeys may serve as intermediate hosts. The mosquito becomes infective about 12 days after it has fed on infected blood. In the human, after an incubation period of 3 to 6 days, either a self-limited, grippelike disease develops, with headache, backache, photophobia and some gastro-intestinal discomfort, or a severe toxic condition evolves, usually with jaundice, in which several organs participate. After an initial *high fever* of 1 week's duration, the temperature returns to normal except for occasional *secondary rises;* in this period bradycardia, severe backache and headache, albuminuria with casts and oliguria dominate the picture. Severe hemorrhagic tendency,

reflected in coffee-ground vomiting, shock and a not necessarily severe jaundice are the attributes of the toxic form, which has a high mortality. Toxic nephrosis and myocardial degeneration are probably the most important causes of death. *The liver is large and flabby* and exhibits a *yellow color,* which becomes apparent when the organ is compressed by a finger or when the blood has leaked out after removal of the liver. The *histologic changes* are very characteristic. Degenerative changes of the liver cells are associated with fatty metamorphosis and spotty as well as midzonal necrosis. In scattered bile-pigmented liver cells, the cytoplasm becomes eosinophilic and the nuclei pyknotic. The final round refractile bodies, described by Councilman, resemble the acidophilic bodies in viral hepatitis, except that the latter are not pigmented or vacuolated. Little is known about the results of hepatic tests.

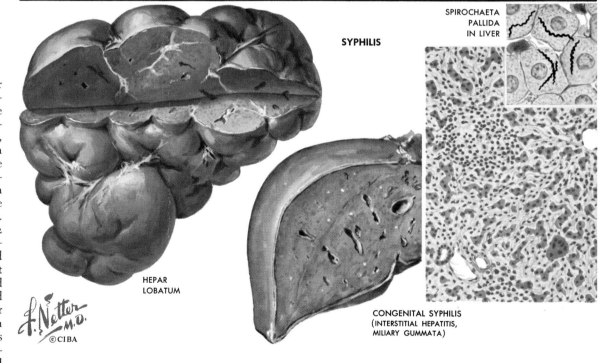

SPIROCHETAL INFECTIONS

Weil's Disease, Syphilis

Weil's disease, infectious jaundice or spirochetal jaundice, is caused by Leptospira icterohaemorrhagiae. The disease has a world-wide distribution. The carriers are wild rats and, to a lesser degree, mice. Both excrete the Leptospira with the urine into stagnant water, where the organisms may survive for months. *Human infection* takes place either through abrasions of the skin or through the mouth. The disease varies in severity. After an incubation period (6 to 12 days), high *fever,* headaches, *abdominal pain, prostration, muscle pain* and *conjunctivitis* appear. Leptospira can at this stage be demonstrated in the blood by *animal inoculation* or dark-field microscopy. About 10 days later the fever subsides, and a toxic stage develops in which renal manifestations, sometimes progressing to uremia, meningitis, myocardial damage, dermal and conjunctival petechiae, epistaxis and skin rashes are conspicuous. Involvement of the liver occurs in about 50 per cent of the cases. When jaundice becomes severe, differentiation from viral hepatitis may present a diagnostic problem, unless azotemia and albuminuria or necroses in muscle biopsy specimens determine the diagnosis. In this period Leptospira are more readily found in urine than in blood. The fever may recur. After the third week a *slow convalescence* sets in, and immunologic tests become positive.

Despite the frequency of hepatic involvement, the liver shows only noncharacteristic changes, such as central or focal necroses, irregular arrangement of the liver cell plates, severe *portal inflamma-*

tory infiltration and swollen Kupffer cells. The hepatic alterations are poorly correlated to the degree of jaundice, part of which is explained by hemolysis. In patients with jaundice, cephalin flocculation and thymol turbidity are frequently abnormal, and the serum activity of alkaline phosphatase is elevated.

Hepatic changes caused by *syphilis* are rapidly decreasing in incidence as a result of the progress in diagnosis and antisyphilitic treatment. Moreover, many cases of hepatic disease in syphilitics are now recognized as incidental to antiluetic therapy; e.g., the viral hepatitis transmitted by syringes (see page 93) previously considered the result of either syphilis itself or of arsenicals or bismuth. Most cases of cirrhosis in syphilitics are now interpreted as the result of other factors, especially nutritional ones (see page 78). The most frequent hepatic alteration of syphilitic etiology at present encountered is the scar forma-

tion following extensive specific coagulation necrosis (gumma), which leads to focal losses of hepatic tissue. The resulting irregular deformation of the liver frequently causes very bizarre shapes and is designated as *hepar lobatum.* Occasionally, however, the deformation with enlargement of the left and shrinkage of the right lobe causes unusual palpatory findings. Only exceptionally, one finds fresh yellow gummatous areas in the depth of the scars. Formerly, the now almost extinct *"brimstone"* liver was frequently found in deeply jaundiced newborns as a characteristic of *congenital syphilis* together with other syphilitic manifestations. The microscopic features are small *miliary necroses* (gummata), diffuse *interstitial hepatitis,* separated and distorted liver cell plates, increased interlobular connective tissue, rich in inflammatory cells, and numerous *spirochetes* readily demonstrable by silver impregnation.

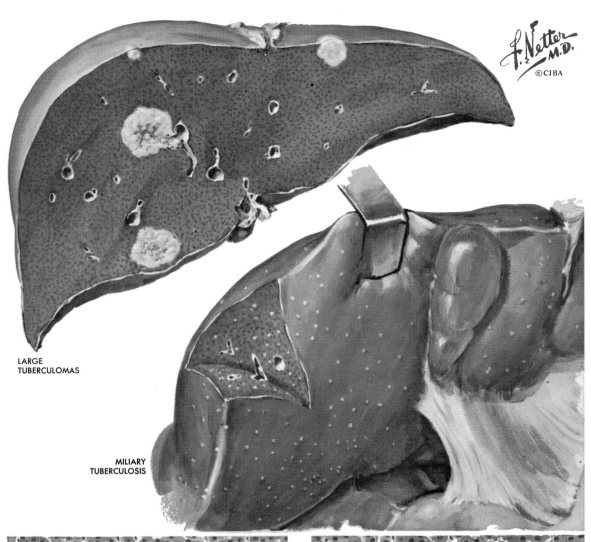

LARGE
TUBERCULOMAS

MILIARY
TUBERCULOSIS

TUBERCULOSIS

Primary hepatic tuberculosis occurs in the extremely rare congenital tuberculosis, but liver involvement secondary to tuberculosis is frequent and of clinical significance, because of its demonstrability by biopsy, which assists in the recognition of the acuity of the process. The most frequent lesion is the small *miliary granuloma* (tubercle), which may be scattered over the liver in all forms of active organ tuberculosis. The granuloma starts with a focal proliferation of Kupffer cells which form small histiocytic nodules located throughout the parenchyma. Subsequently, liver cells surrounded by the histiocytes become necrotic, and in some instances smaller or larger foci of hepatocellular necrosis with little mesenchymal reaction develop. In the nodules some cells become larger and develop into epithelioid cells, the nuclei of which can divide without division of the cytoplasm, resulting in large giant cells (Langhans). On the periphery of the granuloma, lymphocytes create a demarcation against the parenchyma. As the tubercle enlarges, central caseation necrosis may set in. Eventually, the histiocytes transgress into fibroblasts, which form a capsule around the tubercle. Finally, the entire lesion becomes transformed into a nodule of collagenous connective tissue. Such globular scars fail to reveal their etiology. Acid-fast bacilli can hardly ever be demonstrated, and, even with extensive necrosis, tubercle bacilli usually cannot be cultured from liver biopsy specimens.

The morphologic picture of the tubercles is not specific, because other granulomatous diseases may produce similar lesions (see page 101). However, miliary granulomas in the centrolobular zone or

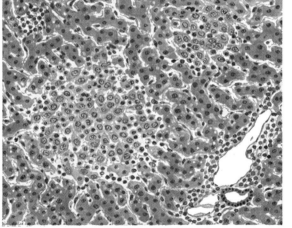

ACUTE MILIARY GRANULOMAS
(SOFT TUBERCLE — CHIEFLY HISTIOCYTES)

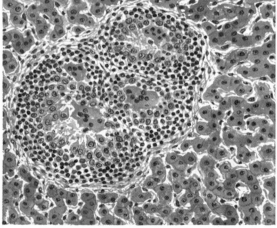

SUBACUTE CONGLOMERATE TUBERCLE
(GIANT CELLS, CASEATION, HISTIOCYTES, SURROUNDED
BY LYMPHOCYTES AND FIBROSIS)

in the wall of the central vein are rarely found in other conditions. Tuberculous granulomas are spread all over the lobule and frequently close to the portal triads, where they show tendency to coalescence.

The flocculation tests frequently yield abnormal results without clear relation to the morphologically demonstrable degree of hepatic involvement. Elevation of serum gamma globulin is somewhat related to the degree of the nonspecific reactive hepatitis present.

In *miliary tuberculosis* the tubercles are densely spread, as is readily seen on gross inspection, and appear as white pinhead-sized nodules which are best recognized through the capsule by inspection of the inferior surface of the left lobe. In early stages of hematogenous dissemination they appear soft, nonsharply limited; as the dissemination becomes older they are firmer, sharply defined and larger, up to 2 mm. in diameter. The hepatic tests yield usually

abnormal results in clinically diagnosed miliary tuberculosis, and some jaundice may be present if the associated nonspecific reactive hepatitis is severe. In view of the fact that in most forms of active tuberculosis elsewhere in the organism tubercle bacilli may be carried into the liver by hematogenous dissemination, a differentiation of organ tuberculosis from generalized miliary tuberculosis with the aid of liver biopsy specimens is at best arbitrary, because it depends largely on the intensity of the seeding, which can hardly be determined in biopsy specimens.

Cases of special interest are on record in which a hepatic miliary tuberculosis anteceded the pulmonary involvement or in which the lungs remained unaffected. In such instances fever may be present for prolonged periods with negative roentgenologic findings in the chest, and only liver biopsy clinches the diagnosis.

SARCOIDOSIS, BRUCELLOSIS, HISTOPLASMOSIS

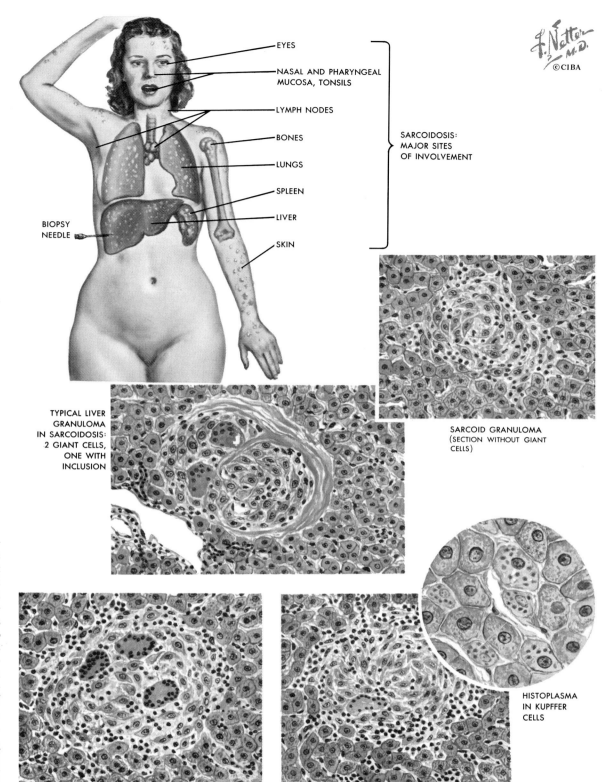

EYES

NASAL AND PHARYNGEAL MUCOSA, TONSILS

LYMPH NODES

BONES

LUNGS

SPLEEN

LIVER

SKIN

SARCOIDOSIS: MAJOR SITES OF INVOLVEMENT

BIOPSY NEEDLE

SARCOID GRANULOMA (SECTION WITHOUT GIANT CELLS)

TYPICAL LIVER GRANULOMA IN SARCOIDOSIS: 2 GIANT CELLS, ONE WITH INCLUSION

HISTOPLASMA IN KUPFFER CELLS

BRUCELLOSIS: LIVER GRANULOMA

HISTOPLASMOSIS: LIVER GRANULOMA

Sarcoidosis of Boeck is a granulomatous disease of unknown etiology. The granulomas resemble tubercles in that aggregated histiocytes are transformed into epithelioid cells, some of which become giant cells with various cytoplasmic inclusions. The Boeck follicle has frequently a lymphocytic rim; it fails to show caseation, but its center zone has sometimes a smudgy appearance, designated as fibrinoid degeneration. Within and around the follicle a hyaline material appears which forms the basis of subsequent partial and complete fibrosis. Such process may involve many organs. It is frequently located in lymph nodes, skin, bones, spleen, in the mucosa of nose, pharynx and tonsils, or in the uveal tract and salivary glands (uveoparotid fever). Wherever the site may be, sarcoid follicles appear frequently in the liver, and this fact makes liver biopsy a valuable tool for diagnosis, especially in the absence of superficial lymphadenopathy or of dermal lesions.

The follicles in the liver are usually near or close to the portal triad, or at least in the vicinity of intralobular cholangioles. They start with proliferation of histiocytes and undergo the same development as in other organs; as a rule, all follicles in the same liver are of similar degree of maturity. In the florid stages the surrounding parenchyma shows nonspecific reactive hepatitis. Coalescence of smaller follicles to larger grapelike bodies occurs. Eventually, all follicles undergo fibrosis. This may lead, occasionally, to perilobular fibrosis and, exceptionally, to cirrhosis.

Hepatic granulomas similar to those in tuberculosis and sarcoidosis are seen in many other conditions. In *brucellosis*, granulomas are irregularly spaced throughout the liver; they vary in size and degree of development and are accompanied by focal necrosis and portal inflammation. In the florid stage the picture is, as a rule, more polymorphous than in other granulomatous diseases, especially when the focal necroses become large and irregularly scattered. Transition into cirrhosis has been claimed but appears to be rare. Positive culture of the biopsy specimen establishes the diagnosis.

In *histoplasmosis*, granulomas, resembling tubercles, occur together with a diffuse proliferation of the Kupffer cells, the cytoplasm of which is sometimes loaded with the fungus Histoplasma capsulatum, best demonstrated in sections stained with the periodic acid-leukofuchsin reagent. Not seldom, the granulomas are the only finding, and in such instances culture of the specimen may be diagnostic. Sometimes the enlargement of the Kupffer cells is so severe as to interfere with sinusoidal circulation, followed by central necrosis and even cirrhosis. In other fungus diseases, such as blastomycosis or coccidioidomycosis, a nonspecific reactive hepatitis is far more frequent than hepatic granulomas. Tularemia, leprosy and beryllium poisoning may also be associated with hepatic granulomas.

The demonstration of hepatic granulomas is one of the most gratifying applications of liver biopsy. A histologic study of the specimen may permit a tentative diagnosis, which becomes definite if the etiologic agent can be demonstrated in the specimen. However, frequently, the etiology of a granulomatous hepatitis must be established on clinical grounds and/or by bacteriologic and biochemical studies.

Amebiasis

Amebiasis, transmitted by the protozoan parasite *Entamoeba histolytica,* is initially and predominantly an intestinal disease, but it involves the liver in one tenth to one third of the cases. The infective, encysted form of the parasite, communicated from man to man, without an intermediate host, by water, food, etc., which has been in contact with fecal human material, enters the intestinal tract by the mouth, passes the stomach and loses its cystic wall in the small intestine. The cyst, 5 to 20 microns in diameter, having matured during its passage, releases there four trophozoites, the vegetative form, which in contrast to the cyst are mobile but do not survive outside the body. The amebae, which have attached themselves to the colonic wall, the major site of the disease, migrate into the crypts and penetrate the epithelium and muscularis. In the submucosa the amebae, living on tissue constituents and red cells, produce small cavities (not abscesses) which eventually communicate with the intestinal lumen and permit the release of trophozoites. Other trophozoites are excreted in the encysted form, maintaining the life cycle.

The described events may proceed asymptomatically, accounting for the "carrier stage", which, upon careful examination of the feces, may be detected in as many as 10 per cent of the population in endemic U.S. areas. Some disturbance of the host-parasite relationship results in amebic colitis or dysentery, characterized by undermined ulcers throughout the colon. The amebae may reach the liver through the portal route in the presence or absence of amebic dysentery. Three forms of hepatic involvement are differentiated:

1. An enlarged liver, which returns to normal size under treatment with nonabsorbable amebicides, is frequently found in intestinal amebiasis. The absence of amebae in the liver suggests a nonspecific reactive hepatitis (see page 91).

2. An attenuated invasion of the liver by amebae leads to amebic hepatitis, the exact morphologic nature of which is not established. Autopsy material being scarcely available, some investigators attribute this hepatitis to multiple small necroses ("micro-abscesses") resulting from histolytic activity of the amebae, whereas others assume nonspecific or hypersensitivity reactions. Fever, pain in the right upper quadrant and a markedly enlarged liver are the clinical signs. Leukocytosis is frequent and jaundice rare. The hepatic tests seldom yield abnormal results. The diagnosis depends upon the demonstration of amebae in the feces and a positive complement fixation test. Antiamebic therapy is usually successful.

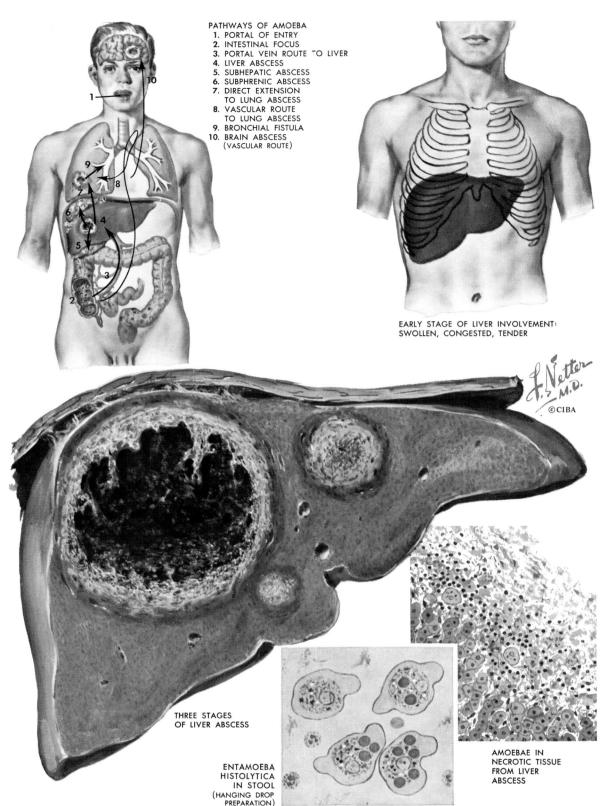

PATHWAYS OF AMOEBA
1. PORTAL OF ENTRY
2. INTESTINAL FOCUS
3. PORTAL VEIN ROUTE TO LIVER
4. LIVER ABSCESS
5. SUBHEPATIC ABSCESS
6. SUBPHRENIC ABSCESS
7. DIRECT EXTENSION TO LUNG ABSCESS
8. VASCULAR ROUTE TO LUNG ABSCESS
9. BRONCHIAL FISTULA
10. BRAIN ABSCESS (VASCULAR ROUTE)

EARLY STAGE OF LIVER INVOLVEMENT: SWOLLEN, CONGESTED, TENDER

THREE STAGES OF LIVER ABSCESS

ENTAMOEBA HISTOLYTICA IN STOOL (HANGING DROP PREPARATION)

AMOEBAE IN NECROTIC TISSUE FROM LIVER ABSCESS

3. The most serious form of hepatic involvement in amebiasis is the development of single or, more frequently, multiple cavities, which have received the unsuitable name "amebic abscesses", although pus is present only in secondary bacterial infections. These lesions are seen in tropical and subtropical zones ("tropical abscesses") but are also frequent in temperate areas. The smaller "abscesses" are circumscribed, necrotic, white and not sharply limited lesions which, when they grow, develop a central cavity with a thin, shaggy yellow membrane surrounding a thick fluid of a brown-to-chocolate color, sometimes described as anchovylike color. The necrotic debris of the inner part of the cavity contains no amebae, which are encountered near normal hepatic parenchyma. The larger "abscesses" are usually located in the right lobe near the dome or near the hepatic flexure of the colon. The diaphragm is fre-

quently fixed to the liver by fibrous and fibrinous adhesions. Severe anorexia, pain, loss of weight, fever, chills, leukocytosis and enlargement of the liver are the foremost clinical manifestations. Fixation of the diaphragm is a roentgenologic characteristic. Hepatic tests are of little diagnostic help. The mortality of "amebic hepatic abscess" is high and rises to over 40 per cent when complications set in. Perforation of an infected or noninfected abscess leads to *subphrenic* or *subhepatic abscess* and, eventually, to diffuse peritonitis. The most typical complication is an extension of the abscess through the diaphragm into the chest cavity, producing first an empyema, eventually a *pulmonary* or *hepatopulmonary abscess,* or sometimes a *hepatobronchial fistula.* A pulmonary abscess may also develop directly by *hematogenous route* from the intestine or from the liver. Even hematogenous brain abscesses occur.

POSSIBLE ROUTES
OF DISSEMINATION
1. DIRECTLY FROM GUT (APPENDIX) TO LIVER
2. VIA PORTAL VEIN
3. EXTENSION FROM LUNG TO LIVER
4. HEMATOGENOUS ROUTE TO LIVER
5. EXTENSION FROM LIVER TO LUNG
6. CUTANEOUS FISTULA

RELATIVELY SMALL ACTINOMYCOTIC ABSCESS

RAY FUNGUS
IN LIVER ABSCESS

LARGE LIVER ABSCESS
PERFORATING INTO LUNG

ACTINOMYCOSIS

Actinomycosis is an infection by an anaerobic fungus, Actinomyces bovis, which is found on many plants and also, frequently, as a harmful saprophytic inhabitant of the oral cavity, especially in peridental structures and on the tonsils. The fungus, on rare occasions, enters the deeper tissues through a break in the mucosa or skin and produces suppuration. The typical initial localizations of the abscesses are the jaws, the lung and the intestine, especially cecum and appendix. From the primary localization the suppuration spreads into the vicinity. Characteristically, actinomycotic abscesses do not respect the natural borders of the organs; they extend in all directions in the form of fistulae which frequently extend from any original site to the body surface. The fistula tracts are multiple, and the skin surface, as well as that of involved organs, assumes a characteristic honeycombed appearance. Only rarely does the actinomycotic infection spread by the hematogenous route, and then metastatic-pyemic abscesses develop; even endocarditis has been reported.

The liver is relatively rarely the site of actinomycotic abscesses. In the majority of such instances, the primary focus is in the proximal colon, especially in the appendix. The liver is reached either by direct spread or through the portal vein. The *liver abscess* may also be a complication of a pulmonary actinomycosis, and then, frequently, a combined pneumopleurohepatic abscess results. However, quite often it is impossible to decide whether the same type of lesion may not result from spread from the liver upward through the diaphragm into the thoracic cage. Actinomycosis and amebiasis are the main causes for hepatobronchial fistulae. The liver rarely becomes involved by the hematogenous route, and then, usually, several abscesses are found. It happens in solitary instances of hepatic actinomycosis that an original site of the infection may not be recognized.

The smaller liver abscess represents an unsharply limited yellow focus which clearly reveals development from coales-cence of even smaller abscesses. The central portions exhibit multiple, partially communicating cavities of different size. In the pus, small yellow granules ("sulfur granules") are found, which consist of concentrically arranged, moderately basophilic, branching filaments with eosinophilic clubbed endings; the arrangement of these filaments, best seen in tissue sections, accounts for the name *"ray fungus"*. In cultures the fungus reveals, in addition to the branching filaments, short single-branched forms, simulating diphtheria bacilli. The ray fungus is surrounded by pus cells which, in turn, are engulfed by granulation tissue earmarked by many fat-containing foam cells. This fat accumulation, characteristic of chronic abscess walls, accounts for the bright yellow color of the lesion. The abscess grows by direct distention until it involves the hepatic capsule, with resulting subdiaphragmatic, subhepatic or perinephritic peri-hepatitis. Eventually, perforation into the surrounding viscus or to the skin takes place. Diffuse peritonitis is rare. The large abscess cavity resulting from the expansion of the smaller lesion is characterized by an extremely shaggy wall. Secondary infection by pyogenic bacteria is a dangerous complication. Clinically, hepatic actinomycosis is a toxic and wasting condition associated with fever, anemia and leukocytosis. The liver is enlarged and tender and abdominal pain develops. Ascites and jaundice are rare, and involvement of surrounding organs as well as multiple cutaneous fistulae contribute to the clinical picture. The hepatic function tests reveal no characteristic alterations except for manifestations of a space-occupying lesion. The prognosis is serious because of the great tendency to suppuration and spreading to other organs. (Nocardia asteroides, an aerobic actinomyces, rarely produces hepatic granulomas.)

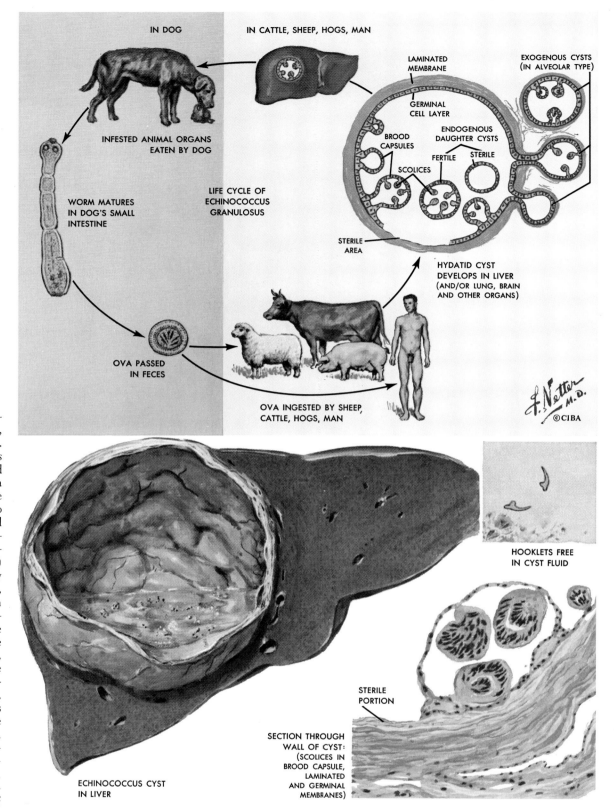

ECHINOCOCCUS CYST

(Hydatid Disease)

The Taenia echinococcus, or Echinococcus granulosus, is a tapeworm which, in the adult stage, is only about 5 mm. long. It lives in the small intestine of *dogs* and other canines that have been infected by ingestion of scolices containing viscera of other animals, mainly sheep. In the canine intestine the scolices develop into the *adult Taenia, i.e.,* a pyriform head with four suckers and numerous hooklets, a short neck and only a few segments, of which the terminal (proglottis) releases the ova. The ova are ingested by the *larval* or *intermediate host,* namely, sheep, cattle and hogs but also human beings (mostly children). In the intestinal tract of the larval host the larvae hatch from the egg and migrate into the liver and, far less commonly, into lungs, brain and other organs, where the larvae develop into a *cyst* with an outer laminated and an inner *germinal layer,* around which a capsule of collagenous tissue is formed. From the cells of the germinal layer evolve embryonal scolices, either directly or after formation of invaginations (*brood capsules*), which eventually become endogenous *daughter cysts.* With successive invagination and subsequent development of generations of cysts, the original unilocular main cyst is eventually filled by hundreds of daughter cysts, varying in size. The main cyst grows through the years, initially symptomless, until it becomes 20 cm. or more in diameter. The daughter cysts are often discharged from the wall and float in the lumen containing the hydatid fluid which, though almost protein-free, is highly irritating. The fluid also contains the *hydatid sand* in which the scolices may be microscopically recognized. Daughter cysts may be seen as outpouchings on the wall of the main cyst or in the surrounding hepatic tissue and, occasionally, implanted in the peritoneal lining of the mesentery. When this asexual production of scolices in the cysts eventually stops, the capsule invades the cyst,

the inner surface, formerly granular, becomes smooth, the wall fibrotic and sometimes calcified and, therewith, roentgenologically visible. Inflammatory reactions in the vicinity of the cyst are rare.

Echinococciasis has its highest incidence in sheep-raising countries, without specific climatic predilections. It was frequent in some parts of Europe, New Zealand and Australia, but sanitary measures, wherever introduced, prompted a reduction. In the United States dogs are hardly ever infected, and echinococciasis is mainly observed in previously infected immigrants. The *cysts,* mostly incidental findings at autopsy in the *right liver lobe,* may deform the organ and lead to unusual palpatory findings. Clinical symptoms are produced by various complications; the most frequent is the rupture of the cysts. Hydatid fluid entering the circulation produces allergic manifestations and, exceptionally, anaphylactic shock. Rupture

of daughter cysts into bile ducts or compression of the main hepatic duct produces jaundice. Secondary bacterial infection of cysts causes fever, chills and leukocytosis. Supposedly, hepatic carcinoma develops around cysts. The alkaline phosphatase activity might be slightly elevated. Eosinophilia is not specific but occurs in one fourth of the cases. A precipitin or complement fixation or intradermal skin test should be performed if the history arouses suspicion.

A very rare variety, the alveolar type of echinococciasis, occurs in Southern Germany, Tyrol and Russia and is characterized by excessive development of innumerable small exogenous daughter cysts; the original cyst also remaining small. These cysts invade the surrounding tissue, so that many years ago this alveolar variety was considered a type of mucus-producing carcinoma. Alveolar echinococciasis has a grave prognosis and produces jaundice and cachexia.

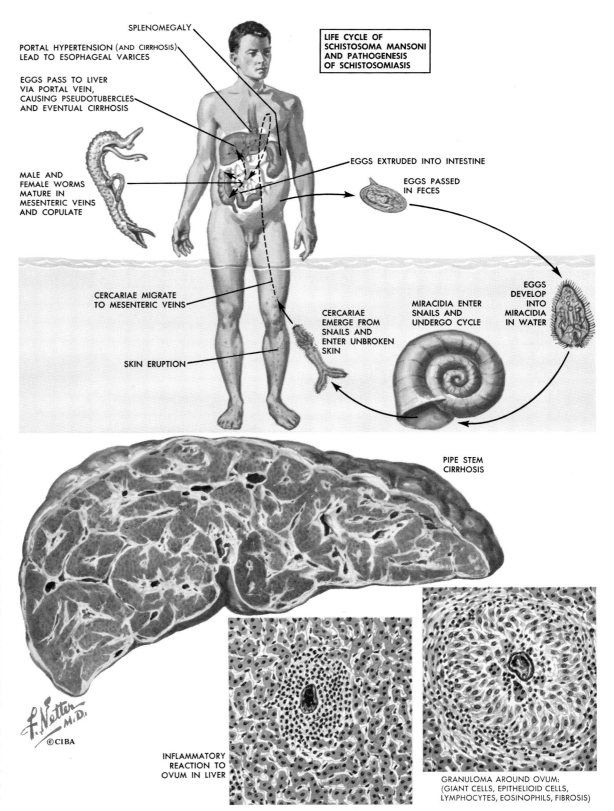

LIFE CYCLE OF SCHISTOSOMA MANSONI AND PATHOGENESIS OF SCHISTOSOMIASIS

SPLENOMEGALY

PORTAL HYPERTENSION (AND CIRRHOSIS) LEAD TO ESOPHAGEAL VARICES

EGGS PASS TO LIVER VIA PORTAL VEIN, CAUSING PSEUDOTUBERCLES AND EVENTUAL CIRRHOSIS

EGGS EXTRUDED INTO INTESTINE

EGGS PASSED IN FECES

MALE AND FEMALE WORMS MATURE IN MESENTERIC VEINS AND COPULATE

CERCARIAE MIGRATE TO MESENTERIC VEINS

SKIN ERUPTION

CERCARIAE EMERGE FROM SNAILS AND ENTER UNBROKEN SKIN

MIRACIDIA ENTER SNAILS AND UNDERGO CYCLE

EGGS DEVELOP INTO MIRACIDIA IN WATER

PIPE STEM CIRRHOSIS

INFLAMMATORY REACTION TO OVUM IN LIVER

GRANULOMA AROUND OVUM: (GIANT CELLS, EPITHELIOID CELLS, LYMPHOCYTES, EOSINOPHILS, FIBROSIS)

Schistosomiasis

Schistosoma is a genus of trematode parasites or blood flukes of which Schistosoma mansoni, japonicum and haematobium are of importance in human pathology. The mansoni variety is found mainly in Africa, in parts of South America and in Puerto Rico, from where, with the increasing immigration, it is imported to the United States. Schistosomiasis japonica is common in the Far East. Schistosomiasis haematobium is found in Africa, especially in Egypt, and in endemic foci in Southern Europe and Asia. The life cycle of these three species is similar, but Schistosoma haematobium predominantly involves the vessels of the urinary bladder. *Eggs of Schistosoma mansoni* and japonicum are excreted with the feces of human carriers; those of haematobium with the urine. Eggs of Schistosoma mansoni, about 140 microns long, exhibit a characteristic lateral spine. They hatch when they fall into fresh water. The larvae or *miracidia* survive only a few hours, unless they can attach themselves to snails, which they penetrate. In the snail's digestive gland the larvae pass through several stages (sporocysts) and develop into *cercariae*, which, having left the snail, propel themselves with a forked tail. They are most active in shallow water exposed to sunlight, where they may attach themselves to wading or swimming human beings, whose unbroken skin or mucous membranes they enter. They reach, eventually, the extrahepatic tributaries and the intrahepatic branches of the portal vein. Here they grow to full sexual maturity, depositing the fertilized eggs, some of which are extruded through the vascular wall into the intestinal lumen, whence they pass with the feces, maintaining the life cycle. Other eggs are carried into the smallest portal radicles in the liver, where they are responsible for the clinical manifestations of hepatic schistosomiasis or Bilharziasis.

Immediately after infestation and during migration, localized or generalized skin reactions occur, accompanied by pruritus (swimmers' itch) and fever. The liver becomes enlarged. In the peripheral blood granulocytosis and eosinophilia (14,000 to 20,000) are found. Within a period of about 6 weeks, symptoms may entirely subside, while in other patients an acute toxic stage may develop, caused by oviposition associated with local reactions, even with abscess formation. This stage is characterized by remittent or intermittent fever, gastro-intestinal symptoms varying from mild discomfort to severe abdominal pain, nausea, vomiting and sometimes persistent cough. The liver is now large and tender and splenomegaly is present. After a variable time interval, chronic colitis, mesenteric lymphadenitis and pulmonary sclerosis may develop, but the most dangerous manifestations occur in the portal system, where worms and ova produce an obstruction of the portal venous blood flow with resulting portal hypertension. The lining endothelium, to which the ova adhere, grows over them. First an *inflammatory reaction* develops, followed eventually by a granuloma, with fibroblasts, epithelioid cells and even giant cells. The ovum becomes necrotic, frequently calcified and may entirely disappear, while the *fibrosing granuloma* persists. The granulomas are demonstrated by liver biopsy, and their etiology can frequently be established by demonstrating the ova or their remnants, but sometimes a nonspecific granuloma or pigment deposition in the macrophages is the only indication in liver biopsy. Although portal fibrosis and *pipe stem cirrhosis* set in, causing severe portal hypertension with all of its sequelae, only exceptionally may postnecrotic cirrhosis develop. Laennec's cirrhosis, if present, has an independent etiology.

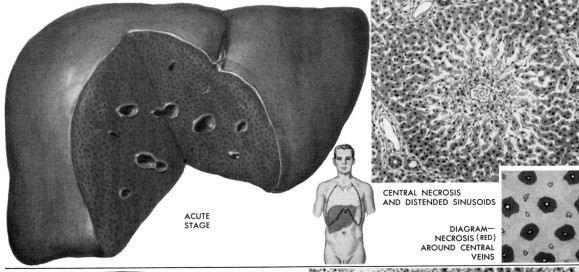

ACUTE
STAGE

CENTRAL NECROSIS
AND DISTENDED SINUSOIDS

DIAGRAM—
NECROSIS (RED)
AROUND CENTRAL
VEINS

CARDIAC LIVER

With the heart so close and being a major blood depot, the liver carries the brunt in passive congestion, whatever its cause. The degree of hepatic involvement has, however, no simple relation to the degree of passive congestion. In some patients the hepatic congestion may be less conspicuous than that of other organs, and vice versa.

In *acute passive congestion* the liver is markedly enlarged, the capsule is tense, the anterior edge is blunt and, on the cut surface, the lobular markings are far more distinct than usual. On closer inspection the zones around the central veins appear dark red and depressed and stand out distinctly against the intermediate and peripheral zones, which, sometimes, exhibit a yellow hue caused by fatty metamorphosis. The hepatic veins are extremely dilated. Histologically, the liver cells in the central zone have disappeared, and the sinusoids, as well as the tissue spaces, are crowded with red cells, as are the dilated branches of the hepatic veins. The *central necrosis* is more marked in necropsy than in biopsy specimens, and it is safe to assume that much of the hemorrhagic necrosis develops in the agonal period, secondary to terminal cardiac failure. Sometimes, in very acute cardiac failure, for instance after rupture of a chorda tendinea, only a small rim of parenchyma is preserved on the lobular periphery. Clinically, the liver appears very large and exquisitely tender, especially in the gallbladder region. Jaundice in the acute stage is not frequent. Increased urinary urobilinogen is found more often than are abnormal results of other hepatic tests, perhaps with the exception of an elevated Bromsulphalein® retention.

In the *subacute stage* the liver is less enlarged, although the edge is still blunt. The lobular architecture in places seems exaggerated but in others appears reversed, in that *bridges* around the portal triads appear to connect the hemorrhagic central zones. Consequently, the original peripheral zone is now surrounded by continuous hemorrhagic areas. Regeneration has led to the formation of small nodules, quite often yellow in color

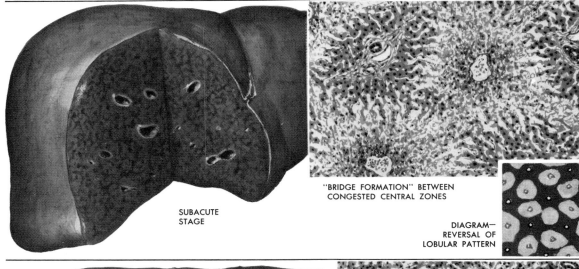

SUBACUTE
STAGE

"BRIDGE FORMATION" BETWEEN
CONGESTED CENTRAL ZONES

DIAGRAM—
REVERSAL OF
LOBULAR PATTERN

CHRONIC
STAGE

ICTERUS,
CYANOSIS,
ASCITES

FIBROSIS OF CENTRAL AREAS
AND "BRIDGES"— REGENERATIVE
NODULE

F. Netter M.D.
©CIBA

because of fatty metamorphosis. The small nodules contribute to the polymorphic appearance of the cut surface, which has led to the term "nutmeg liver". Histologically, the *reversal* of the *lobular pattern* is apparent. On clinical examination the liver feels firm and usually tender; abnormalities in the hepatic tests are more frequent than in the acute form.

In *chronic passive congestion* the liver is smaller than in the acute stages and sometimes even smaller than normal, justifying the connotation "cyanotic atrophy". Its surface is irregular and fine granular; the capsule often is thickened and covered by organized fibrin. On the cut surface *regenerative nodules* are frequent, and, in addition, an increase of connective tissue is reflected in irregularly arranged, gray-white, fine bands. The hepatic veins appear wider than in acute stages. Histologically, the lobular architecture is mostly preserved, but the *central areas*

appear collapsed and fibrosed, and connected with each other by fibrotic bridges, which only exceptionally reach the portal areas. Despite some regenerative nodules, this stage is better designated as *cardiac fibrosis* than cirrhosis. The latter term should be reserved for the infrequent instances in which extensive connections between central fields and portal canals have completely destroyed the lobular architecture. True cardiac cirrhosis is the result of very severe passive congestion, as it occurs in long-standing incompetence of the tricuspid valve or in constrictive pericarditis. In cardiac hepatic fibrosis the firm, non-tender liver appears relatively small. *Ascites* is usually present, and the *cyanotic patients* are slightly and sometimes moderately *jaundiced*. Bromsulphalein retention is usually severe, and the urinary urobilinogen excretion is high; many of the other hepatic tests yield abnormal values.

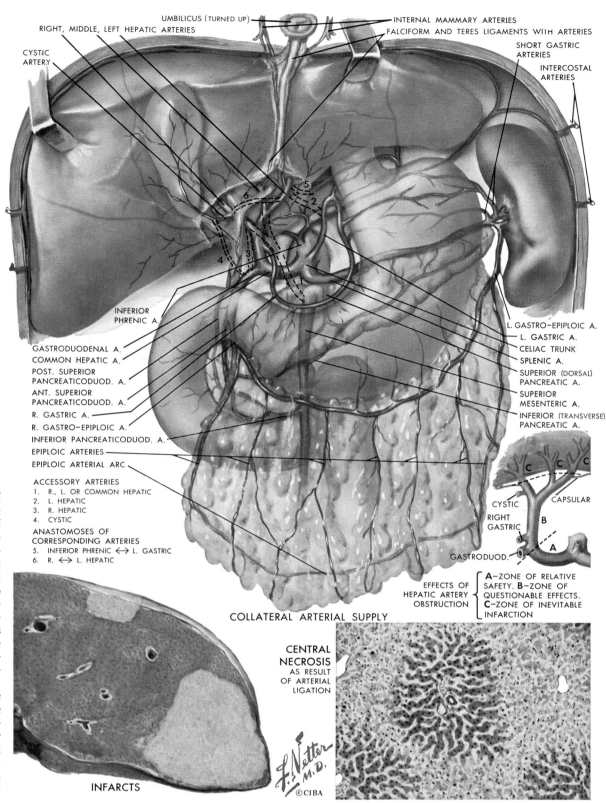

UMBILICUS (TURNED UP)

RIGHT, MIDDLE, LEFT HEPATIC ARTERIES

INTERNAL MAMMARY ARTERIES
FALCIFORM AND TERES LIGAMENTS WITH ARTERIES

CYSTIC ARTERY

SHORT GASTRIC ARTERIES

INTERCOSTAL ARTERIES

INFERIOR PHRENIC A.

GASTRODUODENAL A.
COMMON HEPATIC A.
POST. SUPERIOR PANCREATICODUOD. A.
ANT. SUPERIOR PANCREATICODUOD. A.
R. GASTRIC A.
R. GASTRO-EPIPLOIC A.
INFERIOR PANCREATICODUOD. A.
EPIPLOIC ARTERIES
EPIPLOIC ARTERIAL ARC

ACCESSORY ARTERIES
1. R., L. OR COMMON HEPATIC
2. L. HEPATIC
3. R. HEPATIC
4. CYSTIC
ANASTOMOSES OF CORRESPONDING ARTERIES
5. INFERIOR PHRENIC ⟷ L. GASTRIC
6. R. ⟷ L. HEPATIC

L. GASTRO-EPIPLOIC A.
L. GASTRIC A.
CELIAC TRUNK
SPLENIC A.
SUPERIOR (DORSAL) PANCREATIC A.
SUPERIOR MESENTERIC A.
INFERIOR (TRANSVERSE) PANCREATIC A.

COLLATERAL ARTERIAL SUPPLY

CYSTIC
RIGHT GASTRIC
GASTRODUOD.
CAPSULAR

EFFECTS OF HEPATIC ARTERY OBSTRUCTION

A—ZONE OF RELATIVE SAFETY. B—ZONE OF QUESTIONABLE EFFECTS. C—ZONE OF INEVITABLE INFARCTION

INFARCTS

CENTRAL NECROSIS AS RESULT OF ARTERIAL LIGATION

VASCULAR DISTURBANCES I
Arterial

In the dog dearterialization of the liver, with ligation of all potential collaterals, produces fatal hepatic necrosis, which can be prevented by administration of penicillin because the necroses are the result of an overwhelming spread of anaerobic bacilli normally found in the liver but kept in bound by arterial oxygen. In the human liver such anaerobic organisms are rare, but the oxygen need of the human liver seems apparently to be greater. Incidental or deliberate interference with hepatic arterial blood supply has been tolerated by some patients and not by others, depending upon the site of the interruption and the availability of collaterals able to provide sufficient oxygenated blood to the liver. Unfortunately, the existence and the efficiency of such collaterals cannot be portended in an individual case. An enormous variability has been established by anatomic studies on extensive material (Michels, see also pages 14, 15 and 16).

As a rule, *obstruction of the hepatic artery* between the celiac trunk (see page 14) and the origin of the gastroduodenal artery (*"Zone A"*) is innocuous. The result of an obstruction between the gastroduodenal artery and the hilus of the liver (*"Zone B"*) is unpredictable, but in such instances, quite often, a fatal *necrosis* of the *central* zone of the lobules follows, which is more sensitive to anoxemia than is the peripheral zone. Obstruction of the intrahepatic branches (*"Zone C"*) of the hepatic artery always causes anoxic necrosis (*infarcts*), since here sufficient collaterals do not exist, with the exception of the immediate subcapsular portion.

The *gastroduodenal artery* may bring blood from the splenic via the gastroepiploic, pancreatic and epiploic arteries and from the superior mesenteric via the pancreaticoduodenal arteries. The *right gastric artery* can carry blood shunted

from the *left gastric,* the short gastric (spleen) or the inferior phrenic arteries or through anastomoses with esophageal arteries. The *inferior phrenic artery* may send branches directly to the liver into the fossa for the ductus venosus and into the bare area; it may also shunt blood from the intercostal arteries and from the right superior phrenic artery (branch of internal mammary artery) by anastomoses through the diaphragm and through the intercostal muscles. *Arteries in the falciform and teres ligaments* anastomose with branches of the left and middle hepatic arteries and carry blood from the internal mammary arteries as well as from the abdominal arteries. The arteries for the common bile duct and the *cystic artery* may also supply areas of the liver as does the subcapsular plexus. Anomalous or *accessory arteries* may also provide important collateral arterial supply to the liver. The right or the common hepatic artery may arise

from the superior mesenteric artery (1), or accessory arteries may branch off from this vessel. The *left hepatic artery* or a corresponding accessory artery may take origin from the left gastric artery or vice versa (2). Furthermore, a replaced or *accessory right hepatic artery* may proceed from the gastroduodenal (3), or even from the retroduodenal artery, and an anomalous or *replaced cystic artery* (4) may do likewise. Abnormal anastomoses, such as between left gastric and left hepatic arteries (2), or between inferior phrenic and left hepatic (5), or between right and left hepatic arteries (6) may also become instrumental in supplying arterial blood to the liver.

It deserves emphasis that anemic infarcts of the liver may develop without demonstrable arterial obstruction and sometimes even without obstruction of any vessel, apparently owing to functional reduction of the blood flow.

VASCULAR DISTURBANCES II

Portal Vein

THROMBOSIS OF PORTAL VEIN

CAVERNOUS TRANSFORMATION OF PORTAL VEIN (ALSO INVOLVING SPLENIC, SUPERIOR AND INFERIOR MESENTERIC VEINS)

Sudden complete obstruction of the *portal vein* and its branches by a *thrombus* leads to a clinically dramatic picture dominated by hematemesis, melena with diarrhea, a rapidly developing ascites, abdominal pain, signs of peritonitis, then ileus and, finally, death in coma within the period of a few days. Jaundice is very uncommon. Oliguria and alimentary glycosuria can be observed very regularly. Acute portal vein thrombosis, more frequently seen in men than in women, eventuates after splenectomy or other procedures involving the portal system, in the course of polycythemia vera, in hepatic cirrhosis and, sometimes, without any apparent cause. The wall of the small intestine is thick, edematous and hemorrhagic; the purple-blue serosa is covered by recent fibrin flakes. The spleen is always enlarged, but the liver, in cases without the history of cirrhosis, presents only few uncharacteristic changes. The thrombosis starts either in the portal vein stem itself or extends into it from a splenic or mesenteric vein thrombus or from thrombi in intrahepatic branches of the portal vein. A variety of observations imply that the occlusion of the portal vein per se does not produce the catastrophic manifestations which are much the same when the superior mesenteric vein alone becomes occluded by a thrombus. It appears, therefore, that the clinical picture and course result from simultaneous blockade of portal, mesenteric and splenic veins.

Gradual interruption of the portal circulation is well tolerated in man or experimental animals, because collaterals (see page 18) prevent the fatal portal stasis. The thrombosis may lead either to a cordlike shrinkage of the portal vein or to spongy *cavernous transformation* which is caused by recanalization of the thrombus itself, permitting blood to reach the liver, though some investigators con-

sider this transformation a malformation or an angiomatous tumor. The liver, in slowly progressing portal vein obstruction, presents only little centrolobular fibrosis and, sometimes, atrophy. The clinical picture and the prognosis depend on the efficiency of drainage of the splanchnic area by the collaterals or recanalization. Accordingly, the signs of portal hypertension, with splenomegaly and its sequelae, leukopenia and anemia, vary in intensity. Episodes of aggravation manifest themselves by hematemesis, melena from esophageal varices, gastric hemorrhage and epigastric pain. Ascites is found in about two thirds of the cases, but its sudden onset is always a grave prognostic sign. In the absence of a primary hepatic disease (cirrhosis), jaundice is infrequent. The important causes of chronic portal vein thrombosis are inflammatory processes in the splanchnic system, such as appendicitis, cholelithiasis, pancre-

atitis or cholangitis, or compression of the vein by carcinoma and, also, traumatic lesions.

Considering the amount of blood which the portal vein carries to the liver (under basal conditions about 1.2 lit. per min.), the organ tolerates an interruption or decrease of portal blood supply surprisingly well, a fact explained by the compensatory influx from the hepatic artery. From experiments in which the portal vein blood is diverted into the general circulation (Eck's fistula), it is known that the function suffering from discontinued portal flow is mainly the liver's faculty for regeneration. Whether this inadequate regeneration results from a reduced blood volume or from the lack of material derived from the intestines has not been decided, but it has been observed that regeneration is only partly suppressed when portal and caval blood are transposed so that the liver receives a commensurate volume of nonportal blood.

VASCULAR DISTURBANCES III
Periarteritis Nodosa, Aneurysm

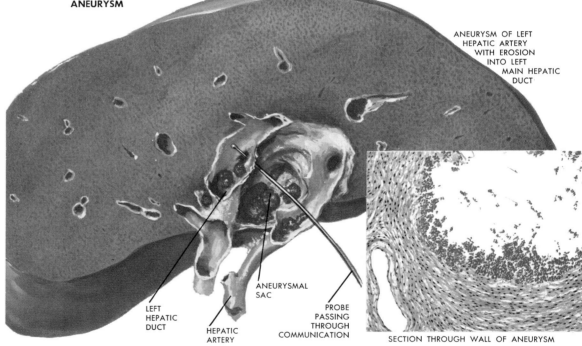

SUBCAPSULAR INFARCTS AND PITTED SCARS ON SURFACE OF LIVER

PERIARTERITIS NODOSA

SMALL BRANCH OF HEPATIC ARTERY: (FIBRINOID DEGENER- ATION OF MEDIA, INFILTRATION OF ADVENTITIA, RUPTURE OF INNER ELASTIC MEMBRANE, INTIMAL PROLIFERATION)

INVOLVEMENT OF LARGE HEPATIC ARTERY BRANCH: (ANEURYSM, THROMBOSIS)

ANEURYSM

ANEURYSM OF LEFT HEPATIC ARTERY WITH EROSION INTO LEFT MAIN HEPATIC DUCT

LEFT HEPATIC DUCT

HEPATIC ARTERY

ANEURYSMAL SAC

PROBE PASSING THROUGH COMMUNICATION

SECTION THROUGH WALL OF ANEURYSM

In *periarteritis* (polyarteritis, panarteritis) *nodosa* the hepatic arteries are involved in about 60 per cent of the cases. Participation of the arteries of the gallbladder is even more frequent. The typical alterations are found in smaller and larger branches (even grossly visible ones) of the hepatic arteries. Segmental *fibrinoid degeneration* of the media, which produces a smudgy appearance somewhat resembling hyalinization, is accompanied in the acute stage by conspicuous *infiltration* by polymorphonuclear leukocytes. Subsequently, *fibrotic proliferation* of the intima sets in, and in the adventitia a severe granulomatous infiltration develops. Finally, the structurally changed and weakened wall of smaller or larger vessels protrudes, forming aneurysms grossly apparent as nodules. The lumen of the arteries becomes obstructed by *thrombi* in organization, which lead to anemic *infarcts* of the liver. These infarcts may heal with *pitted scars,* and are found in approximately one third of the cases of periarteritis. In addition to the arterial lesions characteristic of periarteritis nodosa, the liver is packed with nonspecific inflammatory infiltrations, especially in the portal triads, and nonspecific hepatitis of the parenchyma is seen, apparently a reflection of the toxic manifestations of the disease. However, clinical features pertaining to the liver are not frequently observed in periarteritis nodosa, and hepatomegaly is found in only a small minority. In exceptional cases, the hepatic involvement, with or without jaundice, presents itself as the essential clinical manifestation.

In hypersensitivity angiitis (not illustrated) small hepatic arterial branches are also frequently involved, whereas the portal vein branches, in contrast to typical periarteritis, do not participate in this condition.

Aneurysms of the hepatic artery occur more often in the extrahepatic than in the intrahepatic branches but altogether are rare. They are usually small but may assume cherry size. Their etiology has not yet been clarified, though some develop in the course of a periarteritis or follow a trauma. Arteriosclerosis and various infections (not specifically syphilis) have been held responsible in some instances. The histologic picture usually does not reflect the etiology. The *wall of the aneurysm* is formed by fibrous connective tissue with few elastic fibers; the inner lining is covered by thrombotic material. Most aneurysms are detected as incidental findings at surgical exploration or autopsy. Hardly ever palpable, they are difficult to diagnose. Clinical signs or symptoms manifest themselves if the aneurysm perforates into either the abdominal cavity, the portal vein or the intestine. Most frequently, *perforation* takes place into the *biliary tract,* resulting in gastro-intestinal hemorrhage of puzzling etiology. The cardinal clinical features are: (1) jaundice of obstructive character, due to pressure by the aneurysm upon and blood clots within the bile duct, (2) melena and (3) abdominal pain, colicky in character, when rupture is imminent. The treatment is surgical, either by wiring of the aneurysm or by excision, or, if these are not possible, by ligation of the hepatic artery, as far away from the liver as possible (see page 107).

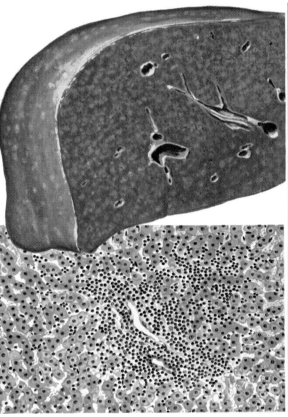

MARGIN OF INFILTRATED
AREA: HEPATOCELLULAR
DEGENERATION, VARIEGATED
INFILTRATE

MULTINUCLEAR
AND LOBULATED
GIANT CELLS
(STERNBERG—REED
CELLS), LYMPHOCYTES,
AND RETICULO-
ENDOTHELIAL CELLS
AND EOSINOPHILS
IN INFILTRATE

HODGKIN'S DISEASE, LEUKEMIA

LYMPHATIC———— LEUKEMIA————MYELOID

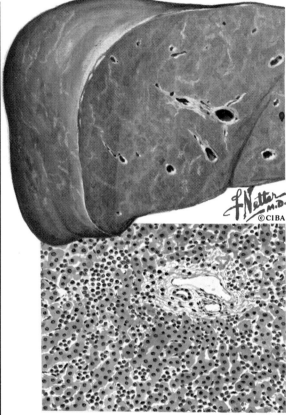

LYMPHOCYTIC INFILTRATION CHIEFLY IN PORTAL
TRIAD BUT ALSO DIFFUSELY IN LIVER

FOCAL AND DIFFUSE INFILTRATION OF
MYELOID CELLS

The liver is involved in almost all hematologic disorders. Anemia may produce such nonspecific effects as centrolobular fat accumulation. Hemolysis may cause increased iron as well as bile pigmentation of the Kupffer cells and bile plugs in the bile capillaries. Intrasinusoidal small nodules, dilating the sinusoids and sometimes resembling granulomas, result from the liver's participation in extramedullary hematopoiesis as it occurs after intoxications from radium, benzol, etc., or in so-called idiopathic myeloid metaplasia. Conspicuous and characteristic changes, sufficiently specific to permit confirmation of the diagnosis by liver biopsy, are seen in lymphomas and leukemias.

The granulomatous and sarcomatous varieties of *Hodgkin's disease* affect the liver in nearly 50 per cent of the cases. In the paragranulomatous form, which has a better prognosis, liver lesions are hardly ever seen. The hepatic alterations range from small, barely visible nodules to irregularly outlined nodules several centimeters in diameter. Usually graywhite and clearly visible through the capsule, the nodules become progressively yellow, mottled and fibrotic, owing to a varying degree of hemorrhage and necrosis. In exceptional cases the liver may be the only site of the disease, but liver, spleen and portal lymph nodes may in some instances ("portal Hodgkin's disease") be the foremost sites of the lesions. A pleomorphism, typical of Hodgkin's disease, manifests itself histologically. The nodules contain neutrophilic and eosinophilic granulocytes, plasma cells, proliferated reticulum cells and the multinucleated, multilobulated giant cells (Sternberg-Reed), the outstanding characteristic of the disease. Later, with a proliferation of the Kupffer cells in the lobular parenchyma and of mesenchymal cells in the portal triad, granulomas develop which coalesce and become necrotic and fibrotic in their center. Perilobular fibrosis and, eventually, cirrhosis emanate from a severe involvement of

the portal connective tissue, and hepatomegaly is a frequent finding in late stages. Jaundice appears in less than 10 per cent of the cases. It originates from degeneration of liver cells rather than from obstruction of intrahepatic or extrahepatic bile ducts.

Tumor nodules of lymphosarcoma are frequently seated in the liver. Varying in size, usually white and homogeneous in appearance, they resemble carcinoma metastases, but they consist, histologically, either of small cells of lymphocytic character or of reticulum cells.

In the *leukemias* the liver is only exceptionally spared. In the *lymphocytic* type, infiltrations are localized mainly in the portal triads, resulting in a white network exaggerating the lobular architecture of the only moderately enlarged liver, the color of which is not significantly changed. The bile ducts are not altered and jaundice, if present, is of parenchymal

origin and is not caused by obstruction.

In typical *myeloid leukemia* the liver is markedly enlarged (over 2000 gm.) and gray-red with gray streaks obscuring the lobular architecture. Myeloid elements from blast cells to segmented granulocytes spread throughout the parenchyma, accumulating focally within sinusoids, the tissue spaces and, to a certain degree, in the portal triads. The maturity of the preponderant cell type depends upon the stage of the disease but does not necessarily reflect the predominant type of cell in the peripheral blood. In monocytic leukemia the liver is usually far less enlarged. The leukemic infiltrations are mainly periportal.

Since the above-described features hold true only for typical cases, the microscopic appearance of liver biopsy specimens is not reliable in the differential diagnosis of leukemia. Moreover, liver biopsy in this condition may be dangerous.

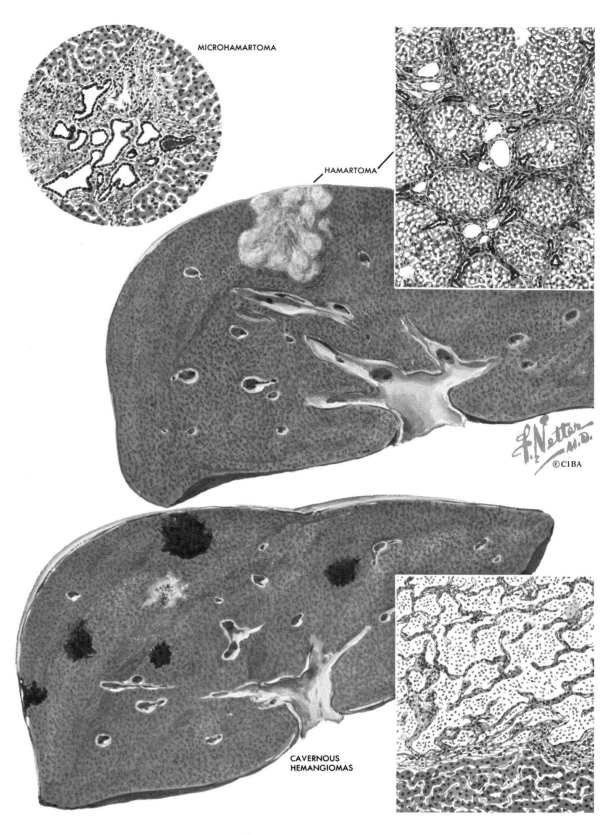

TUMORS I

Hamartomas, Hemangiomas

Hamartomas, resulting from a somehow disturbed correlation between the organizing influences exercised by mesenchyma and epithelium, are found not infrequently in the liver in the form of multiple nodules from pinpoint to child-head size. They exhibit some neoplastic qualities and contain normal structures in abnormal arrangements, which groups them between malformations and tumors. As hepatocellular adenomas consisting of liver cell plates without any bile duct structures are exceedingly rare, the hamartomas are commonly considered to be the benign tumors of the liver, though regenerative nodules in cirrhosis have occasionally been designated as adenomas, in spite of the lack of evidence that they represent neoplastic lesions. The smallest hamartomas, called *microhamartomas* or Meyenberg complexes, are irregular bile duct proliferations surrounded by proliferated connective tissue (see also page 60).

Solid, nodular hamartomas differ in color and architecture from the surrounding parenchyma. With no specific localization, their cut surface appears round if they are small, and irregularly lobulated if they are large. Bulging-outward subcapsular nodules may even become pedunculated. The irregularity of the structural elements (liver cell plates not arranged around a central vein, proliferated bile ducts and connective tissue) and the occasional predominance of one or the other component prompted a variety of descriptive names. They sometimes contain more fat and glycogen than the surrounding liver parenchyma, indicating their metabolic independence. Atrophy of the adjacent liver cells and collapse of the juxtapositional framework occur

when the nodules become large, and their histologic *resemblance to a cirrhotic process* has instigated the term "focal cirrhosis", as well as the assumption that such lesions result from focal disturbances of bile and blood flow. Also, the possibility has been entertained that these nodules may be a precursor of primary hepatic carcinomas in noncirrhotic livers. Otherwise these nodules attain clinical significance only if they become so large that they act as space-occupying lesions.

The *hemangiomas,* pathogenetically probably also belonging to the hamartomas, consist entirely of blood vessels, appear also in varying sizes and, most frequently, are multiple. Thrombosis develops in the dark-red and well-demarcated nodules as they become larger, and the scarred tissue subsequently accepts a brown pigmentation. Histologically, most of the hemangiomas present a *cavernous arrangement* of

blood spaces surrounded by connective tissue septa and, occasionally, capillary sprouts embedded in fibrotic tissue and even budding endothelial cells. Small hemangiomas may come into existence during pregnancy, possibly disappearing afterward, this being one of the features some hemangiomas have in common with the spider nevi of the skin (see page 70). Only exceptionally can they be palpated or act clinically as space-occupying lesions. Still rarer is a life-threatening hemorrhage from large hemangiomas. The also uncommon angiomatosis in children is a diffuse, indistinctly delimited capillary proliferation, which may be associated with similar lesions in other organs. They are probably independent malformations rather than metastases.

True hemangio-endothelial sarcoma of the liver can scarcely be differentiated from anaplastic carcinoma, but it is extremely rare.

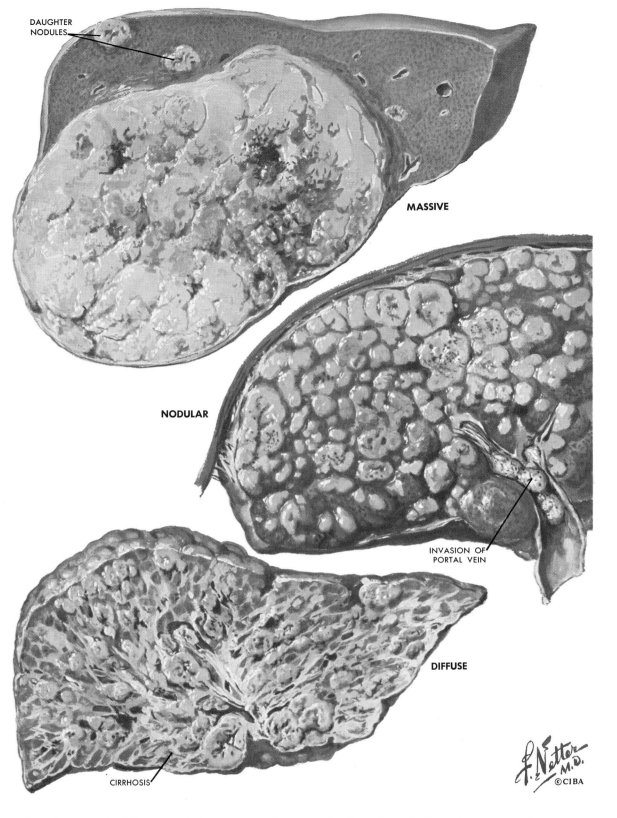

DAUGHTER NODULES

MASSIVE

NODULAR

INVASION OF PORTAL VEIN

DIFFUSE

CIRRHOSIS

TUMORS II

Primary Hepatic Carcinoma

Primary hepatic carcinoma, or hepatoma, consists of epithelial cells derived either from the hexagonal liver cells or from the cholangioles. Formerly, it was customary to differentiate hepatocellular from cholangiocellular carcinoma and group the latter together with bile duct carcinoma. However, it appears more advantageous to combine cholangiocellular carcinoma with hepatocellular carcinoma, because more extensive sampling frequently indicates in a single tumor both hepatocellular and cholangiocellular features with transitions. Moreover, it appears established that liver cells in embryologic development and regeneration are readily transformed into cholangioles. Finally, hepatocellular and cholangiocellular carcinoma have the same biologic characteristics, differentiating them from bile duct carcinoma (see page 114). They occur far more often in the male than in the female, and their incidence is much higher in cirrhotic than in normal livers, especially in far-advanced cirrhosis and in those caused by hemochromatosis. Tumor nodules in a cirrhotic liver are more frequently primary hepatic than metastatic carcinoma, whereas the incidence of metastases in the noncirrhotic liver far exceeds that of primary carcinoma. A high incidence of primary hepatic carcinoma has been observed in the tropical zones, not exclusively, but usually, in areas of malnutrition, apparently as a result of environmental rather than racial influences. In concurrence with this observation and hypothetical conclusion, intoxication and nutritional disturbances, besides other procedures, produce primary carcinoma in livers of experimental animals. Primary hepatic carcinoma, furthermore, represents the most frequent malignant tumor in the first 2 years of life, when it is apparently of congenital origin.

Grossly, primary hepatic carcinoma may appear as a *massive nodule* frequently occupying the right lobe and almost entirely replacing it. On its periphery it usually has a gray-white, slightly granular cut surface, whereas the central portion is mottled yellow and red because of hemorrhage and necrosis, sometimes resulting in central cavity formation. Smaller *daughter nodules,* with a more homogeneous white appearance, are irregularly distributed throughout the

liver, but extensive bile accumulation may sometimes confer on them a dark-green color.

In another, the *nodular form,* small nodules are distributed throughout the liver. They coalesce in advanced stages, are devoid of hepatic architecture and vary from small pinpoint to cherry size. Their color, differing from that of the surrounding tissue, is white to yellow to green, depending upon fatty infiltration and bile production, independent of that of the surrounding normal or cirrhotic parenchyma. The suspicion of a malignant degeneration in cirrhosis must be raised if some regenerative nodules vary from the surrounding tissue by a different yellow or green color as well as by necrosis.

Cirrhosis may accompany any form of hepatic carcinoma, but it is a predominant feature in the third, *diffuse form,* in which the irregular arrangement, color and distribution of tumor and regenerative nod-

ules throughout the liver give an unusual appearance to the cirrhotic organ.

The clinical manifestations of primary hepatic carcinoma, known for their diverse and confusing character, are determined by both the primary lesion and its dissemination, which does not depend on the gross type of lesion in the liver. The manifestations referable to the liver itself, frequently complicating those of cirrhosis, are fever, pain, tenderness and sudden increase in liver size and nodularity, as well as, supposedly, the appearance of a venous hum or bruit over the liver, caused by alteration of the circulation. Jaundice and ascites may develop or be accentuated, and the liver function may deteriorate. The laboratory findings are, as a rule, those of a cirrhosis. Of suggestive value is an increase of alkaline phosphatase out of proportion to jaundice, though that may rarely occur in cirrhosis also.

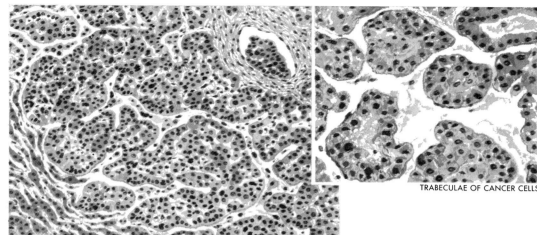

TRABECULAE OF CANCER CELLS

TRABECULAR FORM WITH FOCAL RESEMBLANCE TO LIVER
CELL PLATES AND TRANSITION INTO CHOLANGIOLES

Tumors III

Histology and Spread of Primary Carcinoma

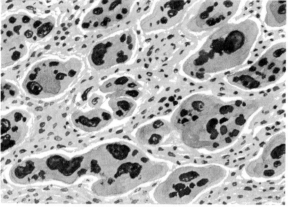

ELONGATED MULTINUCLEAR GIANT CELLS
IN PRIMARY LIVER CELL CARCINOMA

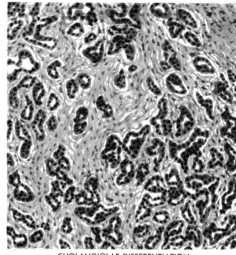

CHOLANGIOLAR DIFFERENTIATION

Histologically, primary hepatic carcinoma may present itself in a great variety of pictures. In the most common kind, the *trabecular form,* several-cell-thick plates or trabeculae are irregularly arranged. The cells more or less resemble the epithelium of normal hepatic plates. They have an abundant eosinophilic cytoplasm and large vesicular nuclei. In the center of the trabeculae a lumen is lined by a refractile membrane, thus resembling a bile canaliculus. The lumen frequently, though not always, exhibits bile plugs, especially if the cytoplasm contains bile-pigmented granules, and when it becomes widened a glandlike acinus forms. The trabeculae are surrounded by sinusoids lined by large endothelial cells that look like Kupffer cells, especially if they exhibit phagocytosis. The connective tissue stroma is very sparse. Sometimes the epithelial cells of the trabeculae are cuboidal and line up in a palisade form, thus imitating cholangioles, though as a rule their cytoplasm is as eosinophilic as that of the other cells.

The carcinoma cells form nodules, which appear to compress the surrounding noncarcinomatous liver cell plates. Moreover, even with small tumors, the neighboring portal vein branches are invaded. In some cases *cholangiolar features* are in the foreground, in that an extensive network of ductules is lined by a cuboidal epithelium with pale cytoplasm and the cells are placed upon a distinct basement membrane. The surrounding stroma is usually more extensive and fibrotic than in the trabecular form, and bile plugs in the lumina are absent. Less frequent are other histologic varieties. The carcinoma cells may reveal extensive fatty metamorphosis not present in the rest of the liver. Sometimes, large *elongated multinuclear giant cells* are present or even predominate the picture. In anaplastic types, sheets or clusters of undifferentiated epithelial cells are noted, and, in such instances, not only is the origin from the liver cell not recognized, but even a sarcomatous character is suggested. In other instances the tumor is exceedingly vascular or extensively necrotic. Occasionally, however, the cells of the primary hepatic carcinoma differ but little from those in hyperplastic and regenerative nodules, and, in such instances, especially if cirrho-

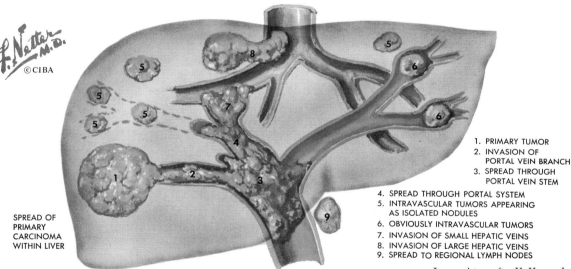

SPREAD OF
PRIMARY
CARCINOMA
WITHIN LIVER

1. PRIMARY TUMOR
2. INVASION OF PORTAL VEIN BRANCH
3. SPREAD THROUGH PORTAL VEIN STEM
4. SPREAD THROUGH PORTAL SYSTEM
5. INTRAVASCULAR TUMORS APPEARING AS ISOLATED NODULES
6. OBVIOUSLY INTRAVASCULAR TUMORS
7. INVASION OF SMALL HEPATIC VEINS
8. INVASION OF LARGE HEPATIC VEINS
9. SPREAD TO REGIONAL LYMPH NODES

Lower picture after H. Hamperl

sis is present, the recognition of the malignant character in biopsy specimens may become difficult. Besides focal anaplasia, invasion of small portal vein branches may be the only clue. The differentiation of primary hepatic carcinoma from metastases to the liver, for instance from hypernephroid carcinoma, presents also a common diagnostic problem. A *trabecular type* of carcinoma and structures which are transitional between hepatic plates and cholangioles are the only convincing indications of primary hepatic carcinoma. Invasion of small portal vein branches in metastatic hepatic carcinoma is relatively rare, but if the portal vein is involved the lesions are found only somewhat distant from the metastatic nodules.

The spread throughout the liver is characterized by *invasion of the portal vein branches.* On gross inspection this may sometimes be quite obvious, but frequently it is not and, then, what appears to be isolated nodules seen on the cut surface actually represents intravascular tumor growth apparent only on histologic study. *Invasion* of tributaries of the *hepatic vein* branches occurs late, and that of the main hepatic veins is usually a terminal event. The *regional lymph nodes* at the hilus of the liver become involved much sooner. Despite the early vascular invasion, metastases to distant organs develop late in many cases. They may be absent at autopsy in the presence of widespread carcinoma throughout the liver. Metastases resemble the primary tumor and may form bile or may contain fat. Besides the regional nodes, lungs and retroperitoneal lymph nodes are most commonly affected. However, any other organ may be the site, and bone metastases are not too infrequent. In some instances the metastatic lesion, for example in bone, lung or brain, may produce the first clinical manifestations.

TUMORS IV
Bile Duct Carcinoma of Liver

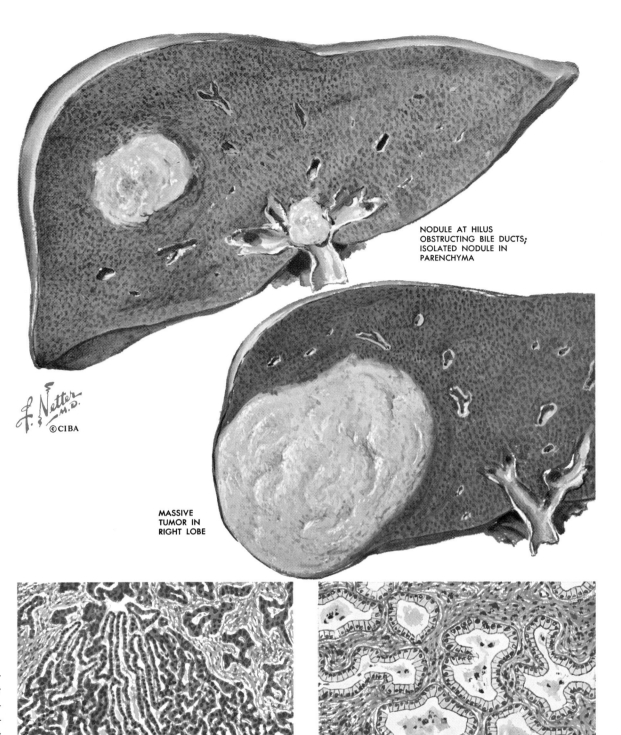

NODULE AT HILUS
OBSTRUCTING BILE DUCTS;
ISOLATED NODULE IN
PARENCHYMA

MASSIVE
TUMOR IN
RIGHT LOBE

PAPILLOMATOUS ARRANGEMENT

DESMOPLASTIC REACTION AROUND
MUCIN–PRODUCING NEOPLASTIC DUCTS

Previously, carcinomas of the intrahepatic bile ducts were considered fairly frequent, because primary hepatic carcinoma with predominant cholangiocellular features was included. The biologic characteristics of carcinomas of the intrahepatic bile ducts differ distinctly, however, from cholangiocellular carcinoma, which resembles biologically hepatocellular carcinoma. It appears, therefore, justified to consider carcinoma developing from the interlobular and larger bile ducts as an independent entity, which is considerably rarer than primary hepatic carcinoma. In biologic characteristics it resembles, rather, carcinoma of the extrahepatic bile ducts and even of the gallbladder. In contrast to primary hepatic carcinoma, it is equally as frequent in males as in females and has no higher incidence in the tropics and no strikingly frequent association with cirrhosis. Invasion of the portal vein is unusual. An association with hepatolithiasis has been claimed.

The tumor typically develops unicentrically and with marked participation of the connective tissue stroma in the form of a *desmoplastic reaction*. It is usually a gray-white, firm node, sharply demarcated from the surrounding parenchyma. The cut surface reveals a homogeneous periphery and mottling in the center, caused by regressive changes. The *tumor* may be found anywhere in the parenchyma and becomes *massive in the right lobe*. Sometimes it is a small, sharply defined *nodule* obstructing one of the main bile ducts. Metastases within the liver in the form of small nodules are rare. Histologically, it is usually a rather mature adenocarcinoma which sometimes assumes distinct *papillomatous arrangements,* also apparent in the rare vascular invasions. Alveoli lined by columnar epithelium, frequently mucus-producing, are seen, and the basement membrane is usually markedly thickened and merges with the fibrotic stroma. Differentiation from metastatic adenocarcinomas, *e.g.*, of the extrahepatic biliary tract, of the gastro-intestinal tract, of the ovary or of a bronchus, is difficult. The cells are the more elongated the closer the tumor is to the hilus of the liver. Metastases develop relatively early in regional lymph nodes and lungs, but survival time is not shorter than in primary hepatic carcinoma. The clinical manifestations are not much different from those of primary hepatic carcinoma. Hepatomegaly, with abdominal swelling and pain, weight loss and ascites, is encountered. Jaundice is as frequent and, generally, as severe as in primary hepatic carcinoma. The tumors located in the large intrahepatic ducts near the hilus exhibit manifestations intermediate between those of primary hepatic carcinoma and carcinoma of the extrahepatic biliary ducts.

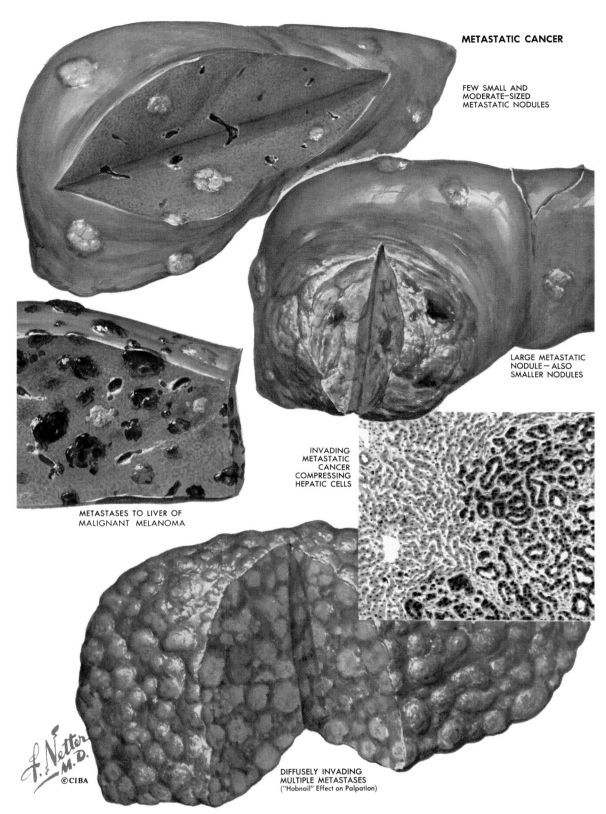

METASTATIC CANCER

FEW SMALL AND
MODERATE—SIZED
METASTATIC NODULES

LARGE METASTATIC
NODULE — ALSO
SMALLER NODULES

INVADING
METASTATIC
CANCER
COMPRESSING
HEPATIC CELLS

METASTASES TO LIVER OF
MALIGNANT MELANOMA

DIFFUSELY INVADING
MULTIPLE METASTASES
("Hobnail" Effect on Palpation)

Tumors V

Secondary, Metastatic

In view of the relative rarity of primary hepatic carcinoma (see page 112) and of the frequency of liver metastases from carcinoma elsewhere, the discovery of liver nodules should suggest secondary carcinoma, unless the nodules are felt in a cirrhotic liver, in which metastases are rare. The liver is the site of predilection for metastases of carcinomas in the stomach, lower part of the esophagus, the colon, pancreas and gallbladder. It is slightly less frequently involved in carcinoma of the breast and lung, still less in carcinoma of the ovary and kidney and relatively rarely in carcinoma of the oral cavity and of the uterus. Melanoblastomas and neuroblastomas metastasize very frequently; sarcomas less frequently to the liver than carcinomas.

Secondary carcinoma of the liver varies greatly from only a few *small white nodules* to *large nodes* of child-head size. The smaller nodes bulge over the surface, when they assume pea size. When they exceed cherry size, a central depression of the elevated portion, "umbilication", develops from necrosis of the tumor center. Neighboring nodules may coalesce and compress the surrounding liver tissue. *Multiple closely spaced nodules* may produce the palpatory feelings of a coarse granular surface. Since different parts of the liver are fairly equally involved, liver biopsy becomes a valuable tool, though negative biopsy findings do not exclude metastatic carcinoma in view of the fact that blind punctures of not distinctly nodular livers yield not more than 30 per cent correct results. A single large secondary carcinoma is found in only one lobe of the liver in exceptional cases.

Because of vascular inadequacies, all larger nodes exhibit central regressive changes reflected in the yellow color of necrosis, the red mottling of hemorrhage and, occasionally, white fibrosis. The marginal zone is of mucoid character in mucus-producing carcinoma; it is granular in squamous cell carcinoma and of grayish appearance in small-cellular carcinoma (*e.g.,* bronchogenic) or sarcomas. Extensive hemorrhagic destruction is particularly noted in choriocarcinomas, hemangio-endothelial sarcoma and also hypernephroid carcinoma. Black color of all or most nodules reflects melanin formation by *malignant melanoma*. Larger tumors interfere with portal vein flow, so as to produce wedge-shaped, hyperemic zones (Zahn infarct).

The microscopic appearance indicates only occasionally the primary site but may narrow the choice, depending upon the presence of malignant glandular structures with or without mucus production, of medullary carcinoma, of squamous cell epithelium, or of various sarcomatous features. Hypernephroid carcinoma frequently resembles primary hepatic carcinoma.

Clinical manifestations entail hepatic enlargement, hepatic pain, abdominal distention with local discomfort, fever, anemia and malaise. When cachexia becomes predominant, ascites and jaundice are frequent. Jaundice, if present, is caused by obstruction of the extrahepatic biliary ducts by the original tumor or by metastases or by toxic hepatocellular injury. Though almost all functional tests may yield abnormal results, only Bromsulphalein® retention and moderate elevation of serum alkaline phosphatase activity are seen, in the absence of jaundice, with sufficient frequency to be of diagnostic significance. Recently, portal venography (see page 54), peritoneoscopy and administration of radio-active serum albumin have been applied in the search for secondary hepatic carcinoma. The characteristic symptoms following metastases of carcinoid tumors are discussed elsewhere (see CIBA COLLECTION, Vol. 3/II, pages 165 and 169).

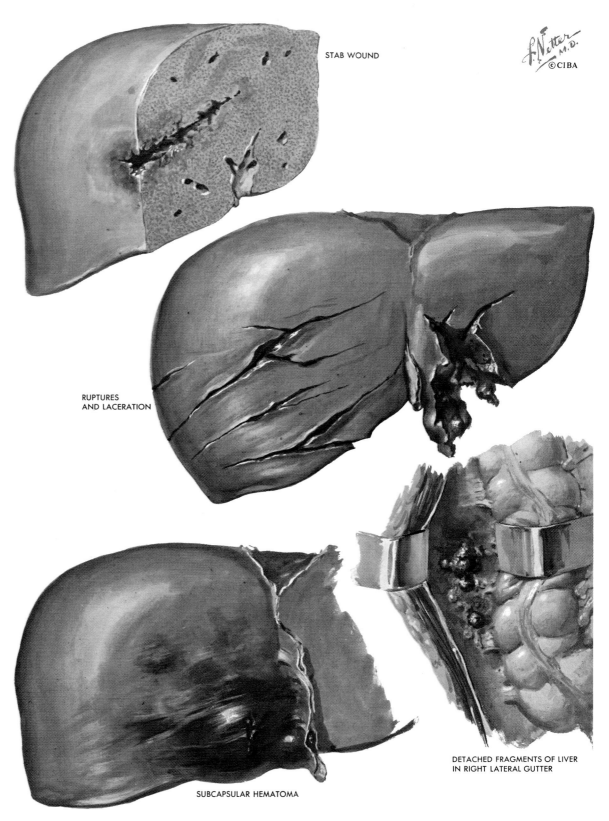

STAB WOUND

RUPTURES AND LACERATION

DETACHED FRAGMENTS OF LIVER IN RIGHT LATERAL GUTTER

SUBCAPSULAR HEMATOMA

Trauma

Because of its size, location and fixation, the liver is frequently subjected to trauma which may be either penetrating or blunt. Next to the brain, it is the organ most commonly hit by blunt violence. Bullet or *stab wounds* penetrate to various depths and produce an intrahepatic canal with a ragged wall and a lumen filled with blood. In more than a fourth of penetrating thoraco-abdominal wounds, the liver is injured. The blunt injuries lead to *ruptures* or *lacerations* varying in size and sometimes in number. They are most commonly the result of automobile accidents or of falls. The lacerations may be inflicted by broken ribs, or the organ may be crushed by impact of the thoracic cage and the resisting spine. Internal stress or counter-coup effects during a blunt injury may set up subcapsular or central lacerations or only a subcapsular hematoma in case of mild impacts.

Rupture, as the consequence of blunt injury, is facilitated if the liver has become more friable or when the capsular tension has increased owing to abscesses, cysts, infectious diseases such as malaria, or to hepatitis and fatty liver. In contrast to the spleen, so-called spontaneous ruptures of a mildly damaged organ are rare. It has been claimed that postprandial hyperemia may predispose to rupture of the liver, and rupture during pregnancy has also been reported.

Except for temporary slight peritoneal irritations from blood oozing into the peritoneal cavity, *subcapsular hematomas* and small lacerations or ruptures usually heal with few clinical manifestations and leave a pigmented or white subcapsular scar. If the hematoma becomes infected, intrahepatic or subphrenic or subhepatic abscesses may complicate the clinical course. Hepatic cysts also may develop, and so do biliary fistulae after laceration of a small bile duct. Rarer complications are portal vein thrombosis or arterial aneurysms. From a forensic point of view, it is interesting that acute hepatitis, including the fulminant variety, and even cirrhosis have been connected causally with a preceding trauma. Centrolobular necrosis may be a consequence of shock. A definite association of trauma with other diffuse hepatic diseases is, however, rather difficult to prove.

Severe lacerations or rupture of the liver have a high mortality rate, more so in military than in civilian practice. Death early after the trauma is caused by hepatic hemorrhage, which is severe and does not stop readily for several reasons: the walls of the valveless hepatic veins are thin, the liver is extremely vascular, the bile admixed to the blood interferes with its clotting and the diaphragm massages the liver. Later, the effects of biliary peritonitis, following laceration of bile ducts or shock or infections, become important causes of death. The so-called hepatorenal syndrome (see page 76), a frequent complication, has been associated with a toxic effect from tissue breakdown products from the liver. However, traumatized, necrotic and even completely separated hepatic tissue has not been convincingly proved to exert a toxic effect different from that of other organs, although it must be admitted that interruption of the blood flow to parts of the liver leads to rapid ischemic necrosis, which, if the patient survives, may be surrounded by a demarcation zone with fibroplasia. On the other hand, completely *detached liver tissue* pieces are well tolerated within the peritoneal cavity and may be even organically attached in the lateral gutter.

The laboratory manifestations of hepatic trauma are surprisingly insignificant. Jaundice is rare and occurs mainly if the gallbladder and bile ducts are ruptured. In later stages it may be the result of liver abscesses or traumatic cholangitis. Foreign bodies, such as bullets, in the liver may eventually migrate into the biliary ducts and produce obstructive jaundice.

The liver is relatively insensitive to external ionizing radiation, and even the effects of internal radiation by radio-active substances accumulating in the liver (*e.g.*, P^{32}) are not severe.

LIVER DISEASE IN PREGNANCY

In normal pregnancy the liver is neither more nor less affected than is any other organ, such as the heart. Hepatic activity and structure are only negligibly influenced, as long as no complications arise. However, if these do appear, serious diagnostic problems may present themselves, sometimes involving the question of interruption of the pregnancy. In *eclampsia* (see CIBA COLLECTION, Vol. 2, pages 235 to 238) hepatic alterations are in the foreground of autopsy findings in at least one half of the cases. Irregularly shaped hemorrhagic areas are distributed over the enlarged, otherwise pale liver, predominantly in the subcapsular portion of the right lobe. *Fibrin* thrombi are found, microscopically, to obstruct the sinusoids of the peripheral zones, and eosinophilic degeneration of the liver cells (see page 62) develops in the adjacent parenchyma. In more advanced stages the liver cells disappear and are replaced by large hemorrhagic zones, in which fibrin has precipitated. These impressive lesions probably develop only shortly before death and, therefore, have little, if any, effect upon the clinical picture, the severity of which is independent of the grade of liver injury. Jaundice, if present, is mild and mainly terminal. The fibrin thrombi, supposedly resulting from an excessive release of thromboplastic material from the placenta, disturb the sinusoidal circulation and probably are the initiating cause of the hepatic lesions. The increased consumption of the circulating fibrinogen causes a coagulation defect which aggravates the hemorrhages. Except for abnormalities of the flocculation tests, due to the serum protein changes in eclampsia, the hepatic tests are not altered significantly. Biopsy specimens obtained from nonfatal cases of eclampsia have revealed similar but more moderate lesions than those encountered at autopsy. The uric acid level of the serum is increased in eclampsia, and this is possibly a reflection of hepatic injury. The liver is not altered in preeclampsia.

Nutritional deficiency as a consequence of *pernicious vomiting* (hyperemesis gravidarum) may eventually produce a fatty liver (see page 78).

In rare instances, shortly before or after delivery, hepatic failure may develop. This is usually fatal and is associated with renal insufficiency. At autopsy, the livers are moderately enlarged and yellow. Histologically, fat has accumulated in liver cells, predominantly in the centrolobular zone. The fat droplets are very small and do not displace the nucleus. Little hepatocellular necrosis or inflammation is noted. Such cases are designated *fatty liver of pregnancy*. (Previously, this was called "toxic hepatitis" because of an

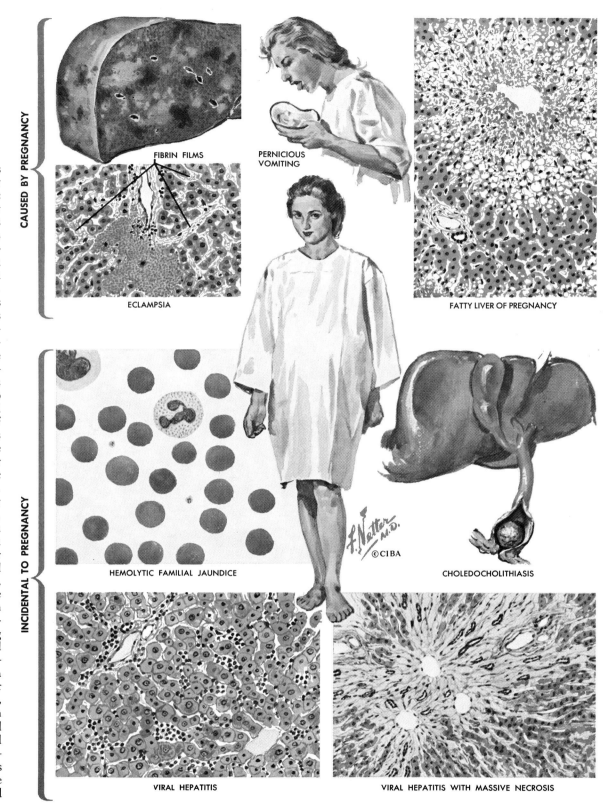

CAUSED BY PREGNANCY

FIBRIN FILMS

PERNICIOUS VOMITING

ECLAMPSIA

FATTY LIVER OF PREGNANCY

INCIDENTAL TO PREGNANCY

HEMOLYTIC FAMILIAL JAUNDICE

CHOLEDOCHOLITHIASIS

VIRAL HEPATITIS

VIRAL HEPATITIS WITH MASSIVE NECROSIS

assumed relation to chloroform anesthesia during delivery.) At present, the etiology of this dangerous complication of pregnancy is unknown, although disturbance of protein metabolism has been postulated.

Under certain conditions jaundice may complicate pregnancy. Since pregnancy predisposes to the formation of *gallbladder stones* (see page 124), signs and symptoms of acute biliary obstruction may appear when a stone passes into the bile ducts. *Familial hemolytic jaundice* (see page 48) may be aggravated during pregnancy. As a sheer coincidence, a gravid woman may acquire *viral hepatitis*. This is usually self-limited, producing only the spotty necrotic type of hepatitis, so that most observers have concluded that its prognosis is not significantly worse than in nonpregnant women. The situation becomes more serious if the woman suffers from nausea or hyperemesis; nevertheless, interruption of the pregnancy

is usually not indicated, and no evidence of damage to the offspring has been disclosed. The hepatitis virus, as a rule, is transmitted not through the placenta from the jaundiced mother with viral hepatitis but, rather, from apparently healthy carriers (see pages 118 and 119).

That pregnancy has an unfavorable influence on the already poor prognosis of the rare *massive necrotic* or fulminant form of viral hepatitis can be readily understood (see page 94).

During each pregnancy, particularly in the last trimester, some women develop jaundice with histologic and laboratory manifestations of intrahepatic cholestasis (see page 97). Clinically, itching may be the most disturbing symptom of this condition, which is designated as "recurrent jaundice of pregnancy". Its etiology is entirely unknown, and no permanent sequelae have been reported.

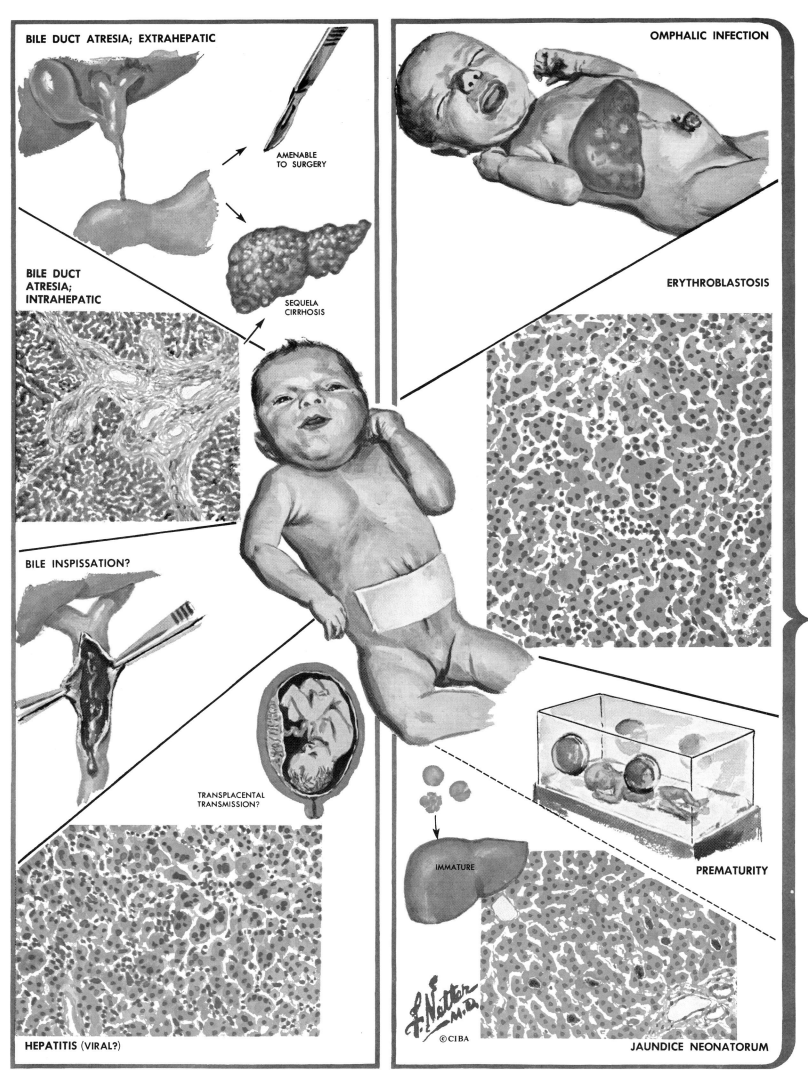

BILE DUCT ATRESIA; EXTRAHEPATIC

AMENABLE
TO SURGERY

SEQUELA
CIRRHOSIS

BILE DUCT
ATRESIA;
INTRAHEPATIC

BILE INSPISSATION?

TRANSPLACENTAL
TRANSMISSION?

HEPATITIS (VIRAL?)

OMPHALIC INFECTION

ERYTHROBLASTOSIS

IMMATURE

PREMATURITY

JAUNDICE NEONATORUM

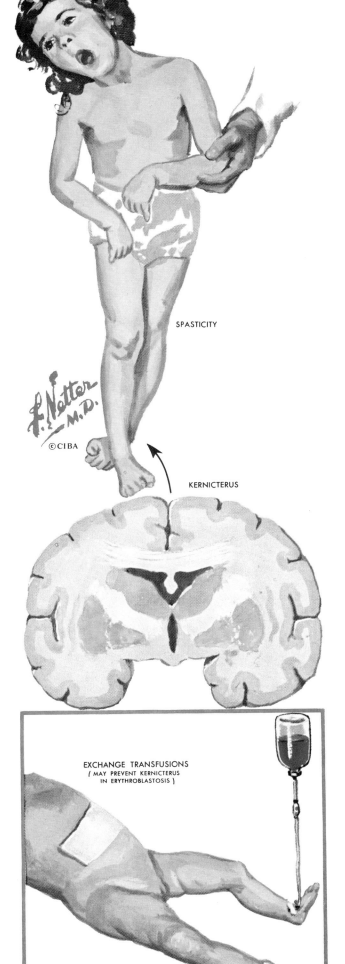

SPASTICITY

KERNICTERUS

EXCHANGE TRANSFUSIONS
(MAY PREVENT KERNICTERUS
IN ERYTHROBLASTOSIS)

JAUNDICE IN THE NEONATAL PERIOD

Jaundice in the first days of life is a common phenomenon. The incidence of 60 to 80 per cent, according to some statistics, gave rise to the impression that "icterus neonatorum" is a more or less physiologic event. This attitude, however, has changed essentially because of scientific advances made in the fields of bilirubin transport and blood-group incompatibilities and in the diagnosis of hemolytic syndromes of newborns. The mechanisms that cause jaundice in infancy are, in principle, the same as those responsible for jaundice in the adult (see pages 48 and 49), although "jaundice with impairment of bile flow" is far less frequent in infants than "jaundice without impairment of bile flow", in contrast to adults.

Congenital atresia or extensive hypoplasia of the *extrahepatic bile ducts* belongs to the group with impairment of bile flow. This results from persistence of the early temporary stage of solid duct anlagen prior to the development of hollow channels. The fibrous cord, which may be found in place of the bile duct or parts thereof, contains no epithelium and may be so fine as to suggest complete aplasia. Obliteration occurs mostly in the lower parts of what should have developed into the common bile duct. Such a situation, if recognized early, may be *amenable to surgery,* because the patent proximal parts of the duct system are dilated, owing to the enormous bile stasis, and may permit the surgical construction of an anastomosis with the intestine. Atresia of the cystic duct alone, which is extremely rare, produces no clinical signs and is no cause for hydrohepatosis, a regular finding in the congenital atresia of the common bile duct. The gallbladder may be absent without disturbance of the well-being of the child. Cystic changes of the bile ducts (choledochal cysts) are developmental anomalies producing intermittent obstructive jaundice, usually more frequent in later childhood than in the neonatal period. With atresia of the distal part of the biliary tract, the gallbladder is enlarged when patency of the proximal duct system permits communication with the liver. Jaundice with duct atresia appears within days or up to a few weeks after birth and deepens rapidly, but, in contrast to experience in older individuals, infants tolerate complete extrahepatic obstruction better and for a considerably longer time. The structural changes in the liver (see page 84) develop much more slowly. Gradually, the effects of bile stasis upon the parenchyma become conspicuous. Eventually, some regenerative nodules and portahepatic venous anastomoses may be found, depending upon how long the patient lives. The prognosis of these chil-

dren with biliary atresia is extremely poor in the majority of instances if surgical reconstruction is impossible. The children live about 1 year, although some are reported to have survived several years. The patients succumb to hepatic failure and the complications of cirrhosis such as bleeding esophageal varices. Owing to disturbed intestinal absorption, they become malnourished and have osteoporosis. The diagnosis rests upon the appearance of jaundice within the first month of life in a child who is born nonicteric but exhibits progressive deepening of skin pigmentation, acholic and sometimes fatty feces, the exclusion of hemolytic or nonhemolytic types of jaundice with only indirect-reacting bilirubin in the blood and the exclusion of hepatitis, which is sometimes possible by liver biopsy. The diagnosis is substantiated by laparotomy and operative cholangiography. The laboratory procedures used in adults for the differential diagnosis of jaundice are of very little help for the diagnosis of obstruction by atresia, as well as for any other type of neonatal jaundice, presumably because many hepatic functions in this period are still immature.

Intrahepatic bile duct atresia, which may or may not be associated with that of the extrahepatic ducts, is a less common occurrence. Jaundice in such instances develops as with extrahepatic atresia, and a similar type of cirrhosis evolves. Liver biopsy may lead to the diagnosis. Hyperlipemia is common, and the children survive longer than with the nonoperable extrahepatic anomaly.

Bile inspissation in extrahepatic bile ducts has been observed in infants either during surgical intervention or at autopsy. Previously, this phenomenon was thought to be the result of a congenital defect in the formation of normal bile ("inspissated bile syndrome"). A thick mucous bile supposedly caused obstruction and, therewith, jaundice. Now the appearance of such inspissated bile is assumed to be the result of cholestasis secondary to neonatal hepatitis or to hemolytic disease, rather than the cause of jaundice. Diffuse hepatitis in the neonatal period is usually characterized by the presence of epithelial giant cells with many nuclei, the cytoplasm of which frequently contains pigment granules and sometimes iron. In addition, moderate inflammatory interstitial reaction and hematopoietic foci are noted and cholestasis is prominent, both histologically and by laboratory tests. Jaundice appears a few days to a few weeks after birth and may persist for months, with high levels of promptreacting bilirubin and considerable bilirubin excretion in the urine. If jaundice appears at birth or shortly thereafter, serum bilirubin is unconjugated because of immaturity of the conjugating system, but by 1 week of age the bilirubin becomes conjugated. In some instances the disease subsides within a few weeks, and the children proceed to develop normally. In other instances the process progresses to *cirrhosis*. Ascites and evidence of portal hypertension appear, and the child eventually succumbs from either hepatic failure or bleeding esophageal varices. The etiology of the lesion is not established. Some

(*Continued on page 120*)

(*Continued from page 119*)

assume that it is a defect in the development of bile canaliculi, others prefer to incriminate a specific metabolic disorder of unknown character, while still another group considers this to be a *neonatal type of viral hepatitis*. This is assumed to be the result of a *transplacental transmission* of virus B (see page 93) from the mother, who is the carrier of the virus rather than a patient with homologous serum hepatitis. The disease has been observed to occur in siblings from apparently healthy mothers. Mothers with obvious viral hepatitis in pregnancy usually have healthy children. The diagnosis of *giant cell hepatitis* (see page 95) is not easy because differentiation from biliary atresia may be particularly difficult. Biopsy seems to be more promising than biochemical investigations. However, giant cells may occur in atresias, and giant cell hepatitis may complicate atresia. Laparotomy is frequently the only means of establishing the diagnosis.

Giant cell formation is noted also in neonatal hepatitis of established etiology such as in cytomegalic inclusion disease as well as in syphilitic hepatitis in which, however, interstitial fibrosis is common (see page 99). The latter disease was previously a rather frequent causative factor of neonatal jaundice, but it has now almost completely disappeared. Other rare types of neonatal hepatitis with extensive necrosis result from toxoplasmosis or herpes simplex infection. Galactosemia (see page 86) occasionally produces jaundice in the neonatal period. The recognition by biochemical tests is important to avoid progression of the disease. A purulent hepatitis with jaundice resulting from an *omphalic infection* is, in this age of chemotherapy, also becoming a rare event.

These conditions of jaundice with impairment of bile flow in which the conjugated or prompt-reacting bilirubin is significantly elevated differ greatly from those without impairment of bile flow in which only unconjugated bilirubin is found. This type of jaundice is more frequent in the early neonatal period.

Mild jaundice is seen, although not regularly, in many newborn infants. This *icterus neonatorum*, if it appears after the second and not later than the fifth day after delivery, and if it remains mild, disappearing within about 10 days, perhaps still merits the designation of "physiologic jaundice". The jaundice may be so faint as to be scarcely visible on the diffusely reddish skin of a newborn.

The main reason for this condition is *immaturity* of the *liver cells,* which are less efficient than normal in taking up unconjugated bilirubin and particularly in conjugating it (see page 180). Inhibition of these functions by maternal steroids is also possible, and a limited functional capacity to excrete conjugated bilirubin into the bile canaliculi cannot be excluded. The newborn must dispose of its fetal hemoglobin, and this process could be related to increased bilirubin production. Recent studies, however, indicate that hemoglobin F disappears slowly and that the hemoglobin F concentration in some children may, at 1 year of age, be the same as at birth. The bilirubin content of serum in normal full-term newborns averages 2 mg. per 100 ml., rising on the second and third days to 7 mg. per 100 ml. and then dropping rapidly. No constant relationship between the appearance and degree of jaundice and bilirubinemia has been established. This type of neonatal jaundice is not present at birth (in contrast to other types) and is not associated with splenomegaly or anemia.

The incidence of jaundice in *prematurely delivered children* is higher than in those born at term. The tendency of the icterus to become more severe is also greater. The immaturity of liver functions is only one facet of the unpreparedness of these infants for extra-uterine life. Jaundice in prematurity appears earlier and persists longer. It is more likely to cause kernicterus (see below). Severe bile stasis has been observed in the livers of such prematurely born children, as have many hematopoietic foci, but no hepatocellular degeneration has been seen except, occasionally, in the left hepatic lobe, which quite suddenly loses its supply of oxygenated blood after interruption of the placental circulation (see page 3). Permanent immaturity of the bilirubin conjugating system occurs in the Crigler-Najjar syndrome.

The most significant type of neonatal jaundice is associated with the hemolytic disease of the newborn, *erythroblastosis fetalis*. The cause of this condition — known long before its pathogenesis was clarified less than 25 years ago — in most cases is iso-immunization of the mother with Rh negative blood by the erythrocytes of an Rh positive fetus who inherited this factor from the paternal side. Fetal erythrocytes passing through the placenta elicit the formation of maternal antibodies, which, in turn, enter the fetus and destroy the red blood cells carrying the Rh blood group. Such a situation cannot always be recognized before the child is born, but determination of the blood groups of the parents and the immune titer of the mother permits anticipation, with a high percentage of probability, of the delivery of an erythroblastotic child. The bilirubin content, the degree of hemolysis and the blood groups in samples of blood from the umbilical vein at the time of delivery will establish the diagnosis beyond doubt. The condition may run a fatal course in utero (see CIBA COLLECTION, Vol. 2, page 233). Children of Rh negative mothers and Rh positive fathers do not always suffer from erythroblastosis. If the father's Rh positive trait happens to be heterozygous, the child may possess the mother's Rh negative characteristic and, thus, will not be exposed to hemolysis of its red blood cells. During a first pregnancy, in most instances, the mother does not produce enough antibodies to damage the fetus, provided she has not received Rh positive blood prior to her first pregnancy. Rh factor incompatibility is the predominant cause of hemolytic disease, but ABO blood-group incompatibilities have recently been noted to produce hemolytic disease in many instances. A child with hemolytic disease, if born alive without hydrops, is usually anemic, has an enlarged liver and spleen and is icteric shortly after birth or develops an icterus within the first 24 hours. This latter fact differentiates jaundice of erythroblastosis from other types of neonatal jaundice, with the exception of sepsis and some of the causes mentioned before. The serum bilirubin in these children exceeds 10 mg. per 100 ml. at birth or shortly thereafter and it is indirect-reacting. The urinary urobilinogen is high. Anemia and splenomegaly progress rapidly, and the children may die within the first 10 days, particularly if not treated. Only children whose jaundice is very mild and whose blood contains little, if any, demonstrable antibodies survive without treatment. The signs of hemolysis may disappear within several weeks. In all other cases exchange blood transfusions are indicated and are lifesaving if started early enough and repeated regularly whenever the level of the indirect-reacting bilirubin, determined at frequent inter-

vals, rises. A simple transfusion of blood with the correct blood groups is sufficient in the mild form of erythroblastosis, but *exchange transfusion* must be used soon after delivery in all infants who are born icteric. Such management has saved the lives of many erythroblastic children and has protected them from the development of fatal or sometimes seriously crippling cerebral aftereffects.

Children exhibiting jaundice in the neonatal period are apt to become afflicted with a permanent brain injury, but not all the types of jaundice discussed above are equally liable to cause this frightful complication. Icterus resulting from those conditions shown on the left side of Plate 56 (see page 118) is seldom, if ever, found to have produced brain lesions, probably because of some unknown characteristics of the accumulated bilirubin. In children surviving neonatal viral hepatitis or extrahepatic biliary atresia, the chances of damage in the basal ganglia of the brain are very low, whereas they exist in exceptional cases of jaundice following an omphalic infection or of so-called "physiologic jaundice" and particularly in the jaundice of immaturity. However, the predominant offender in this respect is doubtless the icterus attending all cases of erythroblastosis, with icterus of the premature child being second in frequency.

This brain affliction was named *kernicterus* by German pathologists in the latter part of the nineteenth century. The fact that erythroblastosis is by far the most frequent cause of kernicterus has been established only in more recent times. The nuclei ("Kerne") in the basal ganglia are severely pigmented and degenerated. Sometimes, the cells of Ammon's horn and, rarely, some parts of the cortex are similarly colored and in the process of disintegration. The mechanism of these cellular changes in the central nervous system and the reason for the predilection for the basal ganglion cannot be explained. Abnormal permeability of the barrier between blood and spinal fluid in early postnatal life and damage produced by anoxia, predisposing to the deposition of bile pigment, have been cited as instrumental factors. The relationship between the degree of bilirubinemia and the postmortem finding of kernicterus has been studied, with the result that the level of the indirect-reacting or nonconjugated and therefore lipid soluble bilirubin seems to have a bearing on the cerebral changes, but other factors, such as immaturity, anoxia, anemia and duration of jaundice, also have an influence. Kernicterus develops rarely when the level of the indirect-reacting bilirubin is kept below 20 mg. per cent by means of exchange transfusions.

The brain complications of neonatal jaundice may become clinically recognizable within the first week of life. The infants become drowsy, vomit and refuse to take food. Irregularities in respiration, instability of circulation, muscular twitchings, spasticity and opisthotonus may be observed. A certain shrillness of the baby's cry has been considered a characteristic sign, as has the appearance of an abnormal Moro reflex. The majority of children who develop kernicterus die within a short time, usually from 1 to 10 days after showing the first signs. The minority — perhaps 25 to 30 per cent — survive, with permanent brain damage. Their mental development may be retarded, and their ability to walk is delayed or is never acquired. Speech difficulties or inadequate muscle coordination occur, and the children remain physically helpless. Kernicterus is not the only cause of cerebral palsy but is one of the most frequent.

Section XVIII

DISEASES OF THE GALLBLADDER AND BILE DUCTS

by

FRANK H. NETTER, M.D.

in collaboration with

DONALD D. KOZOLL, M.D.
Plates 9-12, 16

HANS POPPER, M.D.
Plates 1-8, 13-15

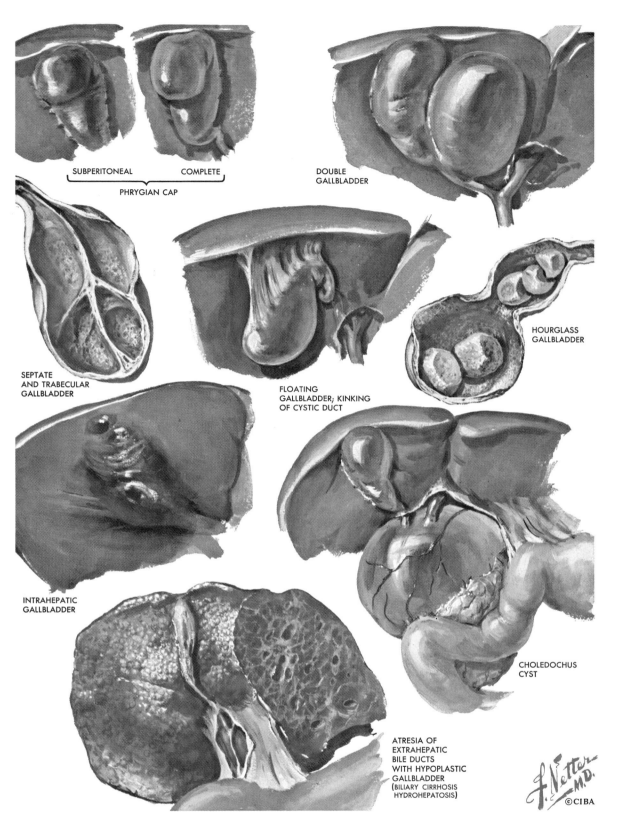

SUBPERITONEAL   COMPLETE

PHRYGIAN CAP

DOUBLE GALLBLADDER

SEPTATE AND TRABECULAR GALLBLADDER

FLOATING GALLBLADDER; KINKING OF CYSTIC DUCT

HOURGLASS GALLBLADDER

INTRAHEPATIC GALLBLADDER

CHOLEDOCHUS CYST

ATRESIA OF EXTRAHEPATIC BILE DUCTS WITH HYPOPLASTIC GALLBLADDER (BILIARY CIRRHOSIS HYDROHEPATOSIS)

CONGENITAL ANOMALIES

Congenital anomalies of the gallbladder are fairly common. Most of them have little clinical significance and are encountered as incidental findings on roentgenologic examination, surgical exploration or at autopsy. But any aberration from the norm is a potential cause for stasis in the biliary system, which, in turn, may facilitate gallstone formation. Discrepancies in the development of the gallbladder in relation to the liver bed result in a kinking or folding of the gallbladder fundus, a phenomenon described as Phrygian or stocking cap (see page 22). The serosa may cover the indentation or may participate in it. In the former case the *Phrygian cap* is *subperitoneal* and nonconspicuous on exploration; in the latter it is *"complete"*. Even the complete form does not, as a rule, cause clinical symptoms, in contrast to previously held beliefs. Complete *duplication of the gallbladder*, with or without two independent cystic ducts, is merely an anatomic curiosity. Functionally more important are internal subdivisions of the gallbladder, which may take the shape of *septa* or *trabeculae* traversing the lumen. They produce diverticula or pockets in which biliary material may stagnate, favoring development of gallstones. The gallbladder may be *bilobular* or of *hourglass shape*, or may embody congenital diverticula, which cannot always be differentiated from pseudodiverticula resulting from inflammatory processes, but all diverticula predispose to gallbladder perforation. The gallbladder may be located on the left side, in the middle or in a transverse position. In some instances the gallbladder is entirely surrounded by serosa and connected with the liver by a mesentery. This *"floating" gallbladder* predisposes not only to kinking of the cystic duct but also to twists of its mesentery and to hemorrhagic infarction of the gallbladder. In other instances the gall-

bladder is entirely surrounded by hepatic tissue; this *intrahepatic gallbladder*, though emptying poorly, has little clinical significance. The gallbladder may be hypoplastic or, in some rare instances, may be entirely missing, remindful of the normal state of various animals, such as the rat or the horse.

These abnormalities of the gallbladder are frequently associated with abnormalities of the bile duct system which are of greater clinical significance. Congenital hypoplasia, valve formation or angulation of the common bile duct may be the cause of a protracted partial obstruction, which leads to dilatation of a part or of the whole *ductus choledochus,* and subsequently to a partially retroperitoneal *cyst.* The lesion may be responsible for intermittent jaundice associated with colicky pain and may sometimes be palpated as a subhepatic tumor, displacing the stomach to the left and the duodenum downward.

More frequent is *atresia* or *hypoplasia* of the extrahepatic bile ducts, which results in congenital biliary obstruction if located in the common or in the hepatic duct (see also pages 118 and 119). The atretic portion is usually represented by a fine strand which may be hardly recognizable on either autopsy or operation. If the obstruction is located only in the cystic duct, congenital hydrops of the gallbladder develops. In contrast, hypoplasia or atresia of the common and hepatic ducts produces dilatation of the intrahepatic ductal system and hydrohepatosis with subsequent biliary cirrhosis, manifestations which develop more slowly than in complete obstruction in the adult. A few instances of survival for several years have been reported. The majority of children thus afflicted, however, succumb within the first 8 months of life. Surgical correction of the atresia is possible only in a minority of instances.

CHOLELITHIASIS I

Stone Formation

Of the three specific constituents of the bile, bile acids, bile pigment and cholesterol, the second is poorly soluble and the last is almost insoluble in water. These substances are kept in aqueous solutions with the help of the emulsifying bile acids and fatty acids. Consequently, the bile is supersaturated with these compounds. In such a labile solution, precipitation readily sets in. Nevertheless, the physicochemical processes in gallstone formation are still but poorly understood. The causes of cholelithiasis, however, appear well established. One is an increased concentration of one of the crucial substances in the bile. Although the constitution of the bile does not necessarily reflect that of the blood serum, elevation of either serum cholesterol or bilirubin may result in their increase in the bile, with their subsequent precipitation giving rise to stone formation. Hypercholesteremia is a metabolic phenomenon occurring in *obesity, diabetes* and *pregnancy,* and also in hypothyroidism and nephrosis, the first three of which have been said to appear relatively often in the histories of patients with gallstones. *Cholesterol stones* are firm and yellow-gray and have a granular surface, while on the cut surface glistening cholesterol crystals produce a radiating pattern. Even if these stones become large, they are radiolucent. But the incidence of pure cholesterol stones is relatively small, and in the greater percentage of cases some bilirubin or calcium-bilirubin is admixed. Only in the hemolytic or overproduction type of jaundice (see page 48) does hyperchromic bile exist, reflecting the hyperbilirubinemia. Any prolonged hemolytic anemia, sicklemia and thalassemia are associated with *bilirubin stones* in the gallbladder, which are brown, small and irregularly shaped. Pure bilirubin stones are soft and are found mostly in the bile ducts as irregular masses or as casts of the ducts. Calcium salts, precipitated in the gallbladder, usually contribute to the composition of these stones and make them radiopaque.

Biliary stasis, brought on by spasms of the sphincter of Oddi, by faulty bladder emptying, by organic obstruction, by a stone in the cystic duct or by some malformations of the gallbladder (see page 123), is another instigating factor for stone formation. The *stagnation of bile in the gallbladder* leads to high concentrations of cholesterol and bile pigment because of excessive *absorption of water*

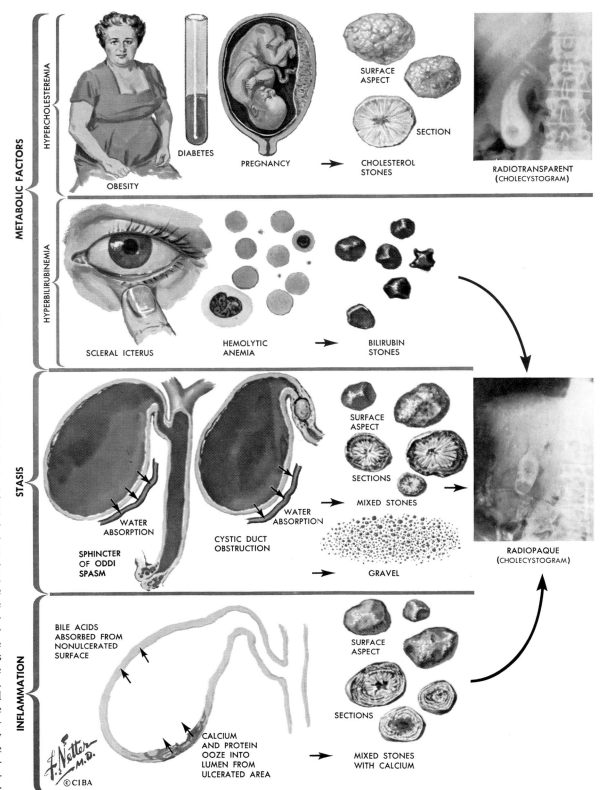

and easily soluble salts. Precipitation under these circumstances leads to *mixed stones,* the most common type. They are of variable size, faceted if multiple, brown, and especially dark on their edges. On the cut surface, as a rule, a dark center is noted, surrounded by a glistening radiating layer which is frequently followed by a harder, more homogeneous shell. Sufficient calcium is generally contained in these bilirubin-cholesterol stones to make them opaque on X-ray examination. Sometimes the stones are small enough to appear as *gravel*.

The third important cause of stone formation is *inflammation of the gallbladder* or bile ducts, sometimes brought about by bacterial infection (see page 128). It results in an altered constitution of the bile. The inflamed gallbladder mucosa permits, in contrast to normal mucosa, absorption of bile acids with subsequent reduction of the solubility of cholesterol.

Moreover, from the inflamed mucosa, especially if ulcerated, *calcium salts diffuse* into the bile in excessive amounts to add calcium bilirubinate to the developing cholesterol stone. In addition, protein oozes from the surface to provide a nucleus for stones. The mixed stones in inflammation are rich in calcium and harder than other stones; they appear whiter and are distinctly radiopaque.

Pure cholesterol or bilirubin stones are rare. The vast majority of stones are mixed, quite independently of their pathogenesis, the mixture reflecting simultaneous or consecutive presence of several of the factors listed. Stones, originally pure, soon receive admixtures of other constituents. For this reason the *cut surface* of most stones shows a variegated picture, reflecting different layers of precipitation. Sometimes gallstones seem to form very rapidly, possibly in a matter of weeks.

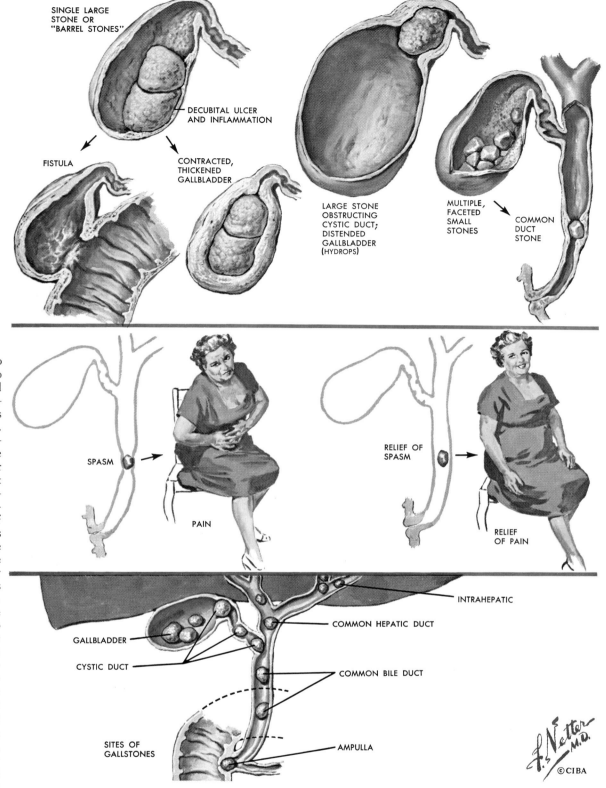

SINGLE LARGE STONE OR "BARREL STONES"

DECUBITAL ULCER AND INFLAMMATION

FISTULA

CONTRACTED, THICKENED GALLBLADDER

LARGE STONE OBSTRUCTING CYSTIC DUCT; DISTENDED GALLBLADDER (HYDROPS)

MULTIPLE, FACETED SMALL STONES

COMMON DUCT STONE

SPASM

PAIN

RELIEF OF SPASM

RELIEF OF PAIN

INTRAHEPATIC

COMMON HEPATIC DUCT

GALLBLADDER

CYSTIC DUCT

COMMON BILE DUCT

SITES OF GALLSTONES

AMPULLA

Cholelithiasis II

Clinical Aspects

Cholelithiasis has been reported to occur in about 10 per cent (according to other observers up to 25 per cent) of all persons examined at necropsy. The incidence rises with age. Occasionally, stones have been encountered even in children. Though the consequences and complications of cholelithiasis, once existent, are the same in both sexes, gallstones are far more frequent in women, to a great extent owing to the contribution of pregnancy, which predisposes to hypercholesteremia and disturbances in emptying of the gallbladder. The enlarged uterus may be another contributive factor. The incidence of gallstones is greater in the white man than in either the Negro or Oriental race. Evidence that the diet has a significant influence is not convincing. The majority of stones are found in the gallbladder itself, but calculi are also detected in the extra- and intrahepatic bile ducts and even in abscess cavities within the liver. Many stones in the gallbladder fail to elicit clinical manifestations and are "silent", while ductal stones produce jaundice in at least 65 per cent of the cases. Ductal concretions are either muddy material or gravel or calculi, which may form directly in the ducts, e.g., after cholecystectomy. But, in general, choledocholithiasis results from movement of stones from the gallbladder into the duct (see page 126).

The consequences of gallstone formation depend upon the location and configuration of the stones. The main complications which transform "silent" cholelithiasis into cholelithiasis disease are inflammation, obstruction and spasm. Large stones, either single or two in contact with each other, produce a mechanical pressure effect upon the underlying mucosa, which develops a decubital ulcer and becomes inflamed. Eventually, large mixed stones lead to chronic cholecystitis and a contracted gallbladder (see also page 130), with fibrous thickening of its wall. If the chronically inflamed calculous gallbladder is adherent to a neighboring portion of the intestine, an internal biliary fistula may develop. Through

it a large stone can escape directly into the intestine (see page 132) and may produce gallstone ileus. Occasionally, middle-sized stones, up to 2 cm. in maximal diameter, obstruct the cystic duct (see page 127) by being located in the neck of the gallbladder. Whereas otherwise the large stones characteristically cause cholecystitis, multiple small stones tend to produce biliary obstruction. The number of small stones can be high, and figures over 100 are not unusual. These small stones are the ones which may pass into the cystic duct and through it into the common duct, where they may be the cause of biliary obstruction and jaundice (see page 82). In most instances the obstruction soon becomes incomplete or the stone is expelled into the duodenum. Nevertheless, in view of the usual multiplicity of the small stones producing biliary obstruction, the chances that another stone may reach the extrahepatic biliary ducts from the gall-

bladder are high. Therefore, once calculous obstruction has produced jaundice, surgical intervention is indicated to prevent a repetition of the episode. It deserves emphasis, however, that in one third of choledocholithiasis cases, jaundice does not appear.

The colicky pain characteristic of the cholelithiasis attack is the result of a spasm primarily of the sphincter of Oddi and to a lesser degree of the sparse ductal muscles. This spasm can be elicited by irritation of the gallbladder mucosa or by impaction of a stone in the cystic or the common duct. The extremely painful attack with the well known "doubling up" of the patient subsides if the spasm is relieved spontaneously or as a result of therapy. However, this does not necessarily indicate subsidence of the mucosal inflammation or relief of the obstruction. Temporarily silent stones may thus be responsible for a variety of significant or even dangerous pathologic conditions.

CHOLELITHIASIS III

Pathologic Features, Choledocholithiasis

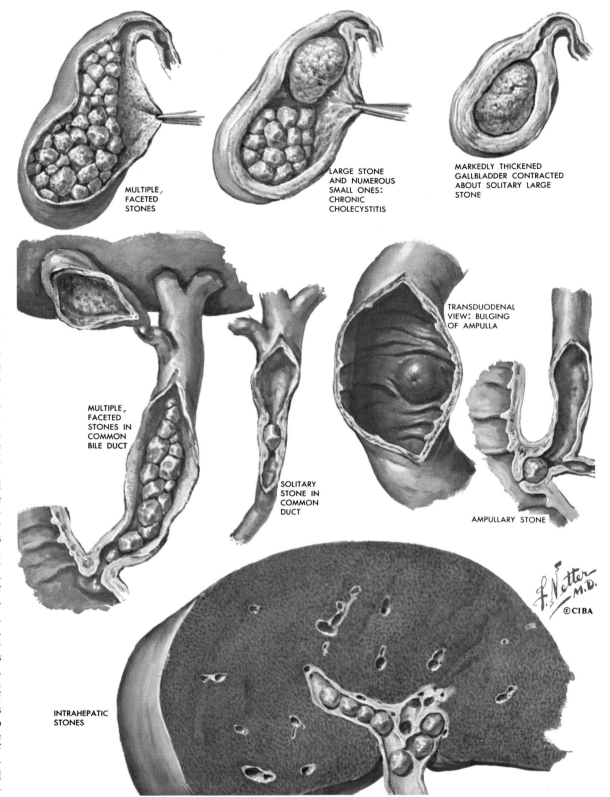

MULTIPLE, FACETED STONES

LARGE STONE AND NUMEROUS SMALL ONES: CHRONIC CHOLECYSTITIS

MARKEDLY THICKENED GALLBLADDER CONTRACTED ABOUT SOLITARY LARGE STONE

MULTIPLE, FACETED STONES IN COMMON BILE DUCT

SOLITARY STONE IN COMMON DUCT

TRANSDUODENAL VIEW: BULGING OF AMPULLA

AMPULLARY STONE

INTRAHEPATIC STONES

The pathologic manifestations of cholelithiasis vary greatly. One or two small stones may exist in an otherwise normal gallbladder, or the entire lumen may be filled with numerous *small, faceted stones* up to 1 cm. in diameter, with little bile between them. Together with the small stones, one *large*, frequently *barrel-shaped, stone* may be noted, while in other cases only one solitary stone between 1 and 5 cm. in diameter is found. In the presence of a large stone, the color and consistency of the bile are usually altered. The accompanying inflammation and *cystic duct obstruction* lead to admixture of mucus and reduction of the bile pigment content. Cholelithiasis may or may not be associated with reactive changes of the *gallbladder,* such as *enlargement,* recognized by palpation, or inflammatory changes of the wall, reflected in tenderness. As a result of accumulation of stones within the lumen and especially of cystic duct obstruction (see page 127), the gallbladder may enlarge moderately, and sometimes tremendously. Enlargement and inflammation stimulate fibrous adhesions with surrounding structures, (duodenum, hepatic flexure of the colon and omentum). The inflammation, if chronic, may vary from a slight fibrous thickening of all layers of the wall to a diffuse scarring with destruction of the epithelial lining and transformation of the wall into thick white scar tissue contracting the lumen. Although acute and chronic cholecystitis can cause stone formation (see pages 128 and 130), the stones may also produce acute cholecystitis, varying from a diffuse inflammatory reaction of the mucosa to circumscribed decubital ulcers, or empyema, gangrene, perforation, pericholecystic abscesses and, exceptionally, also internal and external biliary fistulae.

Gallstones in the bile ducts lead regularly to clinical and pathologic consequences and thus have a graver prognosis than bladder stones. Calculous obstruction of the cystic duct results in elimination of the function of the gallbladder (storage, concentration and pressure-regulating activities) and produces hydrops or empyema (see page 127). Stones in the common duct (choledocholithiasis) are more often *solitary* than multiple. Stones, having passed through

the cystic duct into the common bile duct, may enlarge in the latter and cause acute or chronic inflammation of its wall, with fibrosis and scarring and decubital ulcers, though, in the presence of stones, the choledochal wall is less frequently involved than the gallbladder wall. As a result of the cholangitis, the bile may be discolored and sometimes purulent or, in other instances, may become mucous and white and may lack bilirubin. With an ascending infection, bacterial hepatitis and cholangitic abscesses (see page 92) or, after a long period of cholestasis, a biliary cirrhosis (see page 84) may develop. As a rule, the duct is cylindrically dilated, depending upon the degree and duration of the obstruction. The wall is thickened above the obstruction and only rarely thinner than normal. Internal biliary fistulae may result from decubital ulcers, leading most frequently into the duodenum (sometimes from the distal portion of

the common duct into the stomach and, exceptionally, into the colon, see page 132). The cholangitis may heal with a stricture (see page 133). In some instances a single stone is impacted in the terminal portion of the common duct, where the tapering off of the duct prevents its expulsion into the duodenum. These *ampullary stones* sometimes bulge forward at the papilla of Vater. They almost always produce jaundice. A pancreatic disease occasionally develops, either because of reflux from bile into the pancreas or because of the pancreatic obstruction which the ampullary stone may produce, according to the anatomic situation at the ampulla (see pages 26 and 27). *Stones in the hepatic ducts* outside or within the liver are less frequent and, as a rule, are associated with biliary calculi elsewhere. They also predispose to inflammation and ascending bacterial infection as well as to jaundice.

HYDROPS AND EMPYEMA OF GALLBLADDER

A gallstone *obstructing the cystic duct* usually elicits a biliary colic, which subsides sometimes with persistent impaction of the stone either in the cystic duct or in the neck of the gallbladder. If the resulting obstruction remains complete for prolonged periods, the gallbladder gradually enlarges, its wall becoming thin and stretched. In earlier stages the lining *epithelium secretes* an increased amount of mucus. If the obstruction persists, the lining *epithelium atrophies* and *flattens,* the folds disappear and the wall becomes transformed into a fibrous scar tissue, with gradual disappearance of the muscle bundles and obliteration of the distinction between the layers of the gallbladder. Eventually, a very large (up to 20 cm. long) fibrous sac results, in the wall of which calcium may be deposited. As a result of the obstruction in the absence of infection, bile pigment and bile acids are gradually reabsorbed. Since new bile cannot enter and the mucous secretion cannot leave the gallbladder, the enlarged organ becomes filled with a white and mucous fluid; this prompted the designation of *hydrops* or mucocele. Moreover, calcium salts are released into the lumen and produce either a fine precipitation (milk of calcium bile) or calcium stones. The calcium salts may also form a shell around the stone impacted at the orifice of the cystic duct, thereby enlarging it. Exceptionally, if the stone exercises a ball-valve effect, the gallbladder empties temporarily and refills gradually. Clinically, the enlarged gallbladder is readily palpable. If the mass is large enough, it may be confused with mesenteric, pancreatic and, in rare instances, ovarian cysts. Colicky pain or some abdominal discomfort is occasionally present, primarily because the elimination of the gallbladder function interferes with the regulation of the biliary pressure. For the diagnosis it is characteristic that the mass is not tender and that jaundice and leukocytosis are absent.

The anatomic and clinical pictures radically change if prolonged cystic duct obstruction is complicated by bacterial infection. Whether the cystic duct is occluded by a stone or, more frequently, by scarring and sometimes also by acute

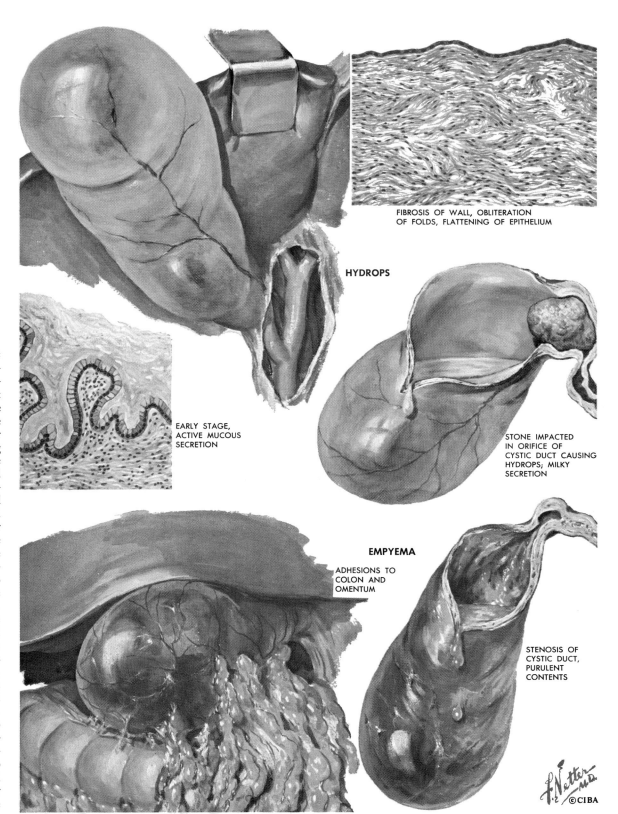

FIBROSIS OF WALL, OBLITERATION OF FOLDS, FLATTENING OF EPITHELIUM

HYDROPS

EARLY STAGE, ACTIVE MUCOUS SECRETION

STONE IMPACTED IN ORIFICE OF CYSTIC DUCT CAUSING HYDROPS; MILKY SECRETION

EMPYEMA

ADHESIONS TO COLON AND OMENTUM

STENOSIS OF CYSTIC DUCT, PURULENT CONTENTS

inflammatory edema, bacteria may invade the gallbladder, and its content then becomes purulent. In the development of such *empyema,* bacteria more frequently reach the bladder by the hematogenous than by the ascending route. The changes depend on the balance between obstruction and bacterial infection, as well as upon the time at which the obstructed bladder is infected. If the infection is strongly virulent and occurs relatively early, the gallbladder is small and contracted and its wall is very thick. If the infection either is mild or eventuates after prolonged obstruction in the presence of a fully developed hydrops, the wall of the large gallbladder is relatively thin, despite the edema in its layers. Under these circumstances the surface is very hyperemic and is not seldom covered by fibrinous exudate which produces *adhesions with* the surrounding organs, especially the *colon.* The omentum often covers the bladder and

must be removed to make the organ visible and accessible surgically. The mucosal surface is dark red and, where ulcerated, is covered by fibrinous purulent or hemorrhagic exudate. The lumen contains brown-to-yellow creamy pus. Diagnostic aids for this condition are diffuse and colicky pain and an extremely tender, somewhat balloting mass palpable through a rigid abdominal wall. Fever and leukocytosis, however, are not necessarily present. Empyema of the gallbladder is sometimes associated with choledocholithiasis or carcinomatous obstruction of the ducts, and then deep jaundice is the rule. But even without involvement of the common or hepatic duct, some icterus may be present because of toxic liver damage.

In the absence of infection and without accumulation of pus cells, empyema of the gallbladder may be simulated by the accumulation of emulsified small cholesterol droplets in the mucus-containing bile.

INTERRELATION OF GALLBLADDER DISEASES

Cholecystitis is associated in about 85 per cent of instances with cholelithiasis. In the majority of instances the stones cause the inflammation by abrasion of, or by their pressure effect upon, the mucosa. The latter mechanism operates mainly in the presence of a large stone and an eventually contracted gallbladder and results in decubital ulcers. However, in a significant number of instances, stones are the consequence rather than the cause of cholecystitis, and in these the etiology of the latter is problematical. Formerly, it was assumed that *bacteria* from the intestine pass from the portal blood circulation into the bile and settle in the gallbladder during stagnation and concentration of bile. This concept is valid for bacterial infections through the systemic arterial route. Salmonella infections, including typhoid fever, predispose to cholecystitis, and carriers are known to lodge bacteria in their gallbladders and to excrete them with the feces. The public hazard created by these carriers is eliminated by cholecystectomy. But the belief that bacteria are the exclusive cause of cholecystitis has recently been found at fault. In the human being, bacterial invasion of the portal vein blood from the intestine is very rare, and cultures of surgical specimens of chronic and even severe, acute noncalculous cholecystitis have proved to be sterile. Because pancreatic enzymes have been demonstrated in the bile, the digesting effect of *pancreatic juice* upon the gallbladder was considered a cause of nonbacterial cholecystitis. However, noncalculous cholecystitis has also been found when the anatomic conditions for reflux of pancreatic juice into the gallbladder do not exist (see page 24). Therefore, one is presently far more inclined to consider the irritating effect of normal or abnormal *biliary constituents* absorbed by the gallbladder mucosa as a causative principle of cholecystitis. *Lipids, especially cholesterol,* have been found within the wall as a result of abnormal absorption. Cholesterol itself, when deposited, may be irritating and, more so, when joined by other bile constituents, especially bile acids. In line with this thinking stands the histologic appearance in acute or chronic cholecystitis, which, as a rule, is rather that of a foreign-body granulation tissue with foam cells around lipids than that of a pyogenic reaction. Bile stasis, brought on either by sphincter of Oddi spasm or calculous obstruction, may sustain all three essential pathogenic principles — chemical factors, bacterial invasion or pancre-

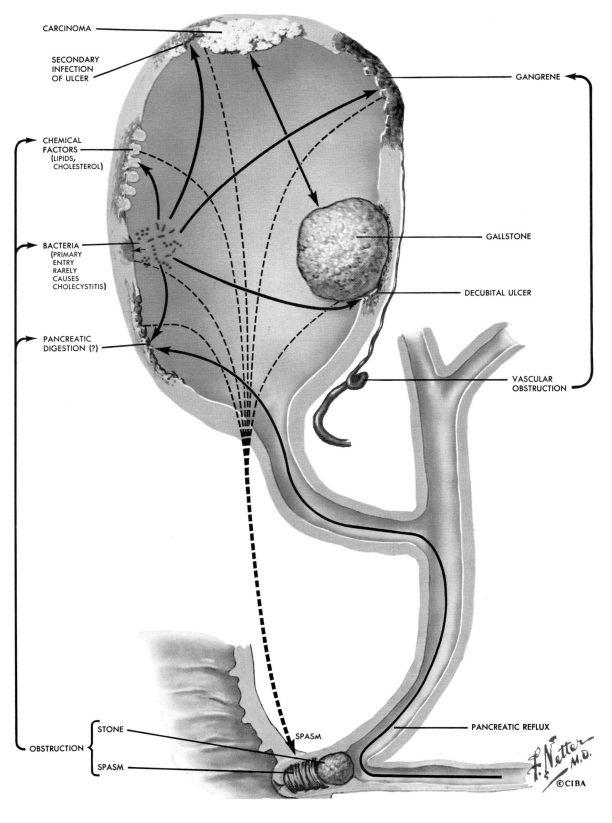

atic digestion — of cholecystitis. Another cause of cholecystitis may be interference with circulation, resulting in gangrene (see page 130). Even if bacteria are not the eliciting cause of cholecystitis, they readily complicate inflammation or even tumor growth instigated by other causes. This explains why usually, especially in chronic cholecystitis, histologic and bacteriologic evidence of infection, especially with E. coli and streptococci, is found.

Cholecystitis, from whatever cause, may in turn not only induce stone formation but may also lead to sphincter of Oddi spasm, with the resulting colicky pain. It also may represent the link between cholelithiasis and carcinoma of the gallbladder. Clinical and pathologic observations have indicated that gallstones are found in at least 65 and up to 85 per cent of cases with carcinoma of the gallbladder. The causative relation between these two disorders is not

established. It is possible that the chronic irritation associated with cancer may lead to stone formation. On the other hand, cases are on record in which gallstones were visualized radiologically years before carcinoma of the gallbladder developed, and many feel that the calculi may act as a chronic irritant which may stimulate carcinoma development. Although the incidence for such happening is low, it is one additional indication for the surgical removal of even "silent" gallstones.

It appears, thus, that any one of the three major disorders of the gallbladder — cholelithiasis, cholecystitis, and muscular spasm (dyskinesia) — may stimulate the development of the two others. All three, therefore, form eventually a common complex from a clinical and pathologic viewpoint, into which, fortunately in only rare instances, carcinoma of the gallbladder also enters.

CHOLECYSTITIS I
Acute and Chronic

A mild structural alteration of the gallbladder, though considered by some an inflammation or at least a precursor of inflammation, is *cholesterolosis,* or *cholesterosis.* From the reddish-green mucosa many irregular-shaped yellow specks protrude, remindful of the seeds of a strawberry, which prompted the name "strawberry bladder". The specks consist of cholesterol dissolved in fat within histiocytes, which give a bright red color in Sudan stains. These histiocytes accumulate in groups within the mucosal folds of the gallbladder, which lose their regularity and normal shape. Such lipid-laden folds may become the nucleus for a cholesterol stone, or a great number of foam cells may extend through the entire mucosa beyond the folds and produce broad yellow plaques. The lesion is considered an expression of unexplained abnormal cholesterol absorption rather than of excretion of cholesterol through the mucosa. Hypercholesteremia, according to experimental evidence, contributes to the development of cholesterolosis. It has also been claimed that inflammation precedes the lipid deposition, but it seems more probable that the abnormal presence of lipids in the wall is rather the stimulus for inflammation. Cholesterolosis, which occurs far more frequently in women than in men, is assumed by some to be associated with clinical manifestations similar to those of chronic cholecystitis. Others feel that cholesterolosis does not cause specific complaints and that those present result from cholelithiasis or other associated diseases.

In *acute cholecystitis* the gallbladder is, as a rule, markedly enlarged and resembles a distended sac, especially when the cystic duct is obstructed either by a stone, or less frequently, by simple swelling of the mucosal duplications (spiral fold or valve of Heister). The gallbladder wall is diffusely thickened and edematous. The mucosa is dark red and irregularly covered by gray-white patches which are frequently confluent. Small or larger ulcerations are covered with fibrinous, partly hemorrhagic, sometimes coalescing exudate. The serosa is also heavily congested, and its redness is interrupted by patches of fibrinous exudate. Edema, as observed microscopically, separates muscle and collagen fibers and broadens the folds. The epithelium in some places is desquamated, in others surprisingly intact. A sprinkling of neutrophilic leukocytes aggregates more in the outer layers. A diffuse phlegmonous infiltration, with segmented leukocytes comparable to acute appendicitis, is seen only exceptionally. In acute and, more so, in subacute stages, little *granulomas* can be found around the larger vessels in the muscular and fibrous layers. They con-

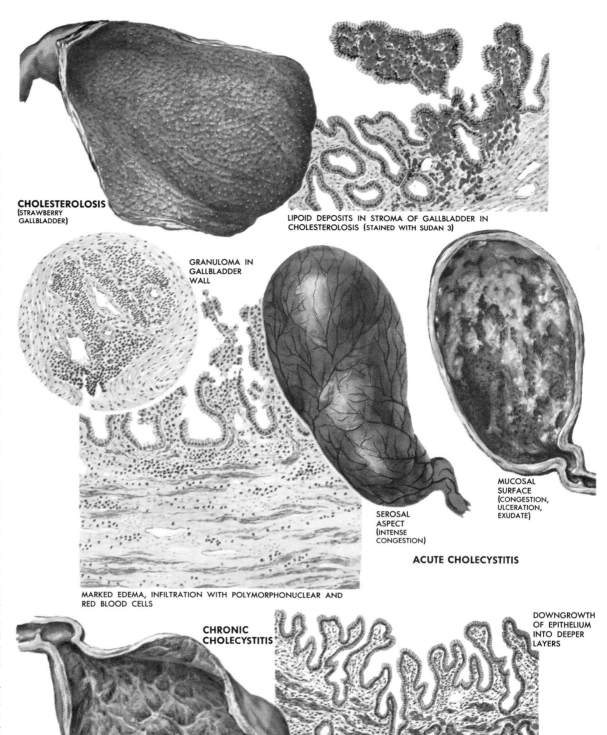

CHOLESTEROLOSIS (STRAWBERRY GALLBLADDER)

LIPOID DEPOSITS IN STROMA OF GALLBLADDER IN CHOLESTEROLOSIS (STAINED WITH SUDAN 3)

GRANULOMA IN GALLBLADDER WALL

MUCOSAL SURFACE (CONGESTION, ULCERATION, EXUDATE)

SEROSAL ASPECT (INTENSE CONGESTION)

ACUTE CHOLECYSTITIS

MARKED EDEMA, INFILTRATION WITH POLYMORPHONUCLEAR AND RED BLOOD CELLS

CHRONIC CHOLECYSTITIS

DOWNGROWTH OF EPITHELIUM INTO DEEPER LAYERS

sist of a variety of cells (segmented leukocytes or histiocytes or foam cells and lymphocytes and, occasionally, eosinophils). Proliferation of capillaries and fibroblasts is more frequent in the subacute stage. All this suggests an inflammatory reaction to an irritating chemical rather than to bacteria.

Acute abdominal symptoms, rebound tenderness in the upper right quadrant and pain, sometimes persistent, sometimes predominant during the night and morning, are, with fever and leukocytosis, the most important clinical features.

Chronic cholecystitis, with or without stones, exhibits a variety of structural changes. The gallbladder may be distended or shrunken; its wall, usually diffusely thickened, appears fibrous on the cut surface, with its layers no longer differentiated. The mucosa may appear normal green, or red, owing to ulcerations. Gray-white scars may crisscross the inner lining

and may result anywhere, in neck or fundus, as thick plaques between which the intact mucosa with exaggerated fold structure may bulge forward. The serosa is irregularly thickened and usually gray-white, frequently revealing fibrous adhesions with surrounding organs. Microscopically, the muscle bundles are more than normally separated from each other by connective tissue which, in addition to scarring, is markedly infiltrated by cellular elements to the point of granuloma formation. Outpouchings of the epithelium extend through the muscular layer, sometimes into the adventitia or fibrous layer. These pseudodiverticula (Rokitansky-Aschoff), to be differentiated from other glandular structures in the adventitial layer (see page 22), develop because of increased intraluminal pressure and because of the destruction of the mucosa. Bacteria or other irritants trapped in them may maintain the chronicity of the inflammation.

CHOLECYSTITIS II

Later Stages and Complications

The anatomic appearance and the sequelae of cholecystitis vary as much as its clinical aspect and course, according to and depending upon the frequent combinations of acute, subacute and recrudescent lesions. Chronic cholecystitis is sometimes reflected only in vague abdominal discomfort and slight tenderness in the gallbladder region but may, at any time, flare up with more severe symptoms of both colicky pain (spasms of sphincter of Oddi) and manifestations of a sudden abdominal condition. The clinical signs also vary in the presence of stones, which produce obstruction as well as pressure effects with erosion (see page 128). Sometimes the stones aggregate in the fundus and are separated by a diaphragm consisting of fibrous tissue from the neck of the gallbladder. Such an *hourglass gallbladder* frequently represents a malformation (see page 123) complicated by cholelithiasis and inflammation, but it is entirely possible that this lesion may be acquired. In chronic cholecystitis the entire wall of the gallbladder is often transformed into fibrous scar tissue, which, in smaller or larger areas, may be calcified. Such plaques are distinctly visible from the outside as well as after opening. The whitish, glistening calcified portion contrasts with the remaining dark-brown tissue and has prompted the name *"porcelain" gallbladder*. A calcified gallbladder is usually functionless and causes surprisingly few clinical symptoms, but it may be palpated as a firm mass or can be detected on X-ray examination.

In *gangrene of the gallbladder,* the edematous and friable wall becomes brown-red. The mucosa is irregularly ulcerated and otherwise dark red and green. The gangrene may involve the entire, as a rule dilated, bladder, or only part of it. In some instances gangrene can be explained by interference with blood supply and/or drainage. Stones are found almost regularly and give rise to cystic duct obstruction; pressure of the calculus upon the cystic vessels also has been held responsible for the lesion. In other instances edema of the wall is supposed to block the blood supply, and in exceptional cases torsion of the gallbladder has been found as a result of an abnormal peritoneal attachment to the liver (see page 123). Not infrequently, however, no anatomic basis for the vascular obstruction can be demonstrated. Bacterial infection, of course, many times complicates gangrene and may facilitate

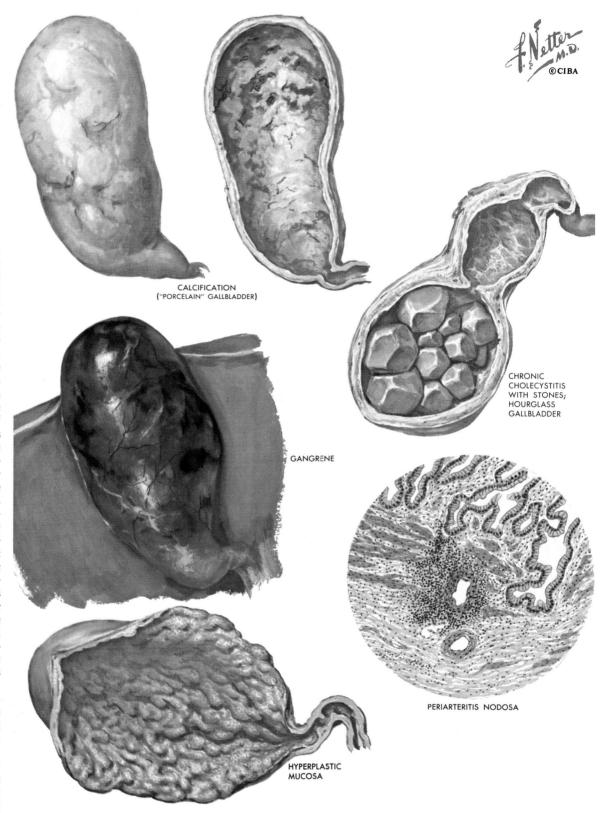

CALCIFICATION ("PORCELAIN" GALLBLADDER)

CHRONIC CHOLECYSTITIS WITH STONES; HOURGLASS GALLBLADDER

GANGRENE

PERIARTERITIS NODOSA

HYPERPLASTIC MUCOSA

perforation. A special but rare variety is primary gas bacillus infection of the gallbladder leading to a rapidly spreading phlegmonous inflammation and disintegration of the wall. Gangrene is seen more frequently in the older age group, where it may become especially treacherous if such alarm signals as fever and leukocytosis fail to appear. Pain in the upper right quadrant with rebound tenderness and with muscular rigidity of the abdominal wall are usually present, but progression of the gangrene is not infrequently associated with subsidence of pain and reduction of tenderness.

Occlusion of arteries in the gallbladder wall occurs in *periarteritis nodosa,* for which the gallbladder represents a site of predilection. One notes segmental fibrinoid degeneration, with leukocytic infiltration, while intima proliferation and thrombi narrow the arterial lumen or may obstruct it. The accumulation of inflammatory cells in the adventitia produces, in addition to some occasional aneurysms, a nodular appearance of the vessel. Circumscribed ischemic necrosis of the mucosa results from this type of vascular occlusion.

In only one form of possible inflammatory gallbladder disease is the radiologic visualization improved and the shadow denser than normal, namely, in *hyperplasia of the mucosa,* in which the normal velvety appearance is exaggerated by a greater thickness of the mucosa thrown into coarse folds. Though the inflammatory character of this hyperplasia is not definitely established, the lesion should be differentiated from the so-called glandular proliferating cholecystitis in which marked downgrowth of the surface epithelium in the form of Rokitansky-Aschoff sinuses, or pseudodiverticula (see page 22), simulates a proliferation of glands.

PERFORATION, SUBPHRENIC ABSCESS

A gross *perforation of the gallbladder* resulting in *generalized peritonitis* occurs in probably less than 1 per cent of patients with acute cholecystitis, because the omentum and serosa of the surrounding viscera seal (see page 127) the gallbladder securely in the early phases, so that a perforation through a gangrenous wall, as happens in about 15 per cent of cholecystitis cases, remains a localized process. Such an event is, as a rule, far less dramatic than with perforation of a peptic ulcer, and it is not seldom that these patients do not have even an antecedent history of gallbladder disease. Those patients with a generalized peritonitis, developing slowly over a period of from hours to days, require immediate operation, at which, usually, a zone of greenish discoloration in the region of the gallbladder comes into sight. In the vast majority of cases, a calculus will be discovered in the neck of the gallbladder, the wall of which is markedly edematous. When no obstructing stone can be found, one must search for other causes (cystic artery thrombosis, arteriosclerosis, typhoid ulcerations, decubital ulceration produced by stones elsewhere in the gallbladder, etc.). With a localized peritonitic abscess, it is the current trend to intervene surgically, when and if signs of a generalized peritonitis become evident.

A pericholecystic abscess or a generalized peritonitis following gallbladder perforation is a more frequent sequela of a biliary disease than is the formation of *subphrenic abscesses*. These, too, may be initiated by a frank perforation but, more often, they are the result of a slow leakage through the pseudodiverticula or sinuses of Rokitansky-Aschoff (see page 22). This mode of escape of gallbladder content can culminate in an abscess of any one of the six subphrenic compartments, which owe their separation to the anatomic position of the various hepatic ligaments.

Thorek has classified* the subphrenic spaces or recesses ("subphrenic" used in the general sense of being between the diaphragm and the transverse mesocolon) into suprahepatic and infrahepatic spaces, the suprahepatic lying between the liver and the diaphragm; the infrahepatic between the visceral surface of the liver and the transverse mesocolon. The suprahepatic space is subdivided into right and left spaces by the falciform ligament (see page 5). He considers the right suprahepatic space to be further subdivided by the coronary ligament into anterior and posterior spaces. Since the coronary ligament is not on the superior aspect of the liver but on the posterior aspect, the "right posterior superior space"

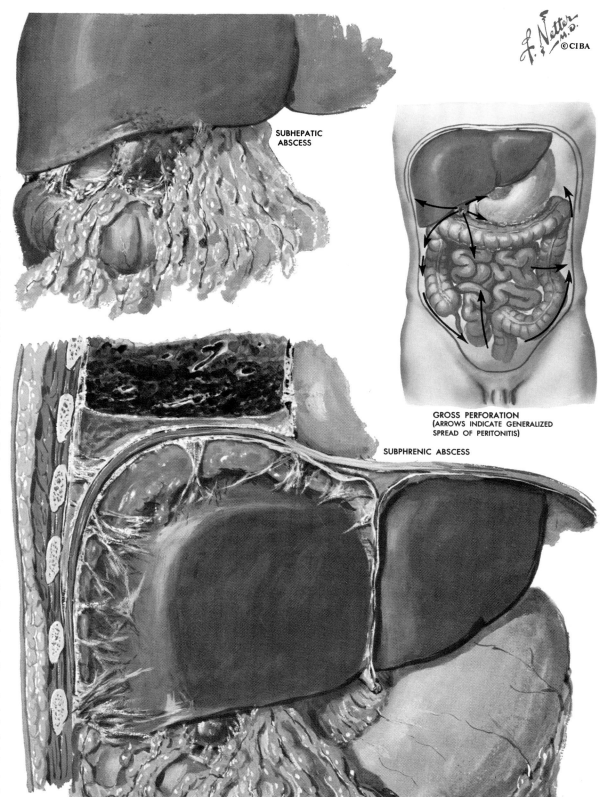

SUBHEPATIC ABSCESS

GROSS PERFORATION
(ARROWS INDICATE GENERALIZED SPREAD OF PERITONITIS)

SUBPHRENIC ABSCESS

is not suprahepatic at all but really retrohepatic.

The infrahepatic space is also subdivided into right and left by the round ligament and the ligament of the ductus venosus. In this case it is the left space which is further subdivided into anterior and posterior by the lesser omentum and the stomach, the left posterior infrahepatic space being the omental bursa. The bare area of the liver, *i.e.*, the area enclosed by the layers of the coronary ligament, constitutes another space, but Thorek does not classify this as a subphrenic space because it is actually extraperitoneal (also retrohepatic: see CIBA COLLECTION, Vol. 3/II, page 193).*

The right superior posterior subphrenic recess (right superior posterior suprahepatic space of Thorek) is the most frequent site of *subphrenic abscesses* which, according to a large series of cases, in 28 per cent are causally related to appendicitis, in 26 per cent to perforation of the stomach or duodenum and in 12 per cent to infections in the liver or biliary tract. Perigastric abscesses most commonly perforate into the left inferior anterior subhepatic recess (also known as the perigastric space), while pancreatic abscesses or pseudocysts may rupture into the omental bursa.

*THOREK'S TERMINOLOGY	TERMS BASED ON NOMINA ANATOMICA
R. sup. ant. space	R. sup. ant. subphrenic recess
R. sup. post. suprahepatic space	R. sup. post. subphrenic recess
L. sup. space	L. sup. subphrenic recess
R. inf. space	Hepatorenal recess
L. inf. ant. space	L. inf. ant. subhepatic recess
L. inf. post. space	L. inf. post. subphrenic recess (omental bursa)

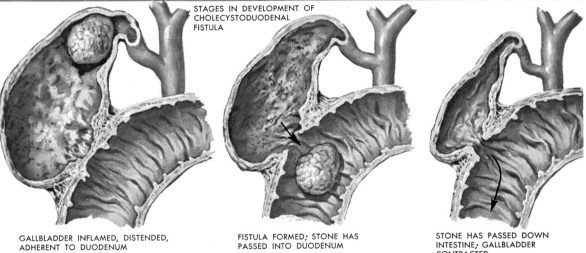

TYPES OF
BILIARY FISTULAE
1. CHOLECYSTODUODENAL
2. CHOLECYSTOCOLIC
3. CHOLECYSTOGASTRIC
4. CHOLECYSTOCHOLEDOCHAL
5. CHOLEDOCHODUODENAL

BILE DUCT FISTULAE

A *cholecystoduodenal fistula* is usually the result of acute cholecystitis with obstruction of the gallbladder neck by a solitary stone too large to pass the cystic duct (see page 127) and a subsequent pericholecystitis (see page 131) developing into an abscess, which, in turn, attaches itself to the duodenum. When such an abscess ulcerates, a fistulous tract of varying length evolves, which is not present when an abscess or gangrene of the gallbladder (see page 130) ulcerates directly into the duodenum. If a stone passes through the fistula, it may obstruct the duodenum in ball-valve fashion, but more often it travels down, usually as far as the narrower terminal ileum, where it becomes arrested, causing a *"gallstone ileus"*. While the removal of the calculus in such a case is mandatory, cholecystectomy need not be considered in elderly patients who are a poor risk, because the gallbladder can, with the obstructing stone gone, empty physiologically, and the fistulous tract will close.

A *choledochoduodenal fistula* forms less often and is usually preceded by an obstructive jaundice, which may disappear when the fistulous tract is completely opened. The rare *cholecystocolic* and still rarer *choledochocolic fistulae* may be first recognized by the recovery of calculi in the feces. Large-bowel obstruction by stones is less likely than severe biliary tract infections with chills and fever, weight loss and jaundice. The latter may ameliorate coincidentally with the appearance of diarrhea. Barium enemas usually reveal the fistula's tract. The essential symptom of a *cholecystogastric fistula* is the vomiting of a gallstone, though such an event could also result from duodenal regurgitation. Occasionally, this type of fistula is encountered with carcinoma of the stomach or pancreas. Fistulae between the various parts of the biliary system (*e.g., cholecystocholedochal*), mostly multiple and secondary to the afore-mentioned fistulae, are infrequent, as are fistulae with other organs (jejunum, ileum, renal pelvis, vagina, pericardium, portal vein, hepatic artery).

Bronchobiliary fistulae are apparently preceded by choledocholithiasis which leads to cholangitis and liver abscesses. These break into the subdiaphragmatic space and rupture into the pleura. After a clinical course of obstructive jaundice,

STAGES IN DEVELOPMENT OF
CHOLECYSTODUODENAL
FISTULA

GALLBLADDER INFLAMED, DISTENDED,
ADHERENT TO DUODENUM

FISTULA FORMED; STONE HAS
PASSED INTO DUODENUM

STONE HAS PASSED DOWN
INTESTINE; GALLBLADDER
CONTRACTED

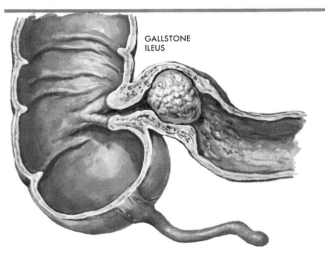

GALLSTONE
ILEUS

SURGICAL
END TO END
FISTULA
("ROUX EN Y")
CHOLECYSTO-
JEJUNOSTOMY

these patients develop the symptoms and signs of a diaphragmatic pleurisy or basal pneumonitis; with the expectoration of a bile-stained sputum or as much as 700 ml. of bile per day, the complication is obvious. Cough is aggravated by the recumbent position. Cure lies in choledochotomy and drainage of a diaphragmatic abscess.

With the surgical treatment of internal biliary fistulae, the patency of the common bile duct must be verified because of a not-infrequent association with a common duct stone that failed to produce jaundice only because the bile had a free outflow through the fistula. Internal biliary fistulae, most commonly between gallbladder and jejunum, may be occasionally created by surgeons to overcome a bile flow obstruction caused by strictures or neoplasms. The *"Roux en Y"* principle is a refinement of such an operation, minimizing the danger of infection, though

the simplest method is preferable, because the survival time after relief of an obstruction from malignant neoplasms is not long enough for the development of cholangitis and its consequences.

Spontaneous external biliary fistulae result when the obstructed and inflamed gallbladder becomes attached to the parietal peritoneum. The fistular tract usually follows the falciform ligament to the umbilicus, where a reddened cutaneous tumor develops, which is easily mistaken for a subcutaneous abscess until incision yields bile or gallstones. A postoperative external fistula may be diagnosed when bile drainage persists more than 10 days after removal of the T tube. The incidence of both spontaneous and postoperative external fistulae has decreased with the advent of modern gallbladder surgery and the replacement of cholecystotomy by cholecystectomy, respectively.

EXTRAHEPATIC CHOLANGITIS, STRICTURES, SURGICAL ACCIDENTS

Infection of the extrahepatic bile ducts can be divided into nonsuppurative and suppurative forms. The former is seen in association with all causes of biliary stasis, in acute and chronic cholecystitis, in silent common duct stones or as a sequel of inflammatory processes in other viscera or generalized infections. Suppurative cholangitis, a more serious disease, follows a variety of pyogenic conditions of the gastro-intestinal tract or biliaryintestinal anastomosis; the sequelae to be feared here are liver abscesses.

Although extrahepatic cholangitis can instigate a spontaneous stricture of the *bile ducts, strictures* are far more often an aftermath of *surgical accidents,* which may occur, *e.g.,* in an effort to arrest hemorrhages from the cystic or hepatic artery. These hemorrhages may happen when the blood vessel, being shorter than the accompanying duct, is torn in case greater retraction is needed, as in obese patients. A too rapid appliance of hemostats may result in a crushing injury of a yet incompletely dissected common bile duct. A retrograde dissection of the gallbladder fundus and displacement of the gallbladder to the left side of the abdomen may impel a similar accident. The type of stricture that develops in such instances is relatively favorable, because only part of the duct is usually involved, permitting surgical repair; clinically suggestive signs of fever, chills and jaundice turn up only after 3 to 4 months, when a commensurate fibrosis has evolved.

A second type of injury, which may cause the development of a *stricture,* may be inflicted when the *common bile duct* is *clamped* under the impression that it is the cystic duct, as may happen in case traction upon the neck of the gallbladder "tents" the common bile duct. Because of the obvious disparity in size of cystic and common bile ducts and because the latter is explored before anything is transected, such an injury rarely occurs with choledochotomy. About 20 per cent of these injuries have been noted after emergency operations for acute cholecystitis, and in a few cases after gastric resection, while the majority come about with elective cholecystectomies for uncomplicated gallbladder disease. This injury many times comprises complete transection of the common bile duct, which will suggest itself by the stellate appearance of the ligated and transected proximal duct. Immediate discharge of bile around the drains, continuing indefinitely, is an indication of what happened, if it is not discovered during operation. As the drainage stops, the patient

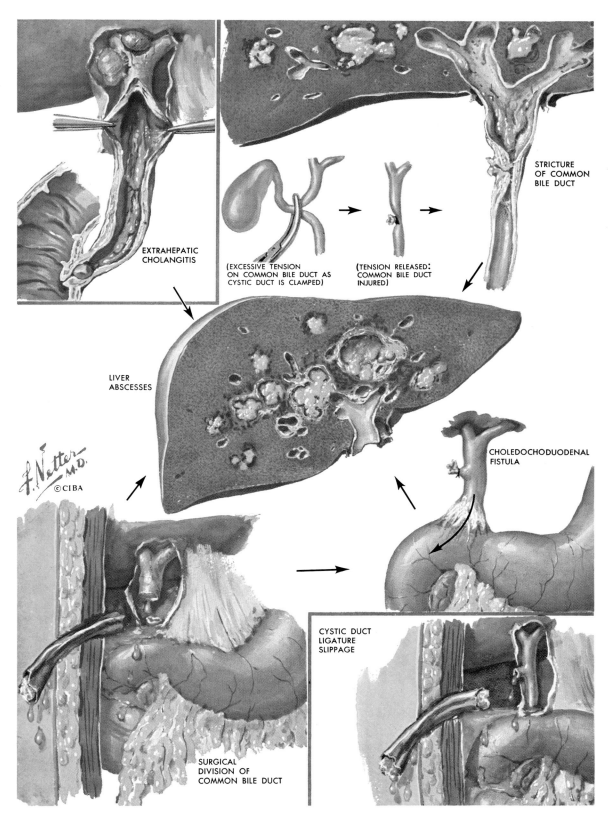

EXTRAHEPATIC CHOLANGITIS

(EXCESSIVE TENSION ON COMMON BILE DUCT AS CYSTIC DUCT IS CLAMPED)

(TENSION RELEASED: COMMON BILE DUCT INJURED)

STRICTURE OF COMMON BILE DUCT

LIVER ABSCESSES

CHOLEDOCHODUODENAL FISTULA

CYSTIC DUCT LIGATURE SLIPPAGE

SURGICAL DIVISION OF COMMON BILE DUCT

becomes icteric and the stools acholic. The subsequent disappearance of jaundice, together with the recurrence of brown stools, means the spontaneous formation of a *choledochoduodenal fistula,* which, however, will often fibrose and stenose.

Transection of anomalous ducts (see page 23) not seldom accounts for the postoperative appearance of bile on the dressings, but this type of fistula usually ceases in a matter of several days. Another source of biliary leakage is a *cystic duct ligature slippage,* when the catgut begins to soften. Bile has lytic qualities and may prevent obliteration of the lumen of the transected cystic duct. With an open common bile duct and if external drainage has been provided, such leakage eventually abates. With all these surgical accidents and no precaution so that the bile will drain to the exterior, the patients, of course, face the dangers of a bile peritonitis. Another feared sequela

of the afore-mentioned fortuitous events is the development of *liver abscesses,* the outcome of which is very dubious. Anemia, gastro-intestinal hemorrhages and severe parenchymal damage of the liver may hasten the inevitable outcome. The liver shrinks, and the spleen enlarges before the patient succumbs to a hepatic coma.

Surgery holds considerable hope for these cases with strictures or fistulae, if performed early and successfully on the first attempt. With each failure of a trial to repair a fistula, the next attempt is much less likely to succeed. The three most frequent causes of postoperative deaths following repair of strictures have been hemorrhages, hepaticocellular failure and peritonitis, all of which have been enormously reduced by the advancements in operative techniques and in pre- and postoperative care adopted in the past few decades.

DIAGNOSIS OF BILIARY TRACT DISEASE

A paroxysmal *pain* originating in the upper right abdominal quadrant and radiating around the right costal margin to the shoulder (see page 21), to the scapular areas and, less often, to the hypochondrium is the most reliable symptom of a diseased gallbladder, although this "biliary colic" is reported in only slightly more than 50 per cent of uncomplicated gallbladder involvement. The incidence approaches, however, 95 per cent in patients with jaundice caused by a stone in the common bile duct. In contrast, with obstruction by a malignant tumor, the incidence of biliary colic is far less (about 25 per cent). A more continuous type of pain, with complaints of localized pressure, fullness or discomfort, though localized in the upper abdominal quadrant and frequently brought on by *dietary indiscretion*, is not pathognomonic for gallbladder disease, because it is encountered with many other gastrointestinal lesions. Generalized abdominal discomfort associated with flatulence is another complaint of a rather small group of patients with disturbance of the gallbladder, and some of them have no pain whatsoever, despite an even advanced biliary disease. Anorexia is more characteristic of liver disease than of extrahepatic tract disorders. Weight loss, though more significant for malignant lesions, can occur even to an extreme degree in benign lesions of the biliary system. Fever and chills, not regular signs of acute cholecystitis, appear frequently with involvement of the common bile duct.

On physical examination the sign most indicative of gallbladder disease is a *palpable mass in the upper right quadrant*. If this mass is tender, an inflammatory process can be assumed, and conservative treatment can be pursued as long as the tenderness remains localized and until it subsides, at which time cholecystectomy becomes mandatory. If the abdominal mass is not tender and the patient is not icteric, the existence of a hydrops of the gallbladder (see page 127) is most likely. The presence of jaundice with a mass, tender or not, points to an obstructive complication, such as a choledochus stone, a tumor or, less often, an extrahepatic cholangitis (see page 133). It should, however, be kept in mind that jaundice is not an obligatory sign of choledocholithiasis (only 65 per cent of the cases are icteric) and that, on the other hand, gallbladder hydrops is often asso-

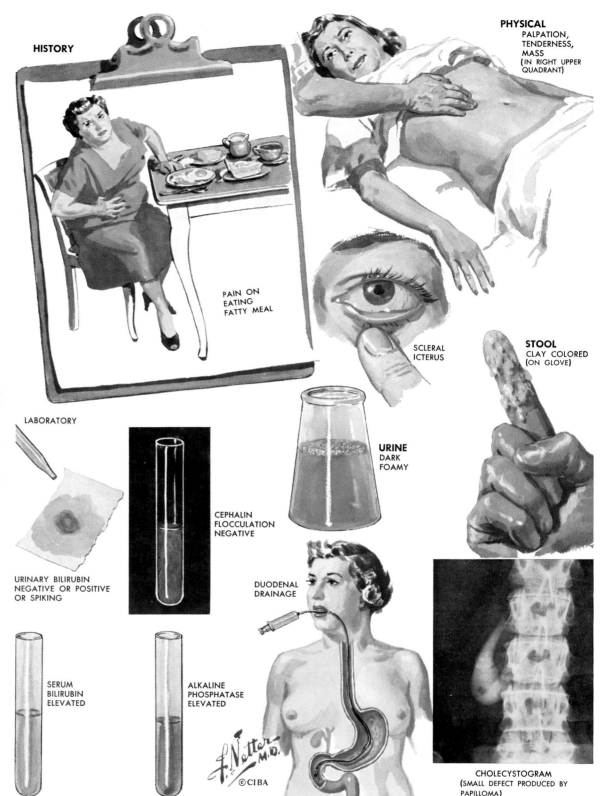

HISTORY

PAIN ON EATING FATTY MEAL

PHYSICAL
PALPATION, TENDERNESS, MASS (IN RIGHT UPPER QUADRANT)

SCLERAL ICTERUS

STOOL
CLAY COLORED (ON GLOVE)

LABORATORY

URINARY BILIRUBIN NEGATIVE OR POSITIVE OR SPIKING

CEPHALIN FLOCCULATION NEGATIVE

URINE
DARK FOAMY

SERUM BILIRUBIN ELEVATED

ALKALINE PHOSPHATASE ELEVATED

DUODENAL DRAINAGE

CHOLECYSTOGRAM
(SMALL DEFECT PRODUCED BY PAPILLOMA)

ciated with a stone in the extrahepatic ducts, so that it is wise to explore the common bile duct whenever the gallbladder is approached surgically.

Though also seen in a great number of cases with medical jaundice, pruritus, particularly when lasting, favors the surgical type, because it is observed in more than 20 per cent of patients with extrahepatic bile duct obstruction due to calculi and in almost 40 per cent of individuals with neoplastic obstruction. Confirmation of an *acholic stool* (see page 49) should always be sought by digital rectal examination, because the patient's description is rarely reliable. The use of laboratory tests for the differential diagnosis of medical and surgical jaundice has been described elsewhere (see page 51). Those most helpful for early clarification of the situation are the *cephalin flocculation test* (see page 38), determination of the *alkaline phosphatase activity* (see page 43) and

measurement of the *bilirubin content of the serum*. Though a *foamy urine* of a mahogany color predicts the presence of abnormal quantities of bilirubin, the semiquantitative Harrison test is sometimes a helpful bedside adjuvant. The addition of a few drops of Fouchet's reagent (trichloracetic acid and ferric chloride) to a filter paper impregnated with barium chloride and moistened with the urine indicates with a bluish-green color the presence of bilirubin. This test is properly supplemented by a quantitative urobilinogen determination.

Biliary drainage (see page 53) is rarely feasible, but the *cholecystogram* (see page 54) has become a standard procedure in nonicteric patients. However, it should be remembered that in the presence of very marked jaundice all cholecystographic techniques (whether oral or intravenous) very seldom yield the desired information.

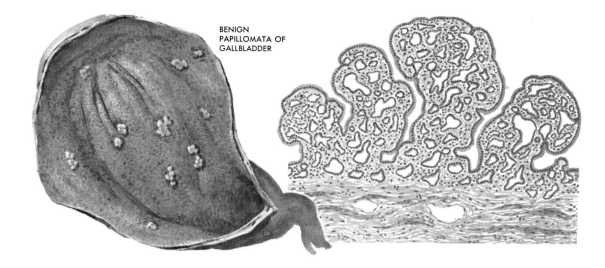

BENIGN
PAPILLOMATA OF
GALLBLADDER

TUMORS OF GALLBLADDER

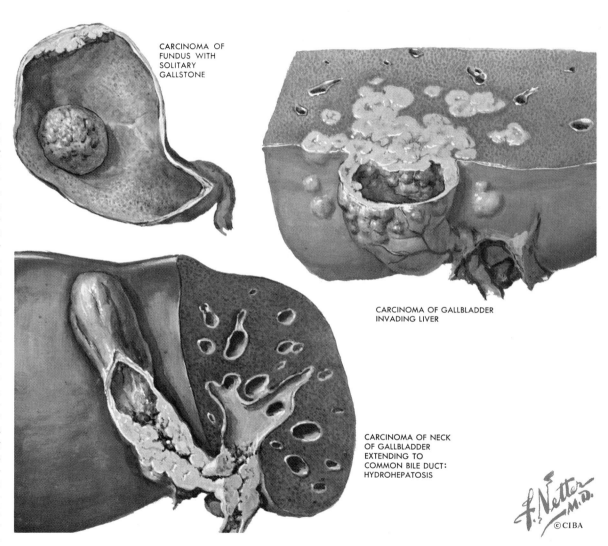

CARCINOMA OF
FUNDUS WITH
SOLITARY
GALLSTONE

CARCINOMA OF GALLBLADDER
INVADING LIVER

CARCINOMA OF NECK
OF GALLBLADDER
EXTENDING TO
COMMON BILE DUCT:
HYDROHEPATOSIS

Papillomatous excrescences, either single or, more commonly, multiple, are not seldom found at cholecystectomy or autopsy. They usually are not larger than a few millimeters in their greatest diameter and project only slightly over the mucosa as yellow, flat, cauliflowerlike lesions. Though they sometimes contain deposited cholesterol, they must be differentiated from the histiocytic eminences in cholesterolosis (see page 129). These papillomas appear histologically as a villous overgrowth of the surface epithelium, with an epithelial lining exhibiting many indentations into a connective tissue stalk of variable thickness. Many times the stalks are found to be infiltrated by inflammatory cells, and it seems that numbers of these papillomatous structures are only inflammatory focal proliferations. Smaller lesions, not large enough to be felt during surgery or to be demonstrated radiologically, show no tendency to malignant degeneration, but this does not hold true to the same degree for larger papillomas that are either polyps with long stalks or flat buttonlike adenomas. The latter give a characteristic picture in cholecystograms and reveal histologically a picture similar to the small papillomas, except that sometimes mucin-producing glands are in the foreground.

Carcinoma of the gallbladder presents itself in several forms. The most common infiltrating type causes thickening and hardening of all layers of the wall and extends in the form of a gray-white, only partially necrotic tumor mass into the surrounding structures, especially into the liver. It consists of anaplastic glandular epithelium, which usually is associated with a marked fibroplasia of the stroma remindful of a scirrhous formation. Its prognosis is rather poor. The less frequent papillomatous type extends cauliflowerlike into the lumen, spreads only relatively little over the surrounding mucosa or into the wall and has a somewhat better prognosis. Ulcers over the projecting area and hemorrhages into the soft tumor mass are customary findings in that type, which consists histologically of carcinomatous epithelium arranged in the form of multiple villi. Still less frequent is the subvariety of an extensively colloid-producing carcinoma. Mixtures of the described three types of adenocarcinoma occur. Relatively rare is squamous cell carcinoma of the bladder. Carcinoma of the gallbladder hardly ever develops in a normal organ. Stones are found in a very high percentage of all carcinoma cases, and the etiologic relation between gallbladder carcinoma and cholelithiasis has elicited much discussion (see page 128). A not unusual scarring seen in the noninvolved part of the bladder suggests a preceding cicatrizing cholecystitis.

The sequelae of carcinoma of the gallbladder depend mainly on location and spread, although perforation is not too rare. *Carcinoma* located *near the neck* of the bladder has a great tendency to *invade the hilar connective tissue* and the *common bile and hepatic ducts,* thus producing obstructive jaundice and hydrohepatosis as well as hepatic abscesses or internal biliary fistulae. *Carcinoma in the fundus spreads* readily *into the liver* or into the peritoneum. All types early involve the regional lymph nodes. Distant metastases are hardly ever absent at autopsy. Sometimes, such metastases produce the first clinical symptoms, whereas the small primary carcinoma is not diagnosed. With a lower incidence than carcinoma of the gastro-intestinal tract, gallbladder cancer occurs in higher ages and has a definite female preponderance similar to that of cholelithiasis and in contrast to carcinoma of the liver or biliary tract. Though the clinical signs — pain, jaundice, a palpable mass, hepatomegaly and sometimes also anemia — are easily attributed to a disorder of the gallbladder and biliary tract, they do not necessarily point to a malignant tumor.

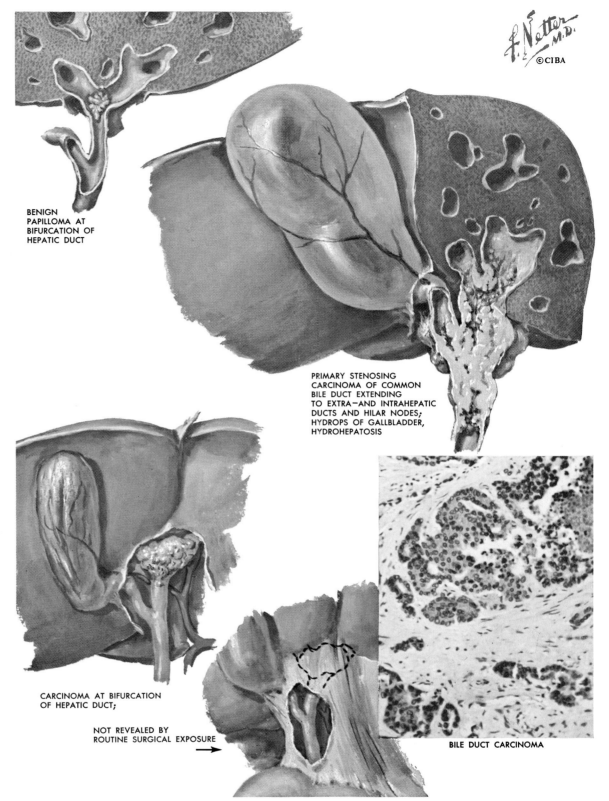

BENIGN
PAPILLOMA AT
BIFURCATION OF
HEPATIC DUCT

PRIMARY STENOSING
CARCINOMA OF COMMON
BILE DUCT EXTENDING
TO EXTRA—AND INTRAHEPATIC
DUCTS AND HILAR NODES;
HYDROPS OF GALLBLADDER,
HYDROHEPATOSIS

CARCINOMA AT BIFURCATION
OF HEPATIC DUCT;

NOT REVEALED BY
ROUTINE SURGICAL EXPOSURE

BILE DUCT CARCINOMA

TUMORS OF BILE DUCTS

In the extrahepatic biliary ducts *papillomas,* polyps or flat, buttonlike adenomas rarely occur. All of them are benign as far as their spread is concerned, but they may cause jaundice by mechanical obstruction. That they are occasionally multiple should be kept in mind at surgical exploration, because it may be just a specifically located single adenoma which must be removed in order to relieve the jaundice. Exceptionally, they undergo cystic degeneration and may become very large. Mesenchymal benign tumors in the larger bile ducts, such as lipomas or fibromas, are seldom seen curiosities.

The far more frequent *carcinomas* of the extrahepatic biliary ducts start as a plaquelike hardening of the wall, which only exceptionally proceeds to a papillomatous intraluminal growth. Usually, such a tumor starts with a diffuse infiltration of the wall by a gray-white firm tissue, which later spreads into the surrounding areolar tissue. The mucosa does not appear ulcerated, so that small and nonspreading carcinomas may closely resemble strictures of the bile ducts. Consequently, provided no operation was performed previously, any stricture of the ducts should be suspected for primary carcinoma of the ducts. Histologically, almost all carcinomas of the bile duct are more or less anaplastic adenocarcinomas, with sometimes conspicuous mucus production and usually severe desmoplastic reaction which causes a scirrhuslike gross appearance. The carcinoma may develop anywhere in the ducts. It may appear as a short annular lesion, but sometimes it spreads along the longitudinal axis of the duct toward the liver and even into the cystic duct, where it then causes hydrops of the gallbladder. If the carcinoma is localized only in the common duct, the gallbladder is markedly dilated but thinwalled (Courvoisier's law, see page 82) because of the unaltered communication between the hepatic and cystic ducts. With a carcinoma located in the main hepatic duct, the gallbladder is small and collapsed. Carcinomas of the cystic duct are rare. The main syndrome, jaundice, is almost always present, because the obstruction is generally complete (see page 82). Hydrohepatosis and cholestasis

in the liver (see page 83), and ascending and descending bacterial infection, ending in bacterial hepatitis and cholangitic as well as pylephlebitic abscesses (see page 92), are the most important consequences. Metastases develop, in the order of incidence, in the liver, regional lymph nodes, pancreas and peritoneum. The lungs are infrequently involved, and generalized spread is rare, possibly because the patient succumbs to the obstructive jaundice before a diffuse spread has set in. The early appearance of jaundice, serving as a warning signal, is the reason that the operating surgeon is less frequently confronted with metastases of bile duct carcinoma than is the case with gallbladder or pancreas cancer.

Carcinoma at the bifurcation of the hepatic ducts at the hilus of the liver may be rather misleading from the diagnostic point of view. With the involvement of both main hepatic ducts, jaundice, of course,

develops early, but, in contrast to all other types of extrahepatic biliary obstruction, the extrahepatic bile ducts *at exploration* appear *not dilated* but rather collapsed. Such an aspect may be taken as a sign of intrahepatic cholestasis of cholangiolitic character (see page 84), unless deep probing or intra-operative cholangiography reveals the nature of the lesion.

The origin of carcinoma of the bile ducts has often been connected with choledocholithiasis and strictures of the ducts, both of which frequently complicate it, but the causal relation is still as dubious as that between carcinoma of the gallbladder and cholelithiasis (see pages 128 and 135).

Jaundice with pruritus but without pain is the first clinical symptom, but pain frequently appears during the course of the disease, probably as a result of an invasion of nerves. Weight loss and cachexia set in sometimes surprisingly late.

AMPULLARY TUMORS

A special variety of the tumors of the bile ducts are those at the papilla of Vater. *Benign papillomas* may develop in the ampullary portion and may sometimes protrude through the papilla into the duodenal lumen, reaching cherry size. Though they are soft, they almost regularly occlude the common bile duct and, depending on the anatomic situation (see page 24), also the pancreatic duct. Extra- and intrahepatic bile ducts and the gallbladder are markedly dilated, and severe jaundice is present. Whether the columnar epithelium forming these papillomas derives from the biliary ducts, from the duodenum or from the pancreatic duct is not clear. Still more difficult is it to determine the origin of *carcinoma of the papilla of Vater,* which involves not only the choledochoduodenal junction but also all the surrounding structures. Many are actually bile duct carcinomas; others are carcinomas of the duodenum, of the pancreatic ducts and even of aberrant or normally located pancreatic tissue (see pages 141 and 148) and of adnexal glands of the ducts. Previously, most of these tumors were considered to be bile duct carcinomas, but many investigators speak of them now as duodenal carcinomas. Whatever the origin, even if small, they form a firm mass which produces an annular stenosis at the papilla. The gray-white, firm cancer tissue usually bulges the papilla of Vater forward and is recognized on transduodenal exposure as an irregularly shaped, fine granular or papillomatous mass. With X-ray visualization the outline of the duodenum is often distorted. The *tumor spreads along the wall of the common bile and pancreatic ducts* and may extend into the head of the *pancreas.* Here the gray-white fibrous or granular tumor tissue may undergo necrosis. It is, as a rule, unsharply demarcated from the intact pancreatic tissue, a fact which makes the differentiation from primary

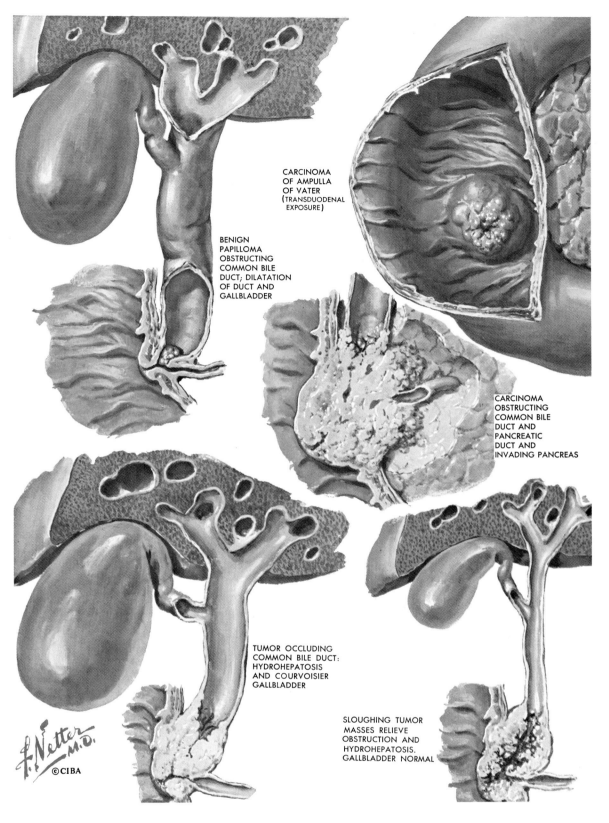

CARCINOMA
OF AMPULLA
OF VATER
(TRANSDUODENAL
EXPOSURE)

BENIGN
PAPILLOMA
OBSTRUCTING
COMMON BILE
DUCT; DILATATION
OF DUCT AND
GALLBLADDER

CARCINOMA
OBSTRUCTING
COMMON BILE
DUCT AND
PANCREATIC
DUCT AND
INVADING PANCREAS

TUMOR OCCLUDING
COMMON BILE DUCT:
HYDROHEPATOSIS
AND COURVOISIER
GALLBLADDER

SLOUGHING TUMOR
MASSES RELIEVE
OBSTRUCTION AND
HYDROHEPATOSIS.
GALLBLADDER NORMAL

carcinoma of the pancreas more difficult. Histologically, the lesions consist of a more or less anaplastic adenocarcinoma, with variable fibrotic reaction and mucus production.

Independent of their histogenesis, the obstruction caused by tumors of the papilla of Vater has the same consequences as has the obstruction of tumors of the common bile duct (see page 136), but, in addition, the main pancreatic duct of Wirsung is always obstructed, even if the common and pancreatic ducts do not have a common terminal pathway. Inevitably, all pancreatic ducts dilate and focal pancreatic and fat necrosis may develop, but, even more frequently, fibrosis replaces within several months the acinar tissue, leaving, as a rule, the islands of Langerhans intact, so that diabetes develops late, if at all. Metas-

tases to the regional lymph nodes are encountered at surgery in more than one third of the cases and, even more often, at the autopsy table. Metastases to liver and distant organs develop relatively early.

The incidence of carcinoma at the ampulla of Vater is greater than in other parts of the bile ducts, but a predominance in males over 50 years of age is common to all of them. Jaundice and pruritus are the leading clinical features. Episodes of partial and complete relief of the obstruction as well as of the jaundice occur (see page 82). Manifestations of pancreatic involvement, with bulky diarrheal stools and elevation of serum amylase (see page 58), as well as the higher incidence and degree of melena caused by bleeding from the tumor at the ampulla, distinguish the latter also from carcinoma of other parts of the biliary tract.

POSTCHOLECYSTECTOMY SYNDROME

Recurrence of preoperative symptoms, but particularly of biliary colic within 2 or more months following cholecystectomy, has been called *postcholecystectomy symptoms* or *syndrome*. Provided the original diagnosis, which presented the indication for surgical intervention, was not erroneous and that no associated illness (osteo-arthritis, hydronephrosis, etc.) complicates the situation, the most frequent cause of these recurrent symptoms is probably one (or more) stone which has escaped exploration of the extrahepatic bile ducts. *Residual stones* are most often hidden in the hepatic duct or in the ampullary portion of the common bile duct. The procurement of cholangiograms (see page 54) during operation has minimized the incidence of overlooked stones. It cannot be denied, however, that stones have formed in the duct some time after surgery.

Anatomic identification of the whole cystic duct and its dissection down to its confluence with the common bile duct is sometimes rather difficult, particularly in the presence of an acutely inflamed gallbladder prompting an emergency operation, and under such circumstances a more or less *excessive cystic stump* remains, which has been shown to give rise to postcholecystectomy symptoms. Though by no means necessarily present, a stone retained in the stump aids materially the manifestations of the syndrome.

Another group of patients with returning pains suffer from *spasms of the sphincter of Oddi,* and rare cases have been seen with actual hypertrophy of the sphincter responsible for a stenosis. Increasing formation of *adhesions constricting the sphincter* may produce a similar effect. The ill-defined diagnostic term "biliary dyskinesia" has been applied to those patients in whom a functional disorder had to be assumed for lack of signs of any organic disorder.

In patients developing jaundice within 6 months following a cholecystectomy, *strictures of the common bile duct* should be suspected. They can emanate from an extrahepatic cholangitis (see page 133) or *adhesions* but are more often the result of some surgical accident, usually at the junction of the common bile duct and common hepatic duct or at the junction with the cystic duct. The differential diagnosis of a stricture and a *carcinoma of the biliary duct* may, in some instances, be rather difficult, but the latter accounts for a not negligible number of cases with postcholecystectomy syndrome. These tumors of both common bile duct and

1. COMMON DUCT STONES
2. EXCESSIVE CYSTIC DUCT STUMP
3. SPHINCTER OF ODDI SPASM (HYPERTROPHY, STENOSIS, DYSKINESIA)
4. STRICTURES OF COMMON BILE DUCT
5. CARCINOMA OF BILIARY TRACT
6. PANCREATITIS
7. AMPUTATION NEUROMA
8. ADHESIONS CONSTRICTING COMMON BILE DUCT

pancreas may be so small at the time of operation that they can easily be overlooked. Even cholangiograms may fail to make such lesions visible. Furthermore, the recovery of a calculus may be wrongly interpreted as the correct and final solution of the patient's diagnostic problem, the fact that gallstones are present in 5 to 30 per cent of cases with a neoplasm being forgotten.

The frequent association of pancreatitis (see page 143) with biliary disease points to the former as a cause of postcholecystectomy symptoms. The detection of an existing *pancreatitis* is not always possible before or during operation, because the serum amylase activity (see page 58) need not always be elevated, nor is the pancreatitis always detectable during operation, because the inflammatory process may be restricted to a portion of the pancreas which remains invisible unless the entire gland can be exposed.

Many patients with pancreatitis are benefited by a cholecystectomy as long as the postoperative paresis of the sphincter of Oddi (see page 52) subsists, but the manifestations of pancreatitis return when, approximately after 2 months, the sphincter regains its tonus. It also happens that the removal of the gallbladder alone does not alleviate the signs and symptoms of the biliary disease in cases of coexisting pancreatitis. Finally, the possibility cannot be denied that excessive instrumentation and intubation of the common bile duct might instigate an inflammatory reaction of the pancreas.

Nodular proliferation of nerves (*amputation neuroma*), representing another cause of the syndrome, has been reported. The nodules develop when a large number of sympathetic nerve fibers are cut, while the cystic duct is stripped down to its junction with the common bile duct.

Section XIX

DISEASES OF THE PANCREAS

by

FRANK H. NETTER, M.D.

in collaboration with

EUGENE E. CLIFFTON, M.D.

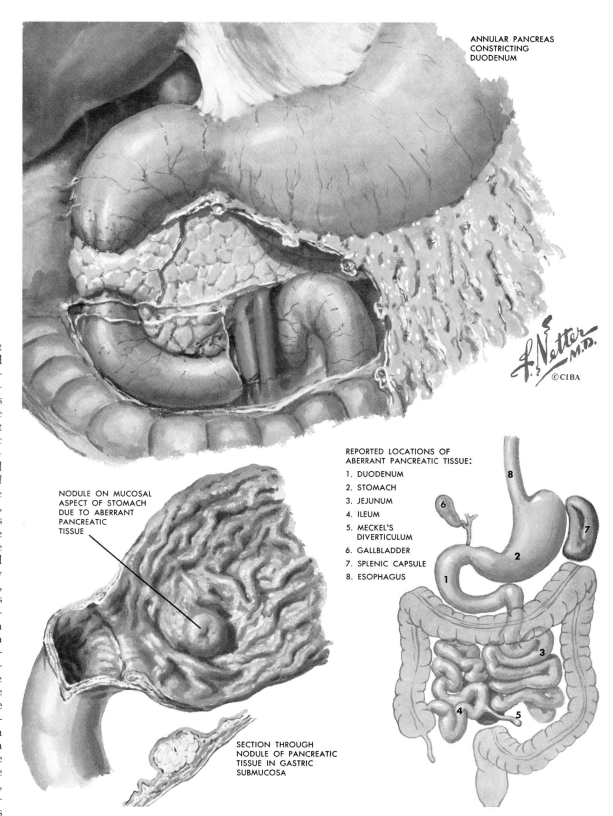

ANNULAR PANCREAS
CONSTRICTING
DUODENUM

NODULE ON MUCOSAL
ASPECT OF STOMACH
DUE TO ABERRANT
PANCREATIC
TISSUE

SECTION THROUGH
NODULE OF PANCREATIC
TISSUE IN GASTRIC
SUBMUCOSA

REPORTED LOCATIONS OF
ABERRANT PANCREATIC TISSUE:

1. DUODENUM
2. STOMACH
3. JEJUNUM
4. ILEUM
5. MECKEL'S
   DIVERTICULUM
6. GALLBLADDER
7. SPLENIC CAPSULE
8. ESOPHAGUS

Congenital Anomalies

The pancreas arises from the foregut just distal to the stomach by ventral and dorsal anlagen (see page 25). The former is frequently derived from the outpouching for the liver and biliary ducts (see page 2). This origin explains the many locations of the most frequent pancreatic anomaly, aberrant or ectopic pancreatic tissue. Nests of *aberrant pancreatic tissue* are most frequently found in the *duodenum, stomach* and *small bowel* but have also been reported in the biliary ducts, *gallbladder,* liver, *spleen,* peritoneum, omentum, colon and organs within the mediastinum, such as the *esophagus.* The favorite site of these aberrant pancreatic nodules is the second portion of the duodenum, followed by the diverticula in the small intestine, such as Meckel's diverticulum. It has even been suggested that these pancreatic cells might be causative agents in diverticulum formation. In more than one half of the cases, the *nodules of pancreatic tissue* are embedded *in the submucosa* or, in other instances, in the muscularis and, least commonly, they are subserosal or involve all layers of the wall. On palpation they may seem polypoid, and characteristically they have a *central dimple.* It is rare that more than a single nodule can be detected. The structure is usually similar to that of the normal pancreas but may become cystic, and instances where the mass was primarily or entirely made up of islet cells have been reported. The ectopic masses are usually small, seldom being over 5 cm., and usually 1 to 2 cm., in diameter. Acute or chronic pancreatitis or tumor, including malignant degeneration, may occur in these ectopic tissues.

Aberrant pancreatic tissues many times give rise to rather bizarre symptoms. They may be the cause of pyloric obstruction or of ulceration when developing in the stomach, or of intussusception when lodged in the intestine, especially in a diverticulum. With a predominance of islet tissue, signs and symptoms of an islet cell tumor may try the ingenuity of the clinician and surgeon, who must search all the common areas of aberrant tissue for the islet tumor if it is not found in the pancreas proper.

In the rare anomaly known as *annular pancreas,* the head of the gland surrounds the second portion of the duodenum (see also page 28). It is more common in males than in females, and all grades from an overlapping of the posterior duodenal wall to a complete ring may be found. If the ring is incomplete, the defect is always on the anterior surface of the duodenum. The pancreatic duct in the annular tissue arises anteriorly and courses laterally to the right and around the duodenum to its posterior wall, terminating in the main pancreatic duct, the common bile duct or the papilla of Vater. The origin of this anomaly rests with a failure of the ventral anlage of the pancreas (see page 25) to migrate normally to the left behind the duodenum.

Annular pancreas may be associated with a complete or partial atresia of the duodenum. The annular portion of the pancreas may fall heir to any of the diseases of the pancreas, such as acute or chronic pancreatitis or tumor. Complete or partial obstruction of the duodenum, with dilatation of the proximal portion and the stomach, is to be expected. Secondary ulceration of the duodenum or stomach, not rare with this anomaly, may lead to the discovery of the lesion. Surgery is, of course, the only treatment of this condition. In view of the inherent complications and the possibility of the existence of a duodenal atresia, some authors recommend gastro-enterostomy or duodeno-duodenal anastomosis around the obstruction in all cases, rather than section of the annular pancreas.

Abnormalities in fusion of the anlage of the gland may result in all degrees of division of the gland, including the presence of two separate glands with individual ducts to the duodenum, known as pancreas divisum. Other anomalies of the gland are extremely rare.

Congenital Cystic Disease

Fibrocystic disease of the pancreas is a genetically determined (recessive gene of both parents?) disease, with no preponderance for sex. Its incidence is approximately 1 in 4 siblings and lies between 1:1000 and 1:10,000 in the total population. Although most attention has been focused on the pancreas and the pulmonary complications, it is a general disease involving all mucus-producing organs, primarily of the alimentary and respiratory tracts. The manifestations of this disease are extremely variable, but the history almost always goes back to early infancy. Death usually occurs in infancy or early childhood, although an occasional patient with mild disease now survives to maturity. In about 20 per cent of the cases, impacted *meconium* causes an intestinal *obstruction* which necessitates ileostomy, at which operation usually a collapsed and empty colon and distended edematous, dark-red, small intestine are encountered. The latter is filled with tenacious, gluelike meconium, which is apparently produced by excessive mucoid secretion of the mucosal cells and which is very difficult to remove by milking or irrigating. If this complication does not occur or if the patient survives this emergency, the patient is found to be underweight or loses weight despite a good or even a ravenous appetite, and the stools will be bulky, fatty and usually with an offensive odor (see also page 57), accentuated by infections. The failure to thrive becomes obvious by the second year of life at the latest. *Abdominal distention* is typical of those patients who survive beyond a few months but is not invariably present, and medical attention is first enlisted usually for acute respiratory infections (bronchitis, bronchiolitis and pneumonitis), which, once they start, recur with increasing residual disability after each attack. Emphysema, chronic pneumonitis, pulmonary fibrosis with reduced respiratory volume, clubbing of fingers, right ventricular stress and, finally, cardiac failure (cor pulmonale) result. The *bronchiectasis* is distinct from the ordinary type, because the dilatation involves the bronchioles and only the most peripheral bronchi. The scant sputum is thick, viscid and mucoid or mucopurulent. The pulmonary disease is the usual cause of death in those children who survive beyond infancy.

Thick, viscid, mucoid material containing little or no trypsin, as obtained

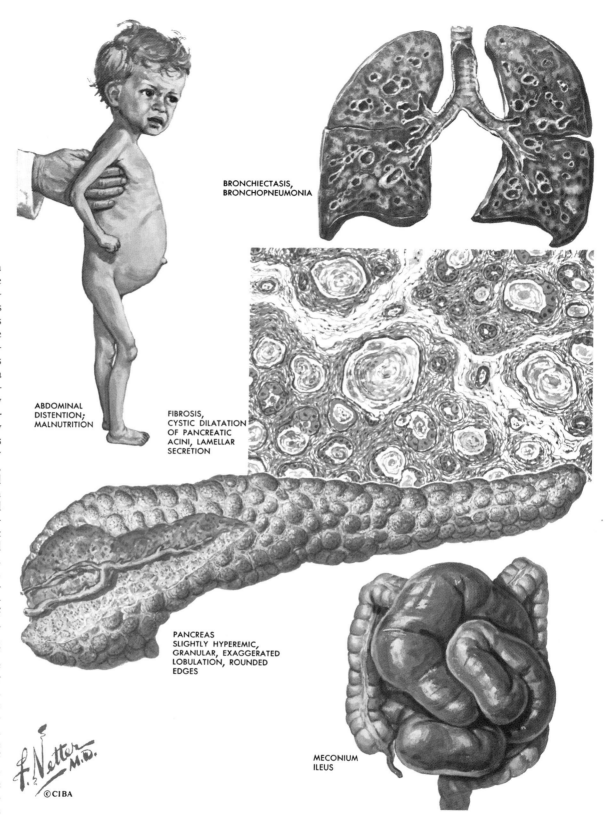

BRONCHIECTASIS, BRONCHOPNEUMONIA

FIBROSIS, CYSTIC DILATATION OF PANCREATIC ACINI, LAMELLAR SECRETION

ABDOMINAL DISTENTION; MALNUTRITION

PANCREAS SLIGHTLY HYPEREMIC, GRANULAR, EXAGGERATED LOBULATION, ROUNDED EDGES

MECONIUM ILEUS

by duodenal drainage, confirms the diagnosis. Determination of fecal trypsin is less dependable.

The pathologic findings at autopsy depend upon the age. They vary from moderate abnormalities in the infant to advanced alterations in the older children. The somewhat lengthened and thinned, *slightly hyperemic pancreas* has a fine *granular appearance.* Its *edges* are *rounded,* and the demarcations between head, body and tail are poorly defined. Cystlike structures can be discerned in the fibrotic substance of the gland. In the early stages the mucus-containing ductules are dilated, and the lobules are atrophied to various degrees. In time the dilatation of ductules and acini, the fibrosis of the interlobular tissue, the flattening of the cells lining the acini and the lamination of the mucoid secretion progress. Ultimately, fatty infiltration results. In the younger children the islets are essentially normal but decrease in number the

longer the child survives. The salivary glands are also affected and produce a viscid mucus which plugs the ducts. Local fibrosis is seen in the liver. A small gallbladder or atrophy and obstruction of the cystic duct are frequently noted. Little more than increased mucus formation is seen in the respiratory tract in the very early stages. Emphysema, areas of pneumonitis, peribronchial inflammation and large quantities of viscid mucus in trachea, bronchi and the dilated bronchioli (tubular type of bronchiectasis) are characteristic of the later stages. Fibrosis of the parenchyma and peribronchiolar tissue develops after numerous pulmonary episodes.

Treatment is directed toward the control of the pulmonary infections (antibiotics) and dietary measures to improve nutrition (high-caloric, high-protein, low-fat diet, vitamins and pancreatic enzymes), but it can, at best, only prolong life.

ACUTE PANCREATITIS

In the *earliest* and mildest *stage* of *acute pancreatitis*, the gland, or portions of it, is *edematous* and pale, with increased prominence of the lobulations and other signs of an acute inflammatory process, such as *congested* vessels. The microscopic structure of the gland, except for the presence of the interstitial fluid accumulation and small cell infiltration, is preserved. The patients complain of epigastric pain, which may radiate to the back, and some tenderness of the epigastric region and muscular resistance may be found. This stage may clear completely but may recur with more severe symptoms and damage to the pancreas. When the process progresses — usually rapidly — to *acute hemorrhagic pancreatitis*, the patients become severely ill, with excruciating pain radiating to the back, and spasm or even boardlike rigidity of the abdomen. Shock is either obvious or insidious. Ileus is common. The gland is grossly inflamed. Hemorrhagic areas alternate with necrotic ones, and complete disruption of the organ can occur. The peritoneal cavity contains bloody fluid. Zones of fat necrosis are spread over the adjacent peritoneum or wherever fat is deposited. The entire gland may slough and may be replaced by liquefied, purulent debris. Large *abscesses* may form, or nothing else than a *gangrenous* mass may be left. Where the process remains localized and if the patient survives, the liquefied necrotic parts may be transformed to cysts. Persisting pain, nausea, vomiting, abdominal tenderness, spasms and ileus dominate the clinical picture during this stage. Edema in the flank and bluish peri-umbilical discoloration due to blood extravasation have been described, but these signs are not specific for acute pancreatitis. The laboratory findings have been discussed on pages 56 and 58. Hypocalcemia and hypokalemia are frequent findings with severe pancreatitis and fat necrosis. Diabetes may become evident during the acute phase, and permanent if patients with necrosis of the gland survive. Edema occluding the common bile duct or, in later phases, scar tissue may cause jaundice. Splenic vein thrombosis and severe hemorrhage with immediate death have been reported as concurrent events. Late complications of acute pancreatitis include abscesses, cysts (see page 145) and fistulae.

Much has been speculated about the causative mechanisms of acute pancreatitis. The anatomic situation at the choledochoduodenal junction, which may make bile regurgitation possible (see pages 24 and 27), the impaction of a stone in the ampulla, spasms of the sphincter of Oddi, obstruction of the

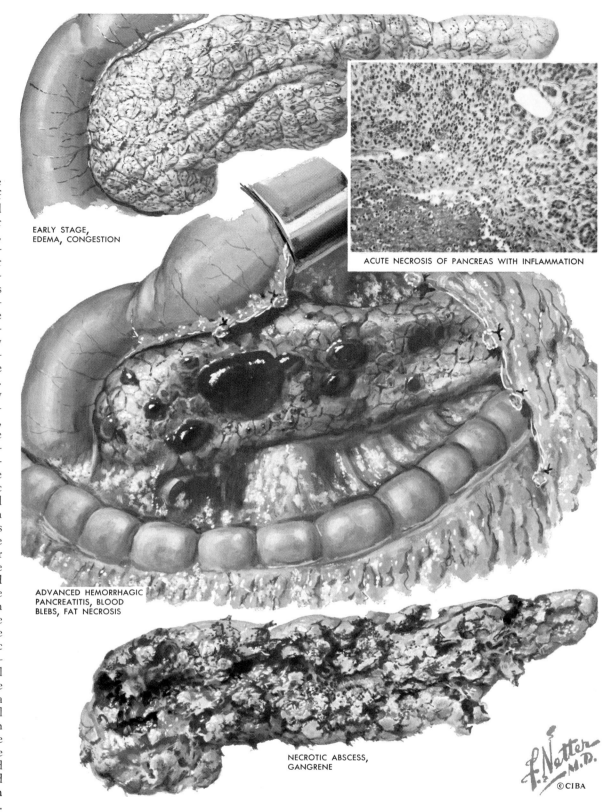

EARLY STAGE, EDEMA, CONGESTION

ACUTE NECROSIS OF PANCREAS WITH INFLAMMATION

ADVANCED HEMORRHAGIC PANCREATITIS, BLOOD BLEBS, FAT NECROSIS

NECROTIC ABSCESS, GANGRENE

pancreatic ducts, especially by epithelial hyperplasia, and vascular spasm have all been implicated as etiologic factors, but so many cases of acute pancreatitis have been carefully examined without detecting any of these conditions that it is difficult to accept them generally as prime movers for this disease. External as well as surgical trauma, especially resection of duodenal ulcers perforating into the pancreas and operative manipulation of the common duct, have frequently been followed by acute pancreatitis. Other observations point to the fact that bouts of alcohol ingestion or a very heavy meal may elicit acute attacks of pancreatitis, a possibility which cannot be denied in view of the acute duodenitis and consecutive sphincter spasm which may follow overindulgence with alcohol and in view of the increased secretin production after heavy meals and its effect on the pancreas (see page 55). Actual infection may be responsible, with inflam-

matory involvement of the duodenum either by direct reflux through the ducts or by the lymphatic connections (see page 30).

With shock in the clinical foreground in acute pancreatitis, fluid and protein replacement becomes mandatory. Since narcotics are of little help (morphine may even aggravate the sphincter spasms), more drastic measures (block of the sympathicus or of the celiac ganglia, epidural analgesia) may be necessary to relieve the pain. Parasympatholytic drugs (spasmolytica) and antibiotics may be tried to inhibit pancreatic secretion and spasms or to control infection, respectively. The presence of diabetes, hypocalcemia, hypokalemia and, particularly, of an ileus requires appropriate measures. Splanchnic nerve or vagus resection or operation for pseudocysts may be indicated if the attack is prolonged, as may be abscess drainage in the early stage.

CHRONIC (RELAPSING) PANCREATITIS

The characteristic sign of chronic pancreatitis, better described as relapsing pancreatitis, is an epigastric pain, with radiation to one or both upper abdominal quadrants and to the back and, in the early stages, very similar to the pain typical of recurrent mild, moderate or even severe acute pancreatitis (see page 143). In later stages the pain becomes more and more persistent. Ingestion of any food may provoke an attack with nausea and vomiting, so that it is not surprising that patients with relapsing pancreatitis become seriously malnourished. In addition, pancreatic secretion is gradually lost, and digestion of fats and proteins suffers, with steatorrhea and a negative nitrogen balance as natural sequelae (see pages 57 and 58). All kinds of gastrointestinal manifestations may emerge. Jaundice may result from a common duct obstruction by the developing pancreatic fibrosis. Diabetes is a late manifestation. Portal hypertension and liver cirrhosis might complicate the course of the disease when a progressing fibrosis seizes the adjacent veins.

The pathologic picture of the gland depends much upon the duration and frequency of the recurrent attacks. The *gland* may be moderately and only partly *involved,* or a *complete fibrosis* of a pale, gray-white, hard or rubbery pancreas may present itself. Within the fibrotic gland may be disseminated some irregular *calcifications* as well as *multiple cysts,* which owe their existence to *obstruction* and *dilatation* of smaller *ducts* at a time when the acini have not yet ceased to function. In the later stages the fibrosis may embrace the common duct with consequences comparable to those after ampullary carcinoma (see page 137) or carcinoma of the pancreas head (see page 148). In the mild cases one sees microscopically interstitial fibrosis and infiltrating inflammatory cells, while islets and acini seem normal in number and appearance. In more advanced cases the acini have disappeared, and a dense fibrous tissue with clustered inflammatory cells surrounds the small ducts and nests of islet cells. If localized, this picture is sometimes difficult to distinguish from scirrhous carcinoma and may lead to a mistaken diagnosis. In still more advanced stages, calcification may have increased, only few islets and only an occasional small cyst remaining; the fibrosis extends to the surrounding structure, especially to the retroperitoneal areolar tissue, and fistulae may have formed. The extension beyond the gland explains the persistent

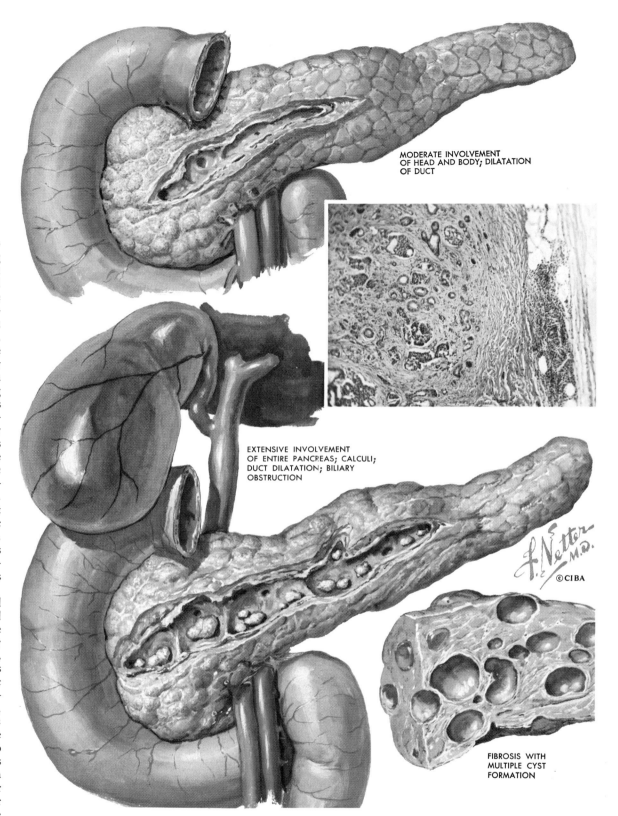

MODERATE INVOLVEMENT OF HEAD AND BODY; DILATATION OF DUCT

EXTENSIVE INVOLVEMENT OF ENTIRE PANCREAS; CALCULI; DUCT DILATATION; BILIARY OBSTRUCTION

FIBROSIS WITH MULTIPLE CYST FORMATION

pain, the complications mentioned and the difficulty in performing pancreatectomy in these patients.

The etiologic mechanism of recurrent pancreatitis is the same as with acute pancreatitis (see page 143) and is as problematic and controversial. Alcoholism is a probable etiologic factor and is said to be disclosed in the history of one third to one half of the cases. During early stages recurrent attacks may be prevented by complete abstinence from alcohol, a bland diet and parasympathetic inhibitors. A great number of operative procedures have been suggested to relieve the pain and the serious sequelae of repeated exacerbations. They run from nerve blocks, splanchnicectomy, celiac ganglionectomy and vagotomy to the formidable procedure of a total pancreatectomy. The neurologic interventions do not prevent further advance of the disease. With the process localized to the head of the pancreas, pancreatoduodenectomy has

offered relief. When an obstruction lies proximal in the main duct, resection of the tail with anastomosis of the proximal end and its duct to the jejunum, giving free drainage to the distal part of the duct, appears logical and has been successful. On the theory that the process is secondary to the obstruction of the main pancreatic duct or of a common channel at the papilla of Vater (see page 24), sphincterectomy has been used with some success, as has also reimplantation of the pancreatic or common bile duct into the jejunum or duodenum. To prevent the hormonal stimulation by secretin and irritation which may cause spasms of the sphincter, partial gastrectomy or pyloric exclusion has been advised, but these measures have not become popular for pancreatic disease without associated gastric or duodenal ulcer. Recently, radiation therapy has been suggested on the basis of its inhibition of secretory function.

Cysts

Cysts of the pancreas are of two types — true cysts and pseudocysts. Both may be either *unilocular* or *multilocular,* although the latter is more common with true cysts.

True cysts may be congenital or acquired. Pseudocysts are always acquired. The former arise from within the substance of the gland, most frequently in the head, and then in the body and tail, in that order. True cysts are distinguished by the presence of lining epithelium, which, however, may be lost with inflammation, making them microscopically indistinguishable from pseudocysts. In practice, the presence of pancreatic enzymes or continuity with a pancreatic duct is considered to indicate a true cyst. To examine for *amylase* the starch-iodine test is used, and the presence of *trypsin* is simply determined by digestion of the gelatin emulsion of a photographic plate.

Pseudocysts result from injuries to the gland or from necroses of acute pancreatitis (see page 143). Peripancreatic collections of pancreatic juice, blood and necrotic debris become encapsulated. Because of the high protein content, osmotic pressure draws more fluid into the cysts which increase in size, and the encapsulating layer is thickened by flattening of adjacent tissues as the cyst expands.

Except for an occasional cyst which gives pain, continuous or intermittent, pancreatic cysts produce few symptoms until they reach large size and become apparent visually or by palpation, or cause symptoms by pressure on other organs. Both types of cysts may protrude in any direction. Pseudocysts most commonly present through the *gastrohepatic (lesser) omentum* in the epigastrium, because leakage from the acutely inflamed or injured organ into the lesser sac occurs easily in view of the broad contact the sac has with the anterior pancreatic surface (see page 28). Other routes of presentation are through the *gastrocolic (greater) omentum,* through the layers of the *mesentery of the colon, below the transverse colon* into the *main peritoneal cavity* and into the *retroperitoneal space* downward and upward behind the left flank of the pancreas tail. True cysts are more common in the head and body and often present somewhat lower than the pseudocysts, through the gastrocolic omentum into the transverse mesocolon or the free peritoneal cavity.

X-ray examination is very helpful in arriving at the diagnosis of pancreatic cyst, because adjacent viscera, stomach and colon are often indented by a smooth

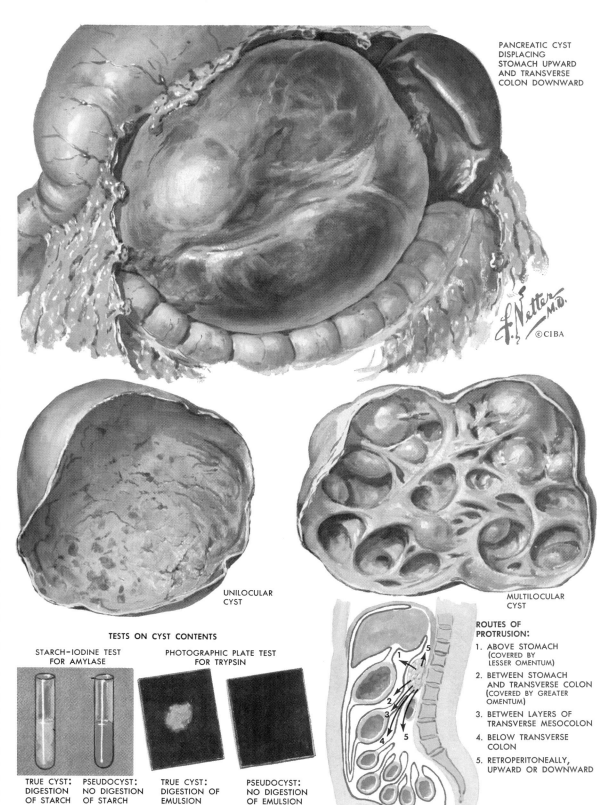

PANCREATIC CYST DISPLACING STOMACH UPWARD AND TRANSVERSE COLON DOWNWARD

UNILOCULAR CYST

MULTILOCULAR CYST

TESTS ON CYST CONTENTS

STARCH–IODINE TEST FOR AMYLASE

PHOTOGRAPHIC PLATE TEST FOR TRYPSIN

TRUE CYST: DIGESTION OF STARCH

PSEUDOCYST: NO DIGESTION OF STARCH

TRUE CYST: DIGESTION OF EMULSION

PSEUDOCYST: NO DIGESTION OF EMULSION

ROUTES OF PROTRUSION:

1. ABOVE STOMACH (COVERED BY LESSER OMENTUM)
2. BETWEEN STOMACH AND TRANSVERSE COLON (COVERED BY GREATER OMENTUM)
3. BETWEEN LAYERS OF TRANSVERSE MESOCOLON
4. BELOW TRANSVERSE COLON
5. RETROPERITONEALLY, UPWARD OR DOWNWARD

rounded mass, pushing the viscus anteriorly and superiorly, inferiorly or laterally, depending upon the position of the cyst. In cysts of the tail, the kidney or spleen may be displaced downward or laterally.

Simple cysts of the pancreas are usually unilocular and surrounded by a thin fibrous tissue capsule, containing a mostly watery fluid which is xanthochromic or brown-colored from old blood or necrotic tissue. True cysts may have thicker walls, at least near the base, arising from the substance of the gland, and the walls may contain pancreatic tissue. Multilocular cysts are distinguished from cystadenomas by the thinner fibrous tissue walls and by their greater uniformity and larger size.

Laparotomy, excision or marsupialization of the cyst's wall is the only treatment. With pseudocysts this may result in complete cure, while a true cyst is replaced by a fistula in most cases, which causes irrita-

tion of the skin and constant drainage. If the cyst is connected with a large duct with proximal obstruction, severe electrolyte imbalance may develop; thus, cystenterostomy has become a favorite surgical technique, because it allows adequate drainage of the pancreatic juice into the bowel. However, the anastomosis may stenose, resulting in a recurrence of the cyst, and, where feasible, complete excision of the cyst and closure of the fistula is considered the procedure of choice. Occasionally, partial pancreatectomy with the cyst may be necessary.

Echinococcus cysts (see also page 104) may occur in the pancreas. They are typically multilocular, with mother and daughter cysts. Calcification may be present. In these lesions complete excision without spillage must be the treatment, to prevent spread of the disease or a severe anaphylactic reaction.

Dermoid cysts are rarely found in the pancreas.

BENIGN TUMORS

Benign tumors of the pancreas are islet cell tumors, cystadenoma, duct cell adenoma, and other infrequent solid tumors. *Islet cell tumors* are the most frequent benign tumors and clinically are the most fascinating because of the development of hyperinsulinism. Hyperinsulinism is present in over 50 per cent of the cases reported and in practically all of those operated upon. The tumors are small, usually 1 to 2 cm. in diameter, ranging from 1 mm. to 15 cm. in size. They may be multiple and may develop in the sites typical for ectopic pancreatic tissue (see page 141). About 80 per cent of islet tumors are benign. Their *microscopic architecture* is the same as that of normal islets (see page 26). Clusters of pale cuboidal to columnar cells with spherical to ovoid nuclei form solid masses, or the cells are arranged in strands or around a small lumen. In hyperfunctioning tumors most of the cells are beta cells. Only about 10 per cent of the islet cell tumors are histologically malignant (see page 147), but these act as if they were benign tumors. The tumors are darker than the surrounding pancreas, are usually umbilicated when on the surface and have a strong vascular supply. The completely benign tumors are well encapsulated, but some of those that are histologically malignant may be poorly encapsulated.

Insulin shock, particularly in a fasting state or with exertion, is the most typical symptom of a functioning islet cell tumor. Psychic disturbances, such as amnesia, confusion, or even mania or coma, are common. Dizziness, nausea and vomiting and signs of shock almost always characterize the history of patients with an islet tumor, and hypoglycemic convulsions are not rare. Blood sugar levels below 50 mg. per cent are significant and confirm the diagnosis, which should be suspected whenever recurrent attacks, as described, are reported. Further confirmation is obtained when the attacks improve with glucose administration and when other conditions which may cause hypoglycemia, responsive to glucose administration (*e.g.,* Addison's disease), can be excluded. The glucose tolerance curve is abnormal, with a slow rise and a peak at about 2 hours, rather than at the normal 30 minutes.

Since a surprisingly high number of these tumors are found in the tail, the exploration for excision is usually begun here. Tumors a few millimeters in diameter have been symptomatic and may not be found in the depth of the gland. Under such circumstances and after exploration of the common sites of aberrant pancreatic tissue, partial pancreatectomy may be performed if the diagnosis seems sure. But even then the tumor may not be removed, and subsequent exploration may become necessary. In some cases more than one hyperfunctioning islet cell tumor may be present, and a few cases of general islet hypertrophy have been reported.

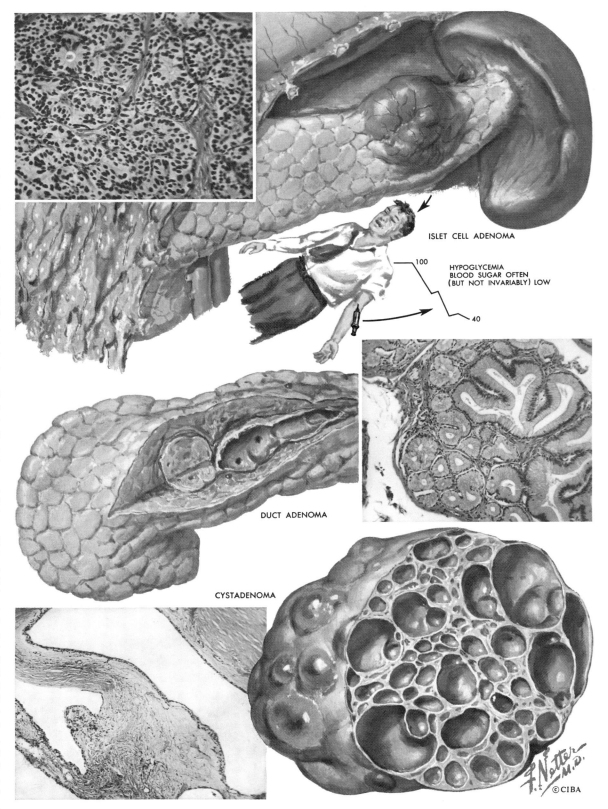

ISLET CELL ADENOMA

HYPOGLYCEMIA
BLOOD SUGAR OFTEN
(BUT NOT INVARIABLY) LOW

DUCT ADENOMA

CYSTADENOMA

Recently, symptoms and signs of intractable peptic ulceration* have been attributed to islet cell tumors of the alpha cell type.

Other benign solid tumors of the pancreas include *duct cell* or acinar cell *adenomas* which may develop in the main pancreatic duct, *causing obstruction.* Microscopically, one sees well-formed glands lined by one or more layers of columnar or cuboidal cells, with occasional goblet cells. These tumors may sometimes be responsible for the appearance of an acute pancreatitis.

Papillomas of the ducts are not uncommon but usually are found in the region of the ampulla (see page 137). They may cause obstruction of both the pancreatic and bile ducts. Other benign solid tumors are very rare.

Cystadenoma is the other common benign tumor of the pancreas. Nine out of ten are found in women. They are coarsely lobulated cystic tumors, generally rounded, with a translucent capsule. They vary in size from 2 to 15 cm. in reported cases. When transected they have an irregular honeycombed appearance, with many cystic spaces varying from microscopic size to more than 1 cm. in diameter in some cases. The fluid is clear, yellow to brown in color and may be mucinous. In general, the cyst walls are thicker and more meaty than the thin membranes between multilocular cysts (see page 145). The cysts are lined by flattened, cuboidal or columnar epithelium. The septa are composed of fibrinous, fibrous or gelatinous stroma, sometimes containing hyalinized areas. Papillary projections into the cystic spaces may occur, but such papillary overgrowth must make one suspicious of malignant change (see page 147).

---

*Characteristic of the Ellison-Zollinger syndrome (see CIBA COLLECTION, Vol. 3/1, page 88; Vol. 3/11, page 99, and Vol. 4).

MALIGNANT TUMORS I

Cystadenocarcinoma, Islet Cell Carcinoma

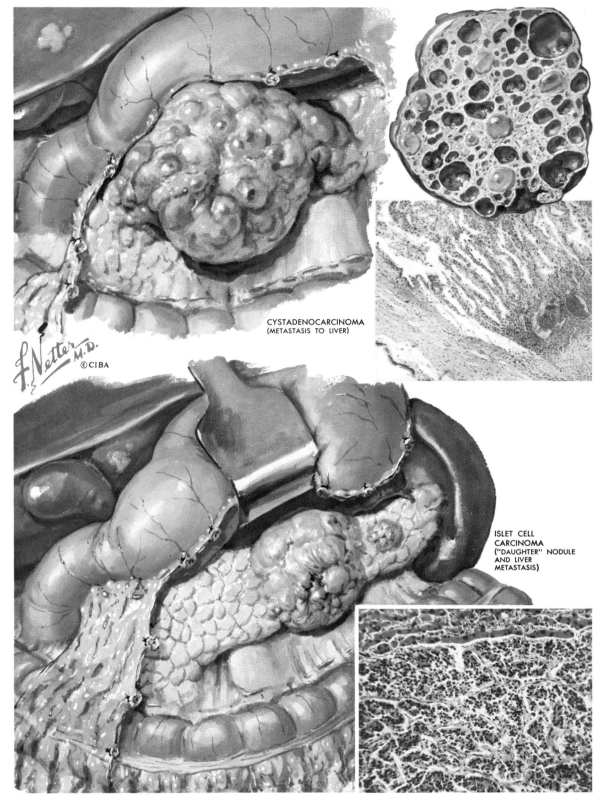

CYSTADENOCARCINOMA
(METASTASIS TO LIVER)

ISLET CELL
CARCINOMA
("DAUGHTER" NODULE
AND LIVER
METASTASIS)

Malignant tumors of the pancreas are not rare, making up over 2 per cent of all reported malignant tumors (Connecticut State Tumor Registry). These include acinar or duct cell carcinoma (see page 148), cystadenocarcinoma, islet cell carcinoma and sarcomas of the pancreas.

Cystadenocarcinoma is not a distinct pathologic entity, since it is difficult to differentiate it from carcinoma arising in a true cyst or cystic degeneration of a solid carcinoma. The adenocarcinoma is an irregular, lobulated cystic tumor, which is blue-red in color. On cross section it appears multiloculated, of irregular size and shape with a thick cellular wall. Papillary infoldings are common and are typical of malignant change, although some papillary projections may occur in benign cystadenomas (see page 146). *Microscopic section* discloses the cellular nature of the tumor, with striking papillary infolding of the tumor lining of the cyst and invasion of the fibrous wall by tumor cells. Solid masses of tumor cells may also be seen, as well as cystic structures lined by irregularly shaped tumor cells. *Metastases* arise most commonly in the lymph nodes and *liver* and, less often and much later, in more distant organs. (The slide illustrated is taken from a liver metastasis.)

The symptoms are those of an increasing tumor mass in the region of the pancreas, with pressure on other organs. The development and growth from benign cystadenoma may be relatively slow, with case histories of known duration of several years not being very uncommon. Several have been reported to develop in a previously marsupialized benign cystic lesion of the pancreas.

Sarcoma of the pancreas (not illustrated) is a rare lesion. It is seen predominantly in children and young adults and may reach a very large size, with local extension, before symptoms or metastases occur. Though carcinomas have been

rarely encountered in children, a malignant tumor of the pancreas in a child can be expected to be a sarcoma. Primary lymphosarcoma, fibrosarcoma and neurogenic sarcoma have also been reported.

Islet cell tumors (see also page 146) are definitely *malignant* in about 10 per cent of the cases and questionably malignant in another 10 per cent. Clinical behavior and appearance of metastases are determining factors in those cases which are questionably malignant or only microscopically malignant. Like the benign islet cell tumors, malignant tumors of this type are relatively more frequent in the tail and body than in the head and are not well encapsulated. *Daughter nodules* in the pancreas itself and metastases, most commonly to the liver or to the lymph nodes and to distant organs, may develop. The questionably malignant lesion shows irregularity of the cells, mitoses and invasion of the capsule, just as do

the proven malignant adenomas. The metastatic nodules in truly malignant islet tumors are often more cellular than the primary, with little tendency toward normal islet cell patterns. (The microscopic section is taken from a metastasis in the liver.)

Hypoglycemia occurs with malignant as well as benign islet cell tumors. Even if the primary tumor is removed, the metastasis will continue to secrete insulin. The cells are poorly radiosensitive, so that radiation therapy has not been successful. Rarely, patients with this type of malignant tumor gain in weight, in contrast to the situation with most malignant tumors, but this weight gain is due to the patient's tendency to overeat out of fear of the hypoglycemic reactions.

Both cystadenocarcinoma and malignant islet cell tumors are slow-growing, by comparison with carcinoma of the pancreas.

MALIGNANT TUMORS II

Carcinoma, Gross Pathology and Clinical Features

Carcinoma of the pancreas is one of the malignant tumors which is most difficult to diagnose and, therefore, usually poorly treated. About 4 per cent of all cancer deaths are due to malignant tumors of the pancreas. The most common site is the *head* where over 40 per cent of the cancers are found. About 20 per cent are diffuse, and the remaining 40 per cent are found in the body and *tail*. A statistically significant preponderance has been found in males, in most series 2:1 or more. The average age of diagnosis is about 55 years.

Except for those lesions arising close to the ampulla or common duct (see page 137), the symptoms of pancreatic carcinoma make their appearance late. The most common symptom is pain, which occurs in about 85 per cent of the cases. Weight loss occurs before the diagnosis is made in about the same percentage, and this weight loss is frequently extreme. Painless jaundice, commonly considered the symptom leading to the diagnosis of carcinoma of the pancreas, is rather seldom a primary sign. As a matter of fact, jaundice, with or without pain, appears in fewer cases before diagnosis is made than do pain and weight loss. Anorexia, present in over half of the patients and mostly associated with nausea and vomiting, is a probable explanation for much of the weight loss. Changes in the stools, with diarrhea or large, bulky stools containing much undigested fat, are fairly characteristic of those patients whose pancreatic duct is obstructed (see page 57). The pain, which may be colicky or intermittent in type, is much the same as with biliary disease (see page 134), including the radiation to the subcapsular areas. It may also radiate diffusely to the back, abdomen or, in paroxysms, to the chest, or it may be a dull, steady aching pain in the midepigastrium boring through to the back, a pain which has been unduly stressed as being typical of pancreatic disease.

Definitive diagnosis before operation is difficult. The presence of jaundice and of a palpable mass pointing to a *dilated gallbladder* is strongly suggestive of carcinoma of the head of the pancreas, major papilla or common duct (Courvoisier's law) (see page 137). The liver may be enlarged in such cases of *common bile duct obstruction* or because of tumor or metastases, but hepatomegaly does not necessarily indicate metastases and is not a sign of inoperability. The pancreatic mass itself is rarely palpable, except in very late cases. A cyst or pancreatitis may occur behind the neoplastic obstruction of the duct. X-ray diagnosis rests upon

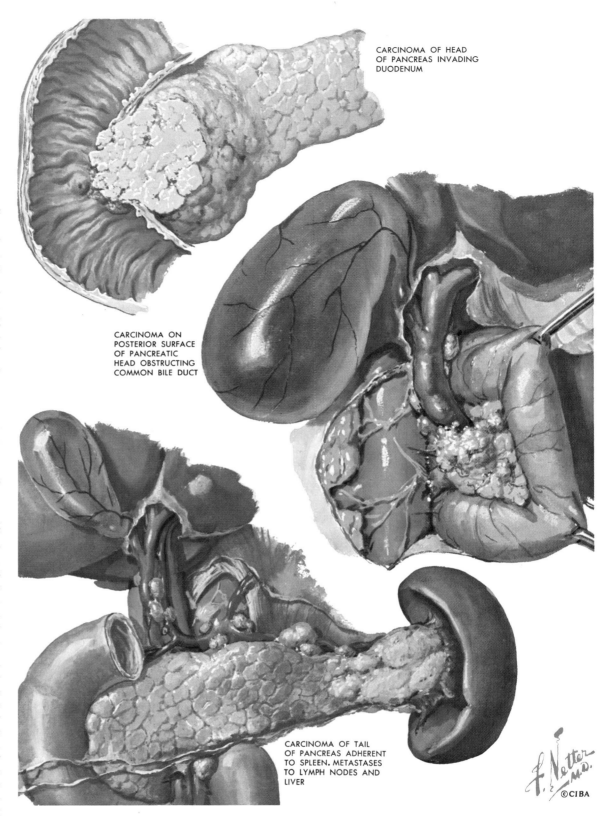

CARCINOMA OF HEAD OF PANCREAS INVADING DUODENUM

CARCINOMA ON POSTERIOR SURFACE OF PANCREATIC HEAD OBSTRUCTING COMMON BILE DUCT

CARCINOMA OF TAIL OF PANCREAS ADHERENT TO SPLEEN. METASTASES TO LYMPH NODES AND LIVER

distortions of adjacent organs which can be visualized, concerning mostly the duodenum and occasionally the gallbladder, stomach or colon. Widening of the duodenal loop has been reported as the diagnostic X-ray sign for a pancreatic tumor, but it is rarely seen in operable lesions. Invasion of the wall of the duodenum or stomach may be visualized as deformities, *e.g.*, an inverted S type of duodenal deformity. Duodenal drainage (see pages 53 and 58), though not often applied, is of particular value for differential diagnosis. With obstruction of the pancreatic ducts, pancreatic enzymes will be absent, or present in only small amounts (see page 57). Cellular cytologic studies may reveal malignant cells, especially in those lesions involving the main ducts.

Even at operation the establishment of the diagnosis of carcinoma may not be easy in early cases. The cancer is ordinarily hard and pale and causes enlargement of the gland, but these features may also be conspicuous in chronic pancreatitis (see page 144). Biopsy will frequently show only chronic pancreatitis in the surrounding tissue, which cannot be distinguished by palpation from the tumor itself. In many instances, resection without a positive pathologic diagnosis will be justified and proved correct, especially if the pancreatic duct distal to the tumor is dilated and if the common bile duct is obstructed.

The only treatment presently available is resectional surgery, but this too is limited because of frequent extension along the pancreatic or common bile ducts, early lymphatic extension in widely separated areas (see page 149) and perineural spread. Despite the difficulties in diagnosis and the extensive surgery involved, 5-year cures of carcinoma of the pancreas are now being reported more frequently than in former years.

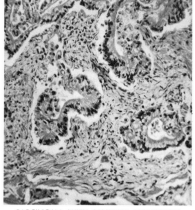

MEDULLARY CARCINOMA

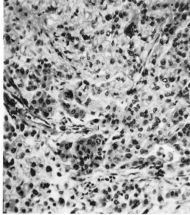

CARCINOMA WITH DUCTLIKE STRUCTURES

ANAPLASTIC CARCINOMA

MALIGNANT TUMORS III

Histology, Metastases

Carcinoma of the pancreas varies a great deal on pathologic examination. It may be a small, localized tumor completely obstructing the common bile and pancreatic ducts, or it may be a large, pale-white, hard tumor mass, filling much of the head (see page 148) of the pancreas but still remaining well localized. When discovered, those in the body and tail are usually extensive, with peritoneal involvement and extension to other sites. Because of the close contact with the duodenum and the lymphatic connection (see page 30), invasion of the duodenum with large tumors is so common that it may be impossible to determine which was the primary site. Extension via the perineural lymphatics occurs early and may partially explain the early appearance of pain in carcinoma of the pancreas. The extensive lymphatic drainage and its quick involvement by the cancer explains, at least in part, the difficulty in obtaining cure by feasible extent of resection. *Extension* beyond the peripancreatic lymphatics involves the regional nodes along the common duct, the peri-aortic nodes, the liver and, via the gastric nodes, the mediastinum and neck. *Direct spread* also takes place to the stomach, colon, spleen and kidney, and erosion through the surface of the gland and overlying peritoneum permits seeding of either the lesser or general peritoneal cavities. The pancreatic ducts are the most frequent site of origin of the cancer, which explains the increased occurrence of the disease in the head and the frequent obstruction of the main duct even by small tumors.

Microscopically, the pancreatic malignant tumors are primarily adenocarcinomas of several types. Epidermoid carcinoma does occur as a primary tumor in the pancreas, but it is rare. *Medullary carcinoma* grows in solid sheets and banks of cells, arranged in a haphazard manner but rather uniform in size, shape and staining quality. In some areas they form ill-defined acini. The well-differentiated *duct cell carcinoma* grows as irregular ductlike or glandular structures formed by one or more layers of cuboidal

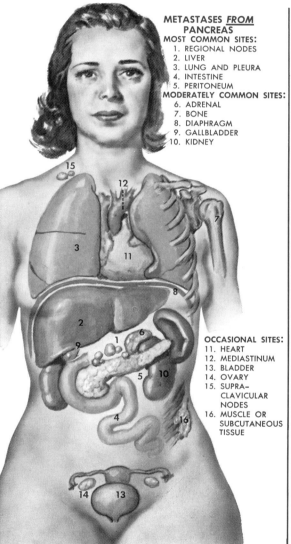

METASTASES *FROM* PANCREAS
MOST COMMON SITES:
1. REGIONAL NODES
2. LIVER
3. LUNG AND PLEURA
4. INTESTINE
5. PERITONEUM
MODERATELY COMMON SITES:
6. ADRENAL
7. BONE
8. DIAPHRAGM
9. GALLBLADDER
10. KIDNEY

OCCASIONAL SITES:
11. HEART
12. MEDIASTINUM
13. BLADDER
14. OVARY
15. SUPRA-
    CLAVICULAR
    NODES
16. MUSCLE OR
    SUBCUTANEOUS
    TISSUE

METASTASES *TO* PANCREAS
COMMON SOURCES:
1. LUNG
2. BREAST
3. THYROID
4. KIDNEY
5. MELANOMA (SKIN)
OCCASIONAL SOURCES:
6. OVARY
7. UTERUS
8. PAROTID GLAND
9. PROSTATE

DIRECT EXTENSION:
10. STOMACH
11. KIDNEY
12. COLON
13. LYMPH NODES
14. DUODENUM
15. COMMON
    BILE DUCT
16. ADRENAL

or columnar cells, separated by abundant fibrous tissue. At times, these may be difficult to distinguish from chronic pancreatitis (see page 144). *Anaplastic carcinoma,* as is characteristic of this type in other organs, is made up of irregular masses of cells which vary considerably in size, shape and staining qualities. The nuclei are usually hyperchromatic, with large nucleoli and frequent mitoses. The cytoplasm is abundant, eosinophilic and, in some cases, vacuolated.

Metastases from carcinoma of the pancreas to distant organs other than by lymphatic spread are, in order of frequency, the liver, lungs, intestine, suprarenal, bone, diaphragm, gallbladder, kidney, heart, mediastinum, bladder, ovary and muscle, skin or subcutaneous tissue.

Metastatic carcinoma to the pancreas from other organs has received little attention. It does occur with some frequency and, at times, may cause difficulty in

differential diagnosis between primary and metastatic cancer. The lung is the most common source of primary carcinoma, and here we have a particularly difficult differential diagnosis, because anaplastic carcinoma is found in both organs. Metastatic melanoma is next in frequency, then breast, kidney, thyroid, ovary, uterus, prostate and, perhaps, parotid gland carcinoma. Metastatic sarcoma is also encountered.

The pancreas is frequently invaded by direct extension of a carcinoma in the stomach, kidney, colon, duodenum, the major papilla and the common bile duct, in which case the original tumor may actually arise in an intrapancreatic position. Lymphatic tumors, such as Hodgkin's disease or lymphoma, involving the regional lymph nodes, may also extend directly into the pancreas. These instances of direct extension can be easily understood from the topographic relations of the organ (see page 28).

REFERENCES

General References

BELL, E. T.: *A Textbook of Pathology*, Lea and Febiger, Philadelphia, 1952.

BOYD, W.: *Textbook of Pathology*, Lea and Febiger, Philadelphia, 1954.

CECIL, R. L., AND LOEB: *Textbook of Medicine*, W. B. Saunders Company, Philadelphia, 1955.

GRAY, H.: *Anatomy of the Human Body*, Lea and Febiger, Philadelphia, 1948.

HARRISON, T. R., ADAMS, BEESON, RESNIK, THORN AND WINTROBE: *Principles of Internal Medicine*, The Blakiston Company, New York, 1954.

LICHTMAN, S. S.: *Diseases of the Liver, Gallbladder and Bile Ducts*, Lea and Febiger, Philadelphia, 1949.

POPPER, H., AND SCHAFFNER: *Liver; Structure and Function*, Blakiston Division of McGraw-Hill Book Company, New York, 1957.

SCHIFF, L.: *Diseases of the Liver*, J. B. Lippincott Company, Philadelphia, 1956.

SHERLOCK, S.: *Diseases of the Liver and Biliary System*, Blackwell Scientific Publications, Oxford, 1955.

SPELLBERG, M. A.: *Diseases of the Liver*, Grune & Stratton, Inc., New York, 1954.

THOREK, P.: *Anatomy in Surgery*, J. B. Lippincott Company, Philadelphia, 1951.

Section XV

	PLATE NUMBER

ALEXANDER, W. F.: *Innervation of biliary system*, J. comp. Neurol., 72:357, 1940. — 19, 29

ANSON, B. J.: *An Atlas of Human Anatomy*, W. B. Saunders Company, Philadelphia, 1950. — 14, 15

AREY, L. B.: *Developmental Anatomy*, W. B. Saunders Company, Philadelphia, 1954. — 1, 2, 23

BAGLEY, E. H., AND GRAFFLIN: *The mechanism of biliary excretion in mammals*, In: "Liver Injury", Trans. 11th Conference, Macy Foundation, New York, 1953. — 9

BALDWIN, W.: *Pancreatic ducts in man, together with a study of the microscopical structures of the minor duodenal papilla*, Anat. Rec., 5:197, 1911. — 20, 25

BAXTER, J. S.: *Frazer's Manual of Embryology*, Baillière, Tindall and Company, London, 1953. — 1, 23

BENZ, E. J., BAGGENSTOSS AND WOLLAEGER: *Atrophy of the left lobe of the liver*, Arch. Path., 53:315, 1952. — 5

BOYDEN, E. A.: *An analysis of the reaction of the human gallbladder to food*, Anat. Rec., 40:147, 1928. — 22

——: *The sphincter Oddi in man and certain representative mammals*, Surgery, 1:25, 1937. — 22

——: *Hypertrophy of the sphincter choledochus; cause of internal biliary fistula*, Surgery, 10:567, 1941. — 22

——: *The anatomy of the choledochoduodenal junction in man*, Surg. Gynec. Obstet., 104:641, 1957. — 22

BRAUS, H.: *Anatomie des Menschen*, Julius Springer, Berlin, 1924. — 7

BRUNSCHWIG, A.: *The Surgery of Pancreatic Tumors*, C. V. Mosby Company, St. Louis, 1942. — 25

CAIN, J. C., GRINDLAY, BOLLMAN, FLOCK AND MANN: *Lymph from liver and thoracic duct*, Surg. Gynec. Obstet., 85:559, 1947. — 18

Section XV (continued)

	PLATE NUMBER

CHILD, C. G.: *The Hepatic Circulation and Portal Hypertension*, W. B. Saunders Company, Philadelphia, 1954. — 11-16

CONNOLLY, J. E., AND RICHARDS: *Bilateral splanchnicectomy and lumbodorsal sympathectomy for chronic relapsing pancreatitis*, Ann. Surg., 131:58, 1950. — 29

DEAVER, J. B.: *Surgical Anatomy, Vol. III*, Blakiston Company, Inc., Philadelphia, 1903. — 26

DES JARDINS, A.: *Technique de la Pancreatectomie*, Rev. de Chir., 1:945, 1907. — 27

DETAKATS, G., WALTER AND LASNER: *Splanchnic nerve section for pancreatic pain*, Ann. Surg., 131:44-57, 1950. — 29

DOUBILET, H., POPPEL AND MULHOLLAND: *Pancreatography: Techniques, principles and observations*, Radiology, 64:325, 1955. — 25

DOUGLASS, B. E., BAGGENSTOSS AND HOLLINSHEAD: *Variations in the portal system of veins*, Proc. Mayo Clin., 25:26, 1950. — 18, 19

DRAPIEWSKI, J. F.: *Carcinoma of the Pancreas: A study of neoplastic invasion of nerves and its possible clinical significance*, Amer. J. clin. Path., 14:549, 1944. — 29

EDWARDS, E. A.: *Functional anatomy of the porta-systemic communications*, Arch. intern. Med., 88:137, 1951. — 16, 17

ELIAS, H.: *A re-examination of the structure of the mammalian liver; parenchymal architecture*, Amer. J. Anat., 84:311, 1949. — 7-10

——: *A re-examination of the structure of the mammalian liver; the hepatic lobule and its relation to the vascular and biliary system*, Amer. J. Anat., 85:379, 1949. — 7-10

——: *Origin and early development of the liver in various vertebrates*, Act. hepat., 3:1, 1955. — 1

——: *Morphology of the liver*, In: "Liver Injury", Trans. 11th Conference, Macy Foundation, New York, 1953. — 7, 8, 11, 12

——: *Liver morphology*, Biol. Rev., 30:263, 1955. — 8, 11, 12

—— AND PETTY: *Gross anatomy of the blood vessels and ducts within the human liver*, Amer. J. Anat., 90:59, 1952. — 8-10

—— AND POPPER: *Venous distribution in liver*, Arch. Path., 59:332, 1955. — 8-10

EPPINGER, H., KAUNITZ AND POPPER: *Die Seröse Entzündung*, Julius Springer, Wien, 1935. — 9

EYCLESHYMER, A. C., AND SCHOEMAKER: *A Cross Section Anatomy*, Appleton & Company, 1923. — 26

FARBER, E., WESER, SZANTO AND POPPER: *Correlation between cytoplasmic basophilia and the nucleic acid content of the liver*, Arch. Path., 51:399, 1951. — 6

GOMORI, G.: *Microscopic Histochemistry*, University of Chicago Press, Chicago, 1952. — 6

GRAFFLIN, A. L., AND CORDDRY: *Further studies of hepatic structure and function by fluorescence microscopy*, Bull. Johns Hopk. Hosp., 93:205, 1953. — 9

GRANT, J. C. B.: *An Atlas of Anatomy*, Williams & Wilkins Company, Baltimore, 1951. — 26, 27

Section XV (continued)

	PLATE NUMBER

GRAY, J. H.: *The relation of lymphatic vessels to the spread of cancer*, Brit. J. Surg., 26:462, 1939. — 28

GREEN, R. M., AND AITKEN: *Warren's Handbook of Anatomy*, Harvard University Press, Cambridge, Massachusetts, 1944. — 29

HAMILTON, W. J., BOYD AND MOSSMANN: *Human Embryology*, Williams & Wilkins Company, Baltimore, 1945. — 1, 26

HARTROFT, W. S.: *Accumulation of fat in liver cells and in lipodiastaemata preceding experimental dietary cirrhosis*, Anat. Rec., 106:61, 1950. — 6

HEALEY, JR., J. E., AND SCHROY: *Anatomy of the biliary duct within the human liver; analysis of the prevailing pattern of branchings and the major variations of the biliary ducts*, Arch. Surg., 66:599, 1953. — 8-11

——, —— AND SÖRENSEN: *The intrahepatic distribution of the hepatic artery in man*, J. int. Coll. Surg., 20:133, 1953. — 8, 11

HERING, E.: *Manual of Human and Comparative Histology*, Stricker, Berlin, 1872. — 7

HOWARD, J., AND JONES: *The anatomy of the pancreatic ducts; the etiology of acute pancreatitis*, Amer. J. med. Sci., 214:617, 1947. — 25

HUNTINGTON, G. S.: *The Anatomy of the Human Peritoneum and Abdominal Cavity*, Lea Bros. & Co., Philadelphia, 1903. — 26

IVY, A. C.: *The physiology of the gallbladder*, Physiol. Rev., 14:1, 1934. — 22

JAMISON, J. K., AND DOBSON: *The lymphatic system of the stomach*, Lancet, 1: 1061, 1907. — 28

KUNTZ, A.: *The Autonomic Nervous System*, Lea and Febiger, Philadelphia, 1945. — 19, 29

——: *A Textbook of Neuro-Anatomy*, Lea and Febiger, Philadelphia, 1950. — 19, 29

LAGERSTEDT, D.: *Hepatic histochemistry*, In: "Liver Injury", Trans. 11th Conference, Macy Foundation, New York, 1952. — 6

LANGERHANS, P.: *Contributions to the Microscopic Anatomy of the Pancreas*, Johns Hopkins Press, Baltimore, 1937. — 26

LEWIS, H. P.: *Pain in acute and chronic diseases of the liver*, Ann. intern. Med., 35: 878, 1951. — 19

LICHTMAN, S. S.: *Diseases of the Liver, Gallbladder and Bile Ducts*, Lea and Febiger, Philadelphia (p. 44), 1953. — 16

LIVINGSTON, E. M.: *A Clinical Study of the Abdominal Cavity and Peritoneum*, Paul B. Hoeber, Inc., New York, 1932. — 5, 26

MAEGRAITH, B. G.: *Micro-anatomy of the hepatic vascular system*, In: "Liver Injury", Trans. 10th Conference, Macy Foundation, New York, 1951. — 9, 10

MARKOWITZ, J., AND RAPPAPORT: *The hepatic artery*, Physiol. Rev., 31:188, 1951. — 12, 13

MAXIMOW, A. H., AND BLOOM: *Textbook of Histology*, W. B. Saunders Company, Philadelphia, 1931. — 6, 24

MEHNEN, H.: *Die Bedeutung der Mündungsverhältnisse von Gallen und Pankreasgang für die Entstehung der Gallensteine*, Arch. klin. Chir., 192:559, 1938. — 22, 25

Section XV (continued)

PLATE NUMBER

MEYER, K. A., STEIGMANN, POPPER AND WALTERS: *Influence of hepatic function on metabolism of vitamin A*, Arch. Surg., 47:26, 1943. — 6

MICHELS, N. A.: *Blood Supply and Anatomy of the Upper Abdominal Organs*, J. B. Lippincott Company, Philadelphia, 1955. — 12-15, 26

——: *Variational anatomy of the hepatic, cystic and retroduodenal arteries; statistical analysis of their origin, distribution, and relations to biliary ducts in 200 bodies*, Arch. Surg., 66:20, 1953. — 12-15, 26

——: *Collateral arterial pathways to the liver after ligation of the hepatic artery and removal of the celiac axis*, Cancer, 6:708, 1953. — 14

OBERLING, C., AND GUÉRIN: *Cancer du Pancreas*, Gaston Doin et Cie., Paris, 1931. — 26, 29

OLSEN, L. L., AND WOODBURNE: *The vascular relations of the pancreas*, Surg. Gynec. Obstet., 99:713-719, 1954. — 26

PFUHL, W.: *Die Leber, in Vol. 2 of Möllendorff, Handbuch der mikroskopischen Anatomie des Menschen*, Julius Springer, Berlin, 1932. — 6, 7

PIERSON, J. M.: *The arterial blood supply of the pancreas*, Surg. Gynec. Obstet., 77:426, 1943. — 12, 13

POPPER, H.: *Distribution of vitamin A in tissue as visualized by fluorescence microscopy*, Physiol. Rev., 24:205, 1944. — 6

——: *Significance of agonal changes in the human liver*, Arch. Path., 46:132, 1948. — 18

——: *Liver disease; morphologic considerations*, Amer. J. Med., 16:98, 1954. — 7-9

RICHINS, C. A.: *The innervation of the pancreas*, J. comp. Neurol., 83:223, 1945. — 29

RIENHOFF, JR., W. F., AND PICKRELL: *Pancreatitis; anatomic study of pancreatic and extrahepatic biliary systems*, Arch. Surg., 51:205, 1945. — 20, 25

ROBSON, A. W. M., AND CAMMIDGE: *The Pancreas, Its Surgery and Pathology*, W. B. Saunders Company, Philadelphia, 1907. — 25, 29

SCHAFER, E. A., AND THANE: *Quain's Elements of Anatomy, Vol. III, pt. IV*, Longman's Green and Co., London, 1896. — 26

SCHAFER, P. W.: *Pathology in General Surgery*, University of Chicago Press, Chicago, 1950. — 25

SCHMIEDEN, V., AND SEBENING: *Chirurgie des Pankreas*, Arch. klin. Chir., 148:319, 1927. — 25-27

SIMKINS, S.: *Variations in pancreatic ducts and minor duodenal papilla*, Amer. J. med. Sci., 182:626, 1931. — 25

SUNDERLAND, D. A., McNEER, ORTEGA AND PEARCE: *Lymphatic spread of gastric cancer*, Cancer, 6:987, 1953. — 28

SZANTO, P. B., AND POPPER: *Basophilic cytoplasmic material (pentose nucleic acid); distribution in normal and abnormal human liver*, Arch. Path., 51:409, 1951. — 6

TWISS, J. R., AND OPPENHEIM: *Practical Management of Disorders of the Liver, Pancreas and Biliary Tract*, Lea and Febiger, Philadelphia, 1955. — 29

WATKIN, K. G., AND MANN: *The intrahepatic circulation of blood*, Anat. Rec., 82:233, 1942. — 12

Section XV (continued)

PLATE NUMBER

WOOLSEY, G.: *Applied Surgical Anatomy*, Lea and Febiger, Philadelphia, 1908. — 27, 28

Section XVI

ALTHAUSEN, T. L., LOCKHART AND SOLEY: *A new diagnostic test (galactose) for thyroid disease*, Amer. J. med. Sci., 199:342, 1940. — 6

—— AND UYEYAMA: *A test of pancreatic function based on starch tolerance*, Ann. intern. Med., 41:563, 1954. — 22, 23

ANDERSEN, D. H., AND EARLY: *Method of assaying trypsin suitable for routine as in diagnosis of congenital pancreatic deficiency*, Amer. J. Dis. Child., 63:891, 1942. — 23

BAYLISS, W. M., AND STARLING: *Mechanism of pancreatic secretion*, J. Physiol., 28:325, 1902. — 20

BEST, C. H., HARTROFT AND SELLERS: *The protection of the liver by dietary factors*, Gastroenterology, 20:375, 1952. — 2

BODANSKY, A.: *Phosphatase studies; determination of serum phosphatase. Factors influencing accuracy of determination*, J. biol. Chem., 101:93, 1933. — 8

BODANSKY, M., AND BODANSKY: *Biochemistry of Disease*, Macmillan Company, New York, 1952. — 20-23

BONDY, P. K.: *Carbohydrate metabolism.* Abstract of paper read at 6th Ann. Meet. Assoc. for the Study of Liver Disease, Amer. J. Med., 21:128, 1956. — 6

BOYDEN, E. A., BERGH AND LAYNE: *An analysis of the reaction of the human gallbladder and sphincter Oddi to magnesium sulfate*, Surgery, 13:723, 1943. — 17, 18

CANTAROW, A., AND SCHEPARTZ: *Textbook of Biochemistry*, W. B. Saunders Company, Philadelphia, 1954. — 2

—— AND TRUMPER: *Clinical Biochemistry*, W. B. Saunders Company, Philadelphia, 1949. — 8

CARTER, R. F., AND GILLETTE: *Immediate cholangiography. Indications, technic and illustrative cases*, J. Amer. med. Ass., 143:951, 1950. — 19

CHERRY, I. S., AND CRANDALL: *The specificity of pancreatic lipase; its appearance in the blood after pancreatic injury*, Amer. J. Physiol., 100:266, 1932. — 23

COMFORT, M. W.: *Tests of pancreatic function*, J. Amer. med. Ass., 115:2044, 1940. — 20-23

——, PARKER AND OSTERBERG: *The concentration of pancreatic enzymes in the duodenum of normal persons and persons with diseases of the upper part of the abdomen*, Amer. J. dig. Dis., 6:249, 1939. — 22

DREILING, D. A.: *An evaluation of pancreatic function tests*, N. Y. St. J. Med., 53:671, 1953. — 23

—— AND JANOWITZ: *The secretion of electrolytes by the human pancreas*, Gastroenterology, 30:382, 1956. — 20, 21, 23

EDMONDSON, H. A., BERNE, HOMANN AND WERTMAN: *Calcium, potassium, magnesium and amylase disturbances in acute pancreatitis*, Amer. J. Med., 12:34, 1952. — 21

Section XVI (continued)

PLATE NUMBER

—— AND FIELDS: *Relation of calcium and lipids to acute pancreatitis necrosis*, Arch. intern. Med., 69:117, 1943. — 21

FARBER, S., SHWACHMAN AND MADDOCK: *Pancreatic function and disease in early life. I. Pancreatic enzyme activity and the celiac syndrome*, J. clin. Invest., 22:827, 1943. — 20, 22, 23

FRANKLIN, M., BEAN, PAUL, ROUTH, DE LA HUERGA AND POPPER: *Electrophoretic studies in liver disease. I. Comparison of serum and plasma electrophoretic patterns in liver disease with special reference to fibrinogen and gamma globulin patterns. II. Gamma globulin in chronic liver disease*, J. clin. Invest., 30:718 and 729, 1951. — 4

GILLMAN, T., AND GILLMAN: *A modified liver aspiration biopsy apparatus and technique, with special reference to its clinical applications as assessed by 500 biopsies*, S. Afr. J. med. Sci., 10:53, 1945. — 11

GRAHAM, E. A., AND COLE: *Roentgenologic examination of the gallbladder. Preliminary report of a new method utilizing intravenous injection of tetrabromophthalein*, J. Amer. med. Ass., 82:613, 1924. — 19

GRAY, S. H., PROBSTEIN AND HEIFETZ: *Clinical studies on blood diastase; low blood diastase as an index of impaired hepatic function*, Arch. intern. Med., 67:805, 1941. — 21, 23

—— AND SOMOGYI: *Relationship between blood amylase and urinary amylase in man*, Proc. Soc. exp. Biol., 36:253, 1937. — 21

GUTMANN, A. B.: *In: Advances in Protein Chemistry, Vol. 4*, Acad. Press, New York, 1948. — 3, 4

HANGER, F. M.: *The meaning of liver function tests*, Amer. J. Med., 16:565, 1954. — 15, 16

——: *Serological differentiation of obstructive from hepatogenous jaundice by flocculation of cephalin-cholesterol emulsion*, J. clin. Invest., 18:261, 1939. — 15, 16

HARPER, A. A., AND RAPER: *Pancreozymin, stimulant of secretion of pancreatic enzymes in extracts of the small intestine*, J. Physiol., 102:115, 1943. — 20

HARPER, H. A.: *Review of Physiological Chemistry*, Lange Medical Publications, Los Altos, California, 1955. — 2

HEIFETZ, C. J., PROBSTEIN AND GRAY: *Clinical studies on blood diastase. II. Significance of increased blood diastase*, Arch. intern. Med., 67:819, 1941. — 21, 23

HOWE, P. E.: *The determination of proteins in blood. A micromethod*, J. biol. Chem., 49:109, 1921. — 3

HUERGA, J. DE LA, AND POPPER: *Estimation of serum gamma globulin concentration by turbidimetry*, J. Lab. clin. Med., 35:459, 1950. — 3

——, YESNICK AND POPPER: *Estimation of total serum lipids by a turbidimetric method*, Amer. J. clin. Path., 23:1163, 1953. — 7

INGELFINGER, F. J., BRADLEY, MENDELOFF AND KRAMER: *Studies with bromsulphalein*, Gastroenterology, 11:646, 1948. — 10

Section XVI (continued)

PLATE NUMBER

INNERFIELD, I., ANGRIST AND BENJAMIN: *Antithrombin titer in acute pancreatitis*, Amer. J. Med., 12:24, 1952. — 21

IVY, A. C.: *The physiology of the gallbladder*, Physiol. Rev., 14:1, 1934. — 11

KING, E. J., AND AITKEN: *An intravenous-galactose test*, Lancet, 2:543, 1940. — 6

KNISELY, M. H., BLOCH AND WARNER: *Selective Phagocytosis. I. Microscopic observations on regulation of blood flow through liver and other organs and mechanism and rate of phagocytic removal of particles from the blood*, Det Kongelige Danske Videnskabernes Selskab Biologiske Skrifter, IV, 7, 1948. — 1

KUNKEL, H. G.: *Estimation of alterations of serum gamma globulin by a turbidimetric technique*, Proc. Soc. exp. Biol., 66:217, 1947. — 3

LEVINE, R., GOLDSTEIN, HUDDLESTUN AND KLEIN: *Action of insulin on the "permeability" of cells to free hexoses, as studied by its effect on the distribution of galactose*, Amer. J. Physiol., 163:70, 1950. — 6

LYON, B. B.: *Nonsurgical Drainage of the Gall Tract*, Lea and Febiger, Philadelphia, 1923. — 18

MELLANBY, J.: *The mechanism of pancreatic digestion — The function of secretin*, J. Physiol., 60:85, 1925. — 20

MELTZER, S. J.: *The disturbance of the law of contrary innervation as a pathogenic factor in the diseases of the bile ducts and the gallbladder*, Amer. J. med. Sci., 153:469, 1917. — 17, 18

MENGHINI, G.: *One-second needle biopsy of the liver*, Gastroenterology, 35:190, 1958. — 11

NOTHMAN, M. M., PRATT AND CALLOW: *Studies on urinary lipase. I. On a fat-splitting enzyme in urine and its relation to pancreas*, Arch. intern. Med., 95:224, 1955. — 21

PIRKEY, E. L., DAVIS AND PILLA: *Preoperative and postoperative cholangiography*, J. Amer. med. Ass., 151:266, 1953. — 19

POPPER, H.: *Differential diagnosis of jaundice by laboratory tests*, Rev. Gastroent., 19:826, 1952. — 13-16

—: *In Liver Disease*, A Ciba Foundation Symposium (p. 8), Blakiston Company, Inc., Philadelphia, 1951. — 3, 4

——, BEAN, DE LA HUERGA, FRANKLIN, TSUMAGARI, ROUTH AND STEIGMANN: *Electrophoretic serum protein fractions in hepatobiliary disease*, Gastroenterology, 17:138, 1951. — 4

—— AND FRANKLIN: *Differential diagnosis of hepatitis by histologic and functional laboratory methods*, J. Amer. med. Ass., 137:230, 1948. — 15

——, DE LA HUERGA, FRANKLIN, BEAN, ROUTH AND SCHAFFNER: *Correlation between electrophoretic and chemical partitions of serum proteins*, Amer. J. clin. Path., 20:530, 1950. — 4

——, ——, STEIGMANN AND SLODKI: *Turbidimetric gamma globulin determinations in hepatobiliary diseases*, J. Lab. clin. Med., 35:391, 1950. — 3, 4

——, KOCH-WESER AND DE LA HUERGA: *Serum and hepatic enzymes in experimental liver damage*, J. Mt. Sinai Hosp., 19:256, 1952. — 8

Section XVI (continued)

PLATE NUMBER

—— AND SCHAFFNER: *Hepatic tests*, Advanc. intern. Med., 4:357, 1950. — 12-16

—— AND ——: *Laboratory diagnosis in liver disease*, J. Amer. med. Ass., 15:1367, 1952. — 13-16

—— AND STEIGMANN: *Differential diagnosis between medical and surgical jaundice by laboratory tests*, Ann. intern. Med., 29:469, 1948. — 16

——, ——, MEYER, KOZOLL AND FRANKLIN: *Correlation of liver function and liver structure*, Amer. J. Med., 6:278, 1949. — 16

——, ——, TSUMAGARI AND DE LA HUERGA: *The flocculation tests in the differential diagnosis of jaundice*, Amer. J. dig. Dis., 18:192, 1951. — 3, 4

——, —— AND SZANTO: *Quantitative correlation of morphologic liver changes and clinical tests*, Amer. J. Path., 19:710, 1949. — 15, 16

——, WALDSTEIN AND SZANTO: *Correlation of clinical features of cirrhosis of the liver with findings on biopsy*, Amer. J. clin. Path., 20:724, 1950. — 11

QUICK, A. J.: *The synthesis of hippuric acid: A new test of liver function*, Amer. J. med. Sci., 185:630, 1933. — 9

—: *On the quantitative estimation of prothrombin*, Amer. J. clin. Path., 15:560, 1945. — 5

SCHAFFNER, F., POPPER AND DALLA TORRE: *Structural alterations in the clinical evaluation of cirrhosis*, Gastroenterology, 30:357, 1956. — 15

——, TURNER, ESHBAUGH, BUCKINGHAM AND POPPER: *Hypergammaglobulinemia in pulmonary tuberculosis*, Arch. intern. Med., 92:490, 1953. — 3, 4

SHWARTZ, M. K., BODANSKY AND RANDALL: *Metabolism in surgical patients. I. Nitrogen metabolism in totally gastrectomized patients. II. Fat and mineral metabolism in totally gastrectomized patients*, Amer. J. clin. Nutr., 4:45 and 51, 1956. — 22-23

SILVERMAN, I.: *A new biopsy needle*, Amer. J. Surg., 40:671, 1938. — 11

SMITH, J. L., WALTERS AND BEAL: *A study of choledochal sphincter action*, Gastroenterology, 20:129, 1952. — 17, 19

SOMOGYI, M.: *Diastatic activity of human blood*, Arch. intern. Med., 67:665, 1941. — 20, 23

STEIGMANN, F., POPPER, HERNANDEZ AND SHULMAN: *Flocculation tests in the diagnosis of hepato-biliary disease*, Gastroenterology, 13:9, 1949. — 15, 16

——, —— AND MEYER: *Liver function tests in clinical medicine*, J. Amer. med. Ass., 122:279, 1943. — 13-16

SZANTO, P. B., AND POPPER: *Basophilic cytoplasmic material (pentose nucleic acid); distribution in normal and abnormal liver*, Arch. Path., 51:409, 1951. — 4

TERRY, R.: *Needle biopsy of the liver with special reference to a modified Gillman technique*, Brit. med. J., 1:657, 1949. — 11

—: *Risks of needle biopsy of the liver*, Brit. med. J., 1:1102, 1952. — 11

—: *Needle necropsy*, J. clin. Path., 8:38, 1955. — 11

THANNHAUSER, S. J.: *Serum lipids and their value in diagnosis*, New Engl. J. Med., 237:515, 1947. — 7

TORSOLI, A., RAMORINO, PALAGI, COLA-GRANDE, BASCHIERI, RIBOTTA AND MARI-

Section XVI (continued)

PLATE NUMBER

NOSCI: *Roentgen-cinematographic and electromanometric observations on the motility of the bile ducts*, Sem. Hôp. Paris, 37:790, 1961. — 17

TWISS, J. R., AND OPPENHEIM: *Practical Management of Disorders of the Liver, Pancreas and Biliary Tract*, Lea and Febiger, Philadelphia, 1955. — 21, 22

UNGER, P. N., AND SHAPIRO: *The prothrombin response to parenteral administration of large doses of vitamin K in subjects with normal liver function and in cases of liver disease; a standardized test for the estimation of hepatic function*, J. clin. Invest., 27:39, 1948. — 5

WALDSTEIN, S. S., POPPER, SZANTO AND STEIGMANN: *Liver cirrhosis; relation between function and structure based on biopsy studies*, Arch. intern. Med., 87:844, 1951. — 15

WATSON, C. J., AND HOFFBAUER: *Liver function in hepatitis*, Ann. intern. Med., 26:813, 1947. — 15

WHITE, A., HANDLER, SMITH AND DEWITT STETTEN: *Principles of Biochemistry*, McGraw-Hill Book Company, Inc., New York, 1954. — 2

WOLSTENHOLME, G.: *Ciba Foundation Colloquia on Endocrinology*, vol. 6, *Hormonal Factors in Carbohydrate Metabolism*, J. & A. Churchill Ltd., London, 1953. — 2, 6

ZIFFREN, S. E., OWEN, HOFFMAN AND SMITH: *Simple bedside test for control of vitamin K therapy*, Amer. J. clin. Path., 4 (Suppl.) 13, 1940. — 5

Section XVII

ABALLI, A. J., AND KATO: *Gaucher's disease in early infancy*, J. Pediat., 13:364, 1938. — 24

ARTMAN, E. A., AND WISE: *Hypokalemia in liver cell failure*, Amer. J. Med., 15:459, 1953. — 14

ASH, J. E., AND SPITZ: *Pathology of Tropical Diseases*, W. B. Saunders Company, Philadelphia, 1945. — 40-43

ASHE, W. F., PRATT-THOMAS AND KUMPE: *Weil's disease*, Medicine, 20:145, 1941. — 37

BAGGENSTOSS, A. H., AND STAUFFER: *Post-hepatic and alcoholic cirrhosis*, Gastroenterology, 22:157, 1952. — 19

BANG, J., AND WANSCHER: *The histopathology of the liver in infectious mononucleosis complicated by jaundice*, Acta med. scand., 120:437, 1945. — 36

BEARN, A. G.: *Genetic and biochemical aspects of Wilson's disease*, Amer. J. Med., 15:442, 1953. — 25

—— AND KUNKEL: *Abnormalities of copper metabolism in Wilson's disease and their relationship to the amino-aciduria*, J. clin. Invest., 33:400, 1954. — 25

BENZ, E. J., AND BAGGENSTOSS: *Focal cirrhosis of the liver: its relation to the so-called hamartoma (adenoma, benign hepatoma)*, Cancer, 6:743, 1953. — 49

BERNSTEIN, A.: *Infectious mononucleosis*, Medicine, 19:85, 1940. — 36

BEST, C. H., HARTROFT AND SELLERS: *The protection of the liver by dietary factors*, Gastroenterology, 20:375, 1952. — 15-17

BICKFORD, R. G., AND BUTT: *Hepatic coma: The electroencephalographic pattern*, J. clin. Invest., 34:790, 1955. — 13

BJØRNBOE, M., JERSILD, LUNDBAEK, THAYSEN AND RYSSING: *Incidence of chronic hepatitis in woman in Copenhagen, 1944-45*, Lancet, 1:867, 1948.   33

BLAKEMORE, A. H.: *Portacaval shunting for portal hypertension*, Surg. Gynec. Obstet., 94:443, 1952.   11

BLOOM, W.: *Splenomegaly (type Gaucher) and lipoid-histiocytosis (type Niemann)*, Amer. J. Path., 1:595, 1925.   24

BURMAN, C.: *Primary Carcinoma of the Liver*, Lewis, London, 1951.   50, 51

CHILD, C. G.: *The Hepatic Circulation and Portal Hypertension*, W. B. Saunders Company, Philadelphia, 1954.   7, 10

COCCAN, P., OBERLING AND DIENST: *La maladie de Niemann-Pick*, Rev. franc. Pédiat., 3:789, 1927.   24

COPE, V. Z.: *Human Actinomycosis*, Heinemann, London, 1952.   41

CRAIG, C. F., AND FAUST: *Clinical Parasitology*, Lea and Febiger, Philadelphia, 1940.   40-43

CRAIG, J. M., AND LANDING: *Form of hepatitis in neonatal period simulating biliary atresia*, Arch. Path., 54:321, 1954.   56

DAVIES, J. N. P.: *Kwashiorkor*, In: "Liver Injury", Trans. 9th Conference, Macy Foundation, New York, 1950.   16

DUBIN, I. N.: *Idiopathic hemochromatosis and transfusion siderosis*, Amer. J. clin. Path., 25:514, 1955.   27

EDMONDSON, H. A., AND STEINER: *Primary carcinoma of the liver*, Cancer, 7:462, 1954.   50, 51

EDWARDS, E. A.: *Functional anatomy of the porta-systemic communications*, Arch. intern. Med., 88:137, 1951.   10, 11

FINCH, C. A., HEGSTED, KINNEY, THOMAS, RATH, HASKINS, FINCH AND FLUHARTY: *Iron metabolism. The pathophysiology of iron storage*, Blood, 5:983, 1950.   26, 27

FOLEY, J. M., WATSON AND ADAMS: *Significance of electroencephalographic changes in hepatic coma*, Trans. Amer. neurol. Assn., 75:161, 1950.   13

FRANKLIN, M., SALK, STEIGMANN AND POPPER: *Clinical, functional and histologic responses of fatty metamorphosis of human liver to lipotropic therapy*, Amer. J. clin. Path., 18:273, 1948.   15-18

GRANICK, S.: *Iron metabolism and hemochromatosis*, Bull. N. Y. Acad. Med., 25:403, 1949.   26, 27

HAMPERL, H.: *Lehrbuch der allgemeinen Pathologie und der pathologischen Anatomie*, Julius Springer, Berlin, 1954.   37, 51

HARRIS, H. J.: *Brucellosis; Clinical and Subclinical*, Paul B. Hoeber, Inc., New York, 1950.   39

HARTROFT, W. S.: *Some histological aspects of renal and hepatic acholinopathy*, In: "Liver Injury", Trans. 6th Conference, Macy Foundation, New York, 1947.   14

——: *Accumulation of fat in liver cells and in lipodiastaemata preceding experimental dietary cirrhosis*, Anat. Rec., 106:61, 1950.   6, 15-17

——: *The locus of the beginning of dietary cirrhosis*, In: "Liver Injury", Trans. 8th Conference, Macy Foundation, 1950 (p. 126).   15, 17, 18

—— AND RIDOUT: *Pathogenesis of cirrhosis produced by choline deficiency. Escape of lipid from fatty hepatic cysts into the biliary and vascular systems*, Amer. J. Path., 27:951, 1951.   6, 15-17

HERBUT, P. A.: *Surgical Pathology*, Lea and Febiger, Philadelphia, 1954.   50-52

HERXHEIMER, G.: In: *Henke-Lubarsch, Handbuch der speziellen pathologischen Anatomie und Histologie*, Vol. 5, Julius Springer, Berlin, 1930.   49

HIGGINSON, J.: *Relation of carcinoma of the liver to cirrhosis, malaria and parasitic diseases*, Schweiz. Z. allg. Path. Bakt., 18:625, 1955.   50

——, GERRITSEN AND WALKER: *Siderosis in the Bantu of Southern Africa*, Amer. J. Path., 24:779, 1953.   27

HIMSWORTH, H. P.: *Lectures on the Liver and Its Diseases*, Harvard University Press, Cambridge, Massachusetts, 1947.   5, 31-34, 44

HSIA, D. Y., PATTERSON, ALLEN, DIAMOND AND GELLIS: *Prolonged obstructive jaundice in infancy*, Pediatrics, 10:243, 1952.   56

HUMPHREY, E. M., AND KATO: *Glycogen-storage disease; thesaurismosis glycogenica*, Amer. J. Path., 10:589, 1934.   24

JOHNSON, B. B., AND LUETSCHER: *The possible rôle of aldosterone in edema*, Ann. N. Y. Acad. Sci., 61 (Art. 2), 605, 1955.   12

KALK, H., AND HEINEMANN: *Klinische und anatomische Verfolgung des Krankheitsverlaufs beim Morbus Bang mit besonderer Berücksichtigung der Leberbefunde*, Ztschr. klin. Med., 149:430, 1952.   39

KARSNER, H. T.: *Human Pathology*, J. B. Lippincott Company, Philadelphia, 1942.   37

KIRSCHBAUM, J. D.: *Congenital absence of the gallbladder and the extrahepatic biliary ducts*, Amer. J. Dis. Child., 47:1080, 1934.   56

KLATSKIN, G., AND YESNER: *Hepatic manifestations of sarcoidosis and other granulomatous diseases. A study based on histological examination of tissue obtained by needle biopsy of the liver*, Yale J. Biol. Med., 23:207, 1950-51.   38, 39

KLECKNER, N. S., BAGGENSTOSS AND WEIR: *Hemochromatosis and transfusional hemosiderosis*, Amer. J. Med., 16:382, 1954.   27

KLOTZ, O., AND BELT: *The pathology of the spleen in yellow fever*, Amer. J. Path., 6:655, 1930.   36

KOCH-WESER, D., FARBER AND POPPER: *Fatty liver without necrosis*, Arch. Path., 51:498, 1951.   5

——, DE LA HUERGA, YESNICK AND POPPER: *Hepatic necrosis due to bromobenzene as an example of conditioned amino acid deficiency*, Metabolism, 2:248, 1953.   51

KUNKEL, H. G.: *Factors in mechanisms of ascites*, In: "Liver Disease", A Ciba Foundation Symposium, Blakiston Company, Inc., Philadelphia, 1951.   12

LANGEWISCH, W. H., AND BIGLER: *Disorders of glycogen metabolism, with special reference of glycogen storage disease and galactosemia*, Pediatrics, 9:263, 1953.   24

LEVINE, P., VOGEL AND ROSENFIELD: *Hemolytic disease of the newborn*, In: "Advances

in Pediatrics", Vol. 6, Year Book Publications, New York, 1953.   58

LINTON, R. R., AND ELLIS: *Emergency and definite treatment of bleeding esophageal varices*, J. Amer. med. Ass., 160:1017, 1956.   11

LONGCOPE, W. T., AND FREIMAN: *A Study of Sarcoidosis*, Williams and Wilkins Company, Baltimore, 1952.   39

LUCKE, B.: *The pathology of fatal epidemic hepatitis*, Amer. J. Path., 20:471, 1944.   31-33

——: *The structure of the liver after recovery from epidemic hepatitis*, Amer. J. Path., 20:595, 1944.   34

——: *Lower nephron nephrosis*, Milit. Surg., 99:371, 1946.   46

—— AND MALLORY: *The fulminant form of epidemic hepatitis*, Amer. J. Path., 22:867, 1946.   5, 32

MACMAHON, H. E.: *Biliary xanthomatosis (xanthomatous biliary cirrhosis)*, Amer. J. Path., 24:527, 1948.   35

—— AND THANNHAUSER: *Xanthomatous biliary cirrhosis (A clinical syndrome)*, Ann. intern. Med., 30:121, 1949.   35

MALLORY, T. B.: *The pathology of epidemic hepatitis*, J. Amer. med. Ass., 134:655, 1947.   3

MARKOWITZ, J., AND RAPPAPORT: *The hepatic artery*, Physiol. Rev., 31:188, 1951.   45

MCCULLOUGH, N. B., AND EISELE: *Brucella hepatitis leading to cirrhosis of the liver*, Arch. intern. Med., 88:793, 1951.   39

MEYER, K. A., POPPER AND STEIGMANN: *Biliary hepatitis*, Quart. Bull. Northw. Univ. med. Sch., 23:321, 1949.   22

MILLIKEN, N. T., AND STRYKER: *Suppurative pylethrombophlebitis and multiple liver abscesses following acute appendicitis*, New Engl. J. Med., 244:52, 1951.   30

MOREY, D. A., AND BURKE: *Distinctive nail changes in advanced hepatic cirrhosis*, Gastroenterology, 29:258, 1955.   9

MORRISON, J. E.: *Umbilical sepsis and acute interstitial hepatitis*, J. Path., 56:531, 1944.   56

MOWREY, F. H., AND LUNDBERG: *The clinical manifestations of essential polyangiitis (periarteritis nodosa), with emphasis on the hepatic manifestations*, Ann. int. Med., 40:1145, 1954.   47

OLIVER, J., MACDOWELL AND TRACY: *The pathogenesis of acute renal failure associated with traumatic and toxic injury*, J. clin. Invest., 30:1307, 1951.   14

PHILLIPS, G. B., SCHWARTZ, GABUZDA AND DAVIDSON: *The syndrome of impending hepatic coma in patients with cirrhosis of the liver given certain nitrogenous substances*, New Engl. J. Med., 247:239, 1952.   13

POPPER, H.: *Correlation of hepatic function and structure based on liver biopsy studies*, In: "Liver Injury", Trans. 9th Conference, Macy Foundation, New York, 1951.   3

——: *Interrelation between hepatic lesions and lesions of the biliary tract*, J. int. Coll. Surg., 18:743, 1952.   20

——: *Liver disease — morphologic considerations*, Amer. J. Med., 16:98, 1954.   5, 23

Section XVII (continued)	PLATE NUMBER

——: *Classification of cirrhosis based on clinical pathological correlation,* Amer. J. Gastroenter., in press. — 6, 17-19, 22

—— AND ELIAS: *Histogenesis of hepatic cirrhosis studied by the three-dimensional approach,* Amer. J. Path., 31:405, 1955. — 5, 6

——, —— AND PETTY: *Vascular pattern of the cirrhotic liver,* Amer. J. clin. Path., 22: 717, 1952. — 7

—— AND FRANKLIN: *Viral versus toxic hepatic necrosis,* Arch. Path., 46:338, 1948. — 31-33

——, JEFFERSON AND NECHELES: *Ligation of hepatic artery for portal hypertension,* J. Amer. med. Ass., 153:1095, 1953. — 45

——, —— AND ——: *Survival of the liver after gradual devascularization,* Amer. J. Physiol., 177:444, 1954. — 45

——, —— AND ——: *Survival of dogs after partial or total devascularization of the liver,* Ann. Surg., 140:93, 1954. — 45

—— AND SCHAFFNER: *Nutritional hepatic injury,* Arch. intern. Med., 94:785, 1954. — 15-17

——, SZANTO AND ELIAS: *Transition of fatty liver into cirrhosis,* Gastroenterology, 28: 183, 1955. — 6, 17, 18

——, —— AND PARTHASARATHY: *Florid cirrhosis,* Amer. J. clin. Path., 25:889, 1955. — 17

—— AND VOLK: *Hepatitis with jaundice in children,* In: A. Lewinson Anniversary Volume, *Studies in Pediatrics and Medical History,* Froben Press, Inc., New York, 1949. — 56

POTTER, E. L.: *Pathology of the Fetus and the Newborn,* Year Book Publishers, Inc., Chicago, 1952. — 2, 37, 56

RATNOFF, O. D., AND PATEK: *Postnecrotic cirrhosis of the liver,* J. Chronic Dis., 1: 266, 1955. — 19

ROESNER, E.: *Die Zusammenhangstrennungen der Leber,* In: *Henke-Lubarsch, Handbuch der speziellen pathologischen Anatomie und Histologie,* Julius Springer, Berlin, 1930. — 54

ROUSSELOT, L. M.: *The present status of surgery for portal hypertension,* Amer. J. Med., 16:874, 1954. — 11

SCADDING, J. G., AND SHERLOCK: *Liver biopsy in sarcoidosis,* Thorax, 3:79, 1948. — 39

SCHAFFNER, F., POPPER AND DALLA TORRE: *Structural alterations in the clinical evaluation of cirrhosis,* Gastroenterology, 30: 357, 1956. — 8, 17, 18

SCHECHTER, M. M., AND JONES: *Hepatolenticular degeneration,* Arch. intern. Med., 9:541, 1953. — 25

SHORR, E.: In: *Seminar on hypertension,* Amer. J. Med., 5:783, 1938. — 14

SMETANA, H. F.: *Histogenesis of coarse nodular cirrhosis,* Lab. Invest., 5:175, 1956. — 19

STEIGMANN, F., MEYER AND POPPER: *Severe interference with bile flow in primary hepatitis; its significance in differential diagnosis of jaundice,* Arch. Surg., 59: 101, 1949. — 31, 34, 35

STUMPF, H. H., AND LIBER: *Hepatocellular adenomatosis,* Amer. J. Med., 17:887, 1954. — 49

TERRY, R.: *White nails in hepatic cirrhosis,* Lancet, 1:757, 1954. — 9

Section XVII (continued)	PLATE NUMBER

TESCHAN, P. E., AND McDOWELL: *The artificial kidney,* U. S. armed Forces Med. J., 3:391, 1952. — 14

THANNHAUSER, S. J.: *Lipidoses,* Oxford University Press, New York, 1950. — 35

UNGER, P. N., ZUCKERBROD, BECK AND STEELE: *Study of the disappearance of congo red from the blood of non-amyloid subjects and patients with amyloidosis,* J. clin. Invest., 27:111, 1948. — 23

VILLELA, E.: *Histology of human yellow fever when death is delayed,* Arch. Path., 31:665, 1941. — 36

VOLINI, I. F., AND POPPER: *Saccular aneurysm of the left branch of the hepatic artery,* Surg. Clin. N. Amer. (Case II), p. 267 (Feb.), 1948. — 47

WADSWORTH, R. C., AND KEIL: *Biopsy of the liver in infectious mononucleosis,* Amer. J. Path., 28:1003, 1952. — 36

WALLACH, H. F., AND POPPER: *Central necrosis of the liver,* Arch. Path., 49:33, 1950. — 5, 28, 29, 44

WATSON, C. J., AND HOFFBAUER: *The problem of prolonged hepatitis with particular reference to the cholangiolytic type and the development of cholangiolitic cirrhosis of the liver,* Arch. intern. Med., 25: 195, 1946. — 22, 35

WERNER, S. C., HANGER AND KRITZLER: *Jaundice during methyltestosterone therapy,* Amer. J. Med., 8:325, 1950. — 35

WHITE, A., HANDLER, SMITH AND DeWITT STETTEN: *Principles of Biochemistry,* McGraw-Hill Book Company, New York, 1954. — 26

WYATT, J. P., MIGHTON AND MORAGUES: *Transfusional siderosis,* Amer. J. Path., 26:883, 1950. — 27

Section XVIII

ANDERSON, W. A. D.: *Pathology,* C. V. Mosby Company, St. Louis, 1953. — 2-8

BOYD, W.: *Surgical Pathology,* Macmillan Company, New York, 1947. — 13-15

BUXTON, R. W., RAY AND COLLER: *Acute cholecystitis,* J. Amer. med. Ass., 146:301, 1951. — 7, 8

COLE, W. H.: *Recent trends in gallbladder surgery,* J. Amer. med. Ass., 150:631, 1952. — 9, 11, 16

——, IRENEUS AND REYNOLDS: *Strictures of the common duct,* Ann. Surg., 133:684, 1951. — 11

ELMAN, R., AND GRAHAM: *Pathogenesis of "strawberry" gallbladder (cholesterosis of gallbladder),* Arch. Surg., 24:14, 1932. — 7

GLENN, F.: *Common duct exploration for stones,* Surg. Gynec. Obstet., 95:431, 1953. — 4

GROSS, R. E.: *Congenital anomalies of the gallbladder; a review of 148 cases, with report of a double gallbladder,* Arch. Surg., 32:131, 1936. — 1

HANSER, R., GALLENBLASE AND GALLENWEGE: In: *Henke Lubarsch, Handbuch der speziellen pathologischen Anatomie und Histologie V/2,* Julius Springer, Berlin, 1929. — 1, 5

Section XVIII (continued)	PLATE NUMBER

HERBUT, P. A.: *Surgical Pathology,* Lea and Febiger, Philadelphia, 1953. — 3-6, 13

MacCALLUM, W. G.: *A Textbook of Pathology,* W. B. Saunders Company, Philadelphia, 1942. — 2

MENTZER, S. E.: *A clinical and pathologic study of cholecystitis and cholelithiasis,* Surg. Gynec. Obstet., 42:782, 1926. — 3, 4, 7, 8

ROBERTSON, H. E.: *The preponderance of gallstones in women. An etiological study,* Int. Abstr. Surg., 80:1, 1945. — 2

——: *Silent gallstones,* Gastroenterology, 5: 345, 1945. — 3, 4

ROLLESTON, H., AND McNEE: *Diseases of Liver, Gallbladder and Bile Ducts,* Macmillan Company, London, 1929. — 13, 14

ROTHMANN, M. M.: In Bockus' *Gastroenterology, Vol. 3,* W. B. Saunders Company, Philadelphia, 1946. — 1

STERNBERG, C., LEBER, GALLENBLASE AND GALLENWEGE: *Pankreas in Aschoff, Pathologische Anatomie,* Fisher, Jena, 1913. — 7-9

TWISS, J. R., AND OPPENHEIM: *Practical Management of Disorders of the Liver, Pancreas and Biliary Tract,* Lea and Febiger, Philadelphia, 1955. — 2

WALTERS, W., AND SNELL: *Diseases of the Gallbladder and Bile Ducts,* W. B. Saunders Company, Philadelphia, 1940. — 1, 15

WOMACK, N. A., AND CRIDER: *The persistence of symptoms following cholecystectomy,* Ann. Surg., 126:31, 1947. — 16

Section XIX

ANDERSEN, D. H.: *Cystic fibrosis of the pancreas and its relation to celiac disease,* Amer. J. Dis. Child., 56:344, 1938. — 2

——: *Therapy and prognosis of fibrocystic disease of the pancreas,* Pediatrics, 3:406, 1949. — 2

BAGGENSTOSS, A. H., POWER AND GRINDLAY: *Further studies on pathogenesis of fibrocystic disease of pancreas,* Arch. Path., 51:510, 1951. — 2

BAKER, J. W., AND BOLES: *Observations pertaining to the place of surgery in acute pancreatitis,* Gastroenterology, 28: 536, 1955. — 3

BAUMEL, J., AND PEDOUSSAUT: *Pseudokystes post-nécrotiques du pancréas,* Presse méd., 58:1470, 1950. — 5

BAUMGARTNER, C. J., AND REYNOLDS: *Functioning metastases from an islet-cell tumor of the pancreas; control with corticotropin (ACTH),* Arch. Surg., 70:793, 1955. — 7

BERENS, J. J., BAGGENSTOSS AND GRAY: *Ductal changes in chronic pancreatitis,* Arch. Surg., 128:609, 1954. — 4

BERK, J. E.: *Diagnosis of carcinoma of the pancreas,* Arch. intern. Med., 68:525, 1941. — 7, 8

BODIAN, M.: *Fibrocystic Disease of the Pancreas,* Grune & Stratton, Incorporated, New York, 1953. — 2

BOWERS, R. F., LORD AND McSWAIN: *Cystadenoma of the pancreas; report of 5 cases,* Arch. Surg., 45:111, 1942. — 6

Section XIX (continued)

PLATE
NUMBER

Boyd, W.: *Surgical Pathology,* Macmillan Company, New York, 1947. 3, 4

Brown, R. K., Moseley, Pratt and Pratt: *The early diagnosis of cancer of the pancreas based on the clinical and pathological study of one hundred autopsied cases,* Amer. J. med. Sci., 223:349, 1952. 8, 9

Brunschwig, A.: *The Surgery of the Pancreatic Tumors,* C. V. Mosby Company, St. Louis, 1942. 5-8

Cattell, R. B., and Warren: *Surgery of the Pancreas,* W. B. Saunders Company, Philadelphia, 1953. 5, 7, 8

Cliffton, E. E.: *Carcinoma of the pancreas; symptoms, signs and results of treatment in 122 cases,* Arch. Surg., 65:290, 1952. 8

Coffey, R. J.: *The relationship of acute and chronic cholecystitis to acute pancreatitis,* Sth. Med. J., 47:448, 1954. 3, 4

Comfort, M. W., Gambhill and Baggenstoss: *Chronic relapsing pancreatitis; a study of twenty-nine cases without associated disease of biliary or gastro-intestinal tract,* Gastroenterology, 6:239, 1946. 4

Connolly, J. E., and Richards: *Bilateral splanchnicectomy and lumbodorsal sympathectomy for chronic relapsing pancreatitis,* Ann. Surg., 131:58, 1950. 4

Crain, E. L., and Thorn: *Functioning pancreatic islet cell adenomas,* Medicine, 28:427, 1949. 6

De Castro Barbosa, J. J., Dockerty and Waugh: *Pancreatic heterotopia; review of the literature and report of 41 authenticated surgical cases, of which 25 were clinically significant,* Surg. Gynec. Obstet., 82:527, 1946. 1

Dodd, G. W., and Nafis: *Annular pancreas in the adult,* Amer. J. Roentgenol., 75:333, 1956. 1

Doubilet, H., and Mulholland: *Recurrent acute pancreatitis; observations on etiology and surgical treatment,* Ann. Surg., 128:609, 1948. 3, 4

Dragstedt, L. R., Haymond and Ellis: *Pathogenesis of acute pancreatitis (Acute pancreatic necrosis),* Arch. Surg., 28:232, 1934. 3

Drapiewski, J. F.: *Carcinoma of the pancreas; a study of neoplastic invasion of nerves and its clinical significance,* Amer. J. clin. Path., 14:549, 1944. 9

Duff, G. L., and Murray: *The pathology of islet cell tumors of the pancreas,* Amer. J. med. Sci., 203:437, 1942. 6

DuVal, Jr., M. K.: *Caudal pancreaticojejunostomy for chronic relapsing pancreatitis,* Ann. Surg., 140:775, 1954. 4

Section XIX (continued)

PLATE
NUMEER

Farrar, J. T.: *Pancreatitis, medical aspects,* Med. Clin. N. Amer., 38:1393, 1954. 3

Frantz, V. K.: *Tumors of islet cells with hyperinsulinism; benign, malignant, and questionable,* Ann. Surg., 112:161, 1940. 6

Gruber, G. B.: *Pathologie der Bauchspecheldrüre, in Henke-Lubarsch, Handbuch der speziellen pathologischen Anatomie und Histologie, V/2,* Julius Springer, Berlin, 1929. 1-3

Heacock, C. H., and Cara: *Radiation therapy of pancreatitis,* Radiology, 62:654, 1954. 4

Horgan, E. J.: *Accessory pancreatic tissue,* Arch. Surg., 2:521, 1921. 1

Howard, J. M., Moss and Rhoads: *Hyperinsulinism and islet cell tumors of the pancreas,* Int. Abst. Surg., 90:417, 1950. 6

Judd, E. S., Mattson and Mahorner: *Pancreatic cysts; report of 47 cases,* Arch. Surg., 22:838, 1931. 5

Kemp, R. C.: *Diseases of Stomach, Intestines and Pancreas,* W. B. Saunders Company, Philadelphia, 1917. 3, 4

Kennard, H. E.: *Papillary cystadenocarcinoma of the pancreas,* Surgery, 9:65, 1941. 7

Lehman, E. P.: *Annular pancreas as clinical problem,* Ann. Surg., 115:574, 1942. 1

Mahorner, H. R., and Mattson: *The etiology and pathology of cysts of the pancreas,* Arch. Surg., 22:1018, 1931. 5, 7

Maingot, R.: *Abdominal Operations,* Appleton-Century-Crofts, Incorporated, New York, 1955. 1

Mason, L. W., DeGiorgio and McGrath: *Papillary cystadenocarcinomas of the pancreas,* J. int. Coll. Surg., 22:440, 1954. 7

May, C. C.: *Cystic Fibrosis of the Pancreas in Infants and Children,* Charles C Thomas, Publisher, Springfield, Ill., 1954. 2

McWhorter, G. L.: *Cysts of the pancreas,* Arch. Surg., 11:619, 1925. 5

Miller, J. R., Baggenstoss and Comfort: *Carcinoma of pancreas; effect of histological type and grade of malignancy on its behavior,* Cancer, 4:233, 1951. 9

Oberling, C., and Guerin: *Cancer du Pancreas,* Gaston Doin et Cie., Paris, 1931. 7-9

Opie, E. L.: *Disease of the Pancreas; Its Cause and Nature,* J. B. Lippincott Company, Philadelphia, 1910. 3

Parry, E. W., Hallenbeck and Grindlay: *Pressures in the pancreatic and common ducts,* Arch. Surg., 70:757, 1955. 3

Parsons, W. B.: *Carcinoma of the pancreas and carcinoma of the ampulla of Vater; a re-evaluation,* Bull. N. Y. Acad. Med., 27:339, 1951. 7, 8

Payne, Jr., R. L.: *Annular pancreas,* Ann. Surg., 133:754, 1951. 1

Section XIX (continued)

PLATE
NUMBER

Poppel, M. H.: *Roentgen Manifestations of Pancreatic Disease,* Charles C Thomas, Publisher, Springfield, Ill., 1951. 5

Ray, B. S., and Console: *The relief of pain in chronic (calcareous) pancreatitis by sympathectomy,* Surg. Gynec. Obstet., 89:1, 1949. 4

Rich, A. R., and Duff: *Experimental and pathological studies on pathogenesis of acute haemorrhagic pancreatitis,* Bull. Johns Hopk. Hosp., 58:212, 1936. 3

Richman, A.: *Acute Pancreatitis,* Amer. J. Med., 21:246, 1956. 3

—— and Colp: *Chronic relapsing pancreatitis. Treatment by subtotal gastrectomy and vagotomy,* Ann. Surg., 131:145, 1950. 4

Robson, A. W. M., and Cammidge: *The Pancreas, Its Surgery and Pathology,* W. B. Saunders Company, Philadelphia, 1907. 3, 4, 6

Schmieden, V., and Sebering: *Chirurgie des Pankreas,* Arch. klin. Chir., 148:319, 1927. 5

Schwachman, H., Pryles and Gross: *Meconium ileus; a clinical study of 20 surviving patients,* Amer. J. Dis. Child., 91:233, 1956. 2

Silver, G. B., and Lubliner: *Carcinoma of the pancreas; a clinico-pathologic survey,* Surg. Gynec. Obstet., 86:703, 1948. 8, 9

U. S. Naval Med. School: *Color Atlas of Pathology,* J. B. Lippincott Company, Philadelphia, 1954. 1, 2, 6-9

Warren, K. W.: *Current management of benign and malignant pancreatic tumors,* Arch. Surg., 45:111, 1942. 6-8

——: *Surgical considerations in the management of chronic relapsing pancreatitis,* Surg. Clin. N. Amer., 35:785, 1955. 4

——, Fallis and Barron: *Acute pancreatitis and diabetes,* Ann. Surg., 132:1103, 1950. 3

Whipple, A. O.: *Surgical treatment of carcinoma of the ampullary region and head of the pancreas,* Amer. J. Surg., 40:260, 1938. 8

Willis, R. A.: *The Spread of Tumours in the Human Body,* J. & A. Churchill Ltd., London, 1933. 9

Winslow, S. B.: *Large pancreatic cyst. Case report, general discussion and review of the literature,* J. Mich. med. Soc., 47:1351, 1948. 5

Wissler, H., and Zollinger: *Die familiare kongenitale zystiche Pankreasfibrose mit Bronchiektasien,* Helv. paediat. Acta, 1, Supplem. 1945. 2

Zintel, H. A., Enterline and Rhoads: *Benign cystadenoma of pancreas,* Surgery, 35:612, 1954. 6

peritoneum — *continued*
  mesocolon, 28, 29, 131, 145
  mesoduodenum, 25
  omentum, greater, 6, 28, 145
    lesser, 5, 6, 22, 26, 28, 29, 131,
      145
    pancreas relation, 25, 28, 145
    pancreatic aberrant tissue, 141
peritonitis, biliary, 10, 116, 133
  purulent, 46, 78, 102, 103, 131
pernicious vomiting, 117
phagocytosis, *see* cell, Kupffer
phenol, halogenated, 44
phosphatase, acid, 43
  alkaline, origin, 43
    test, *see* test, hepatic,
      phosphatase
  glucose-6-, 86
phosphatid, *see* phospholipid
phospholipid, 37, 42, 86, 97
phosphorus poisoning, 91
phosphorylase, 36, 86
Phrygian cap, 22, 123
pilocarpine, *see* cholinergic drug
pituitary
  hemochromatosis and hemosiderosis,
    88, 89
  hormone, 41
placental circulation, 3
plant poison, 91
plate theory, 8, 9, 10
pleura, 4, 149
pleuropulmonary suppuration, 85
plexus
  nervous, celiac (anterior and
    posterior), 21, 31
    gastroduodenal, 21, 24
    hepatic (anterior and posterior),
      21, 24
    mesenteric, superior, 31
  venous, vitelline, 2, 3
pneumonia, 51, 78, 91, 97, 142
pneumothorax, 46
polyarteritis, *see* periarteritis nodosa
polycystic disease, 60
polycythemia vera, 108
polyp (gallbladder and bile duct),
  135, 136
porta hepatitis, *see* liver, porta
portal
  Hodgkin's disease, 110
  hypertension, ascites, 70, 71, 74
    children (without cause), 72
    cirrhosis, 68, 69, 70, 72, 73
    clinical manifestation, 70, 71
    obstruction, biliary, chronic, 84
    pathogenesis, 69, 72
    portacaval anastomosis, 18, 69,
      108
    schistosomiasis, 72, 105
    spleen, 69, 70, 71, 72, 73
    surgical relief, 73
    venous thrombosis, 72, 108
  triad and -tract, acute hepatic
    failure, 79
    biliary obstruction, 83, 84
    cholangiolitis, 97
    cirrhosis, 66, 67, 68, 69, 80, 81
    constituent, 8, 9, 10, 11
    granulomatous disease, 100, 101
    hepatitis, 92, 93, 94, 96
    left lobe atrophy, 6
    leukemia, 110

portal — *continued*
  triad and -tract — *continued*
    mononucleosis, 98
    periarteritis, 109
    Weil's disease, 99
  vein, *see* vein, portal
  venogram, 54, 73, 115
postcholecystectomy syndrome, 52,
  138
postnecrotic cirrhosis, *see* cirrhosis,
  postnecrotic
potassium intoxication, 76
pregnancy, cholesterol blood level,
  42, 124
  hemangioma producing, 111
  liver relation, 116, 117
proaccelerin, 40
process, uncinate, *see* pancreas,
  lingula
prostate, 43, 71, 149
protein (*see also* albumin; globulin;
  fibrinogen)
  choleretic effect, 52
  diet, high in (hepatic coma), 75
  digestion, 36, 37, 55, 57
  formation in liver, 7, 35, 36, 37,
    38, 39, 70
  lipotropic action, 37
  metabolism, 36, 37, 38, 55
  serum, ascites, 74
    cirrhosis, 38, 81
    eclampsia, 117
    hepatitis, 92, 93, 94, 95
    metabolic liver disease, 85
    nutritional liver disease, 77, 78
    obstruction, biliary, 92
prothrombin (*see also* test, hepatic,
  prothrombin time), 38, 40, 70
pruritus, 71, 97, 134, 136, 137
pseudocirrhosis, 68, 84
pseudodiverticulum, 22, 123, 129,
  131
pseudosclerosis, 87
putamen, 87
pylephlebitis, 92, 136
pyronine stain, 7, 39
pyruvic acid, 36

Q

quadrate lobe, 5, 6, 13, 18
Quick's prothrombin determination,
  40
quinine, 44

R

radiation, 110, 116, 144, 147
"ray fungus", 103
recess (*see also* space)
  hepatorenal, 131
  subhepatic, 131
  subphrenic, 131
reflux, bile and pancreatic juice, 24,
  27, 28, 29, 126, 128, 143
regenerative nodule, *see* liver,
  regeneration
renal (*see also* kidney; nephrosis)
  impression, 5, 6
  diseases, 76
reticulo-endothelium (*see also* cell,
  Kupffer), 47
retinal changes (lipidosis), 86
rheumatic vascular disease, 72
rheumatoid arthritis, 85

Rh factor, *see* erythroblastosis
ribose, 36
ribs, anatomic relation, 4, 6
rickets, 43
Rickettsial disease, 91
Riedel's lobe, 60
Roentgen ray, *see* radiation
Rokitansky-Aschoff's pseudo-
  diverticulum, 22, 123, 129, 131
rose bengal, 45
Rotor's disease, 48
Roux en Y procedure, 132

S

salivary gland, 58, 142, 149
Salmonella infection, 128
Santorini's duct, *see* duct, pancreatic
sarcoidosis, 38, 68, 101
sarcoma, 82, 110, 115, 147, 149
schistosomiasis, 72, 105
secretin, 31, 55, 58, 143, 148
Sengstaken balloon, 73
septicemia, 48, 51, 91, 92
septum (*see also* cirrhosis,
  morphogenesis)
  secundum, 3
  transversum, 2
serine, 37
shock, 90
shunt operation, 19, 73
sickle cell anemia, 48, 90, 124
siderophilin, 88
Silverman's needle, 46
sinus venosus, 2
sinusoid
  anatomic relation, 8, 9, 11, 12, 20
  bile pigment formation, 47, 48, 49
  cirrhosis development, 68
  development, 2, 3
  endothelial activity, 63
  obstruction, 64
  permeability, 20, 35, 64
  zonal necrosis, 64
situs inversus, 61
skin
  carcinoma, metastatic, 149
  hemochromatosis, hemosiderosis,
    88, 89
  hemorrhages, 99
  rash, 99
  sarcoidosis, 101
sodium
  retention, 71, 74
  sulfate, 52
solvent, organic, 91
space (*see also* recess)
  Disse's, 8, 9, 20
  Mall's, 8, 9, 20
  Morison's, 131
  perisinusoidal, 8, 9, 20
  subphrenic, 131
sphincter
  Oddi, action, 24, 27, 52, 53
    gallbladder removal, 52, 138
    innervation, 21, 52
    resection, 144
    spasm, 82, 124, 125, 128, 130,
      138
  venous (intrahepatic), 12
sphingomyelin, 86
spider nevi, 70, 71, 78, 79, 111
spinal cord, 21, 31
spiral fold, 22, 129

Spirochaeta pallida, 99
splanchnicectomy, 31, 143, 144
spleen (*see also* hypersplenism)
  anatomic relation, 6, 28
  carcinoma (extension), 149
  cirrhosis, 70, 71, 72, 73, 78, 79, 80,
    81
  displacement (pancreatic cyst), 145
  erythroblastosis, 120
  fatty liver, 78
  hemochromatosis, hemosiderosis,
    88, 89
  Hodgkin's disease, 110
  infected, 92
  metabolic liver disease, 86
  obstruction, biliary, 84
  pancreatic, aberrant tissue, 141
  portal hypertension, 69, 70, 71, 72,
    73
    vein thrombosis, 108
  rupture, 98
  sarcoidosis, 101
  schistosomiasis, 105
splenectomy, 73
splenomegaly, *see* hypersplenism; s.,
  cirrhosis; s., portal hypertension
starch, 36, 55, 57
starvation, 37, 77
steatorrhea, 55, 57, 142, 144, 148
stercobilinogen, 47
Sternberg-Reed cell, 110
steroid (*see also* aldosterone;
  androgen; cholesterol; estrogen)
  adrenal, 37, 41, 76
  metabolism, 37
stomach
  anatomic relation, 4, 5, 6, 14, 22,
    26, 28
  carcinoma, 114, 132
  displacement (pancreatic cyst), 145
  fistula, 126, 132
  hemochromatosis, hemosiderosis, 89
  pancreatic aberrant tissue, 141
    tumor extension, 148, 149
  perforation, 131
  resection, 16, 133, 144
stone, *see* cholelithiasis; pancreas,
  stone
stool, *see* fever
sucrose, 36
sugar, *see* glucose
sulfonamide, 44, 91
syndrome
  celiac, 57
  Chiari's, 72
  Cruveilhier-Baumgarten, 69
  Dubin-Johnson, 48
  Fanconi's, 40
  hepatorenal, 76, 116
  "inspissated bile", 120
  postcholecystectomy, 52, 138
syphilis, 4, 68, 72, 99, 119

T

Taenia echinococcus, 104
Talma-Morison omentopexy, 73
Tay-Sachs disease, 86
telangiectasis, 70, 71, 78, 79, 111
Terry needle, 46
test
  Coomb's, 120
  dye excretion, *see* t., hepatic
  Graham-Cole's, 54

THE CIBA COLLECTION OF MEDICAL ILLUSTRATIONS

SUPPLEMENT TO VOLUME 3

DIGESTIVE SYSTEM

PART III

LIVER, BILIARY TRACT AND PANCREAS

A Compilation of Paintings on
New Aspects of Structure, Metabolism,
Diagnostic and Surgical Procedures
Associated with Certain Liver Diseases

Prepared by
FRANK H. NETTER, M.D.

In collaboration with

HANS POPPER, M.D., PH.D.
and
GEORGE T. PACK, M.D.

Edited by
FREDRICK F. YONKMAN, M.D., PH.D.

Commissioned and published by

C I B A

CONTENTS

Printed in U.S.A.

Original Printing by Colorpress, New York, N.Y.
Color Engravings by Embassy Photo Engraving Co., Inc., New York, N.Y.
Offset Conversion by R. R. Donnelley & Sons Company
Current Printing by R. R. Donnelley & Sons Company

INTRODUCTION

In the years that have passed since my original collaboration with Dr. Hans Popper on the preparation of Volume 3, Part III, of the CIBA COLLECTION, our friendship has flourished and my admiration for the man has grown continuously. I have called upon him many times for advice and guidance when confronted with difficult problems. His medical knowledge is great, his urge to help is unlimited and his enthusiasm for this project has been truly stimulating. It was, consequently, with sincere pleasure that I undertook to collaborate with him again on the revision of this book and the preparation of its supplement.

Dr. Popper is a leader on the frontier of investigational medicine, yet he interprets it in relation to the vast panorama of established knowledge which his eyes encompass. It was most inspiring to have him point out the significant features of this combined vista, and I have endeavored to portray these in the illustrations herein contained. The proper selection of new and important topics and the simplification thereof would have been impossible without him. I also wish to thank Dr. Popper's brilliant associates who helped us with advice in their specialized fields; these are

Dr. Tibor Barka, Dr. Sergei Feitelberg, Dr. Fenton Schaffner and Dr. Ferenc Hutterer of The Mount Sinai Hospital, New York City.

One of the major advances in the management of liver tumors, since the original publication of this book, concerns the development, refinement and appropriate application of techniques for segmental and lobar extirpation. Dr. George Pack has been a major contributor to this advance. Dr. J. H. Walton, the editor of *Clinical Symposia* (CIBA), with his characteristic editorial acumen, induced Dr. Pack to contribute an article on this subject to that publication, and I was fortunate to have had the opportunity to illustrate the article. Luckily, this occurred at the time when the present supplement was in preparation, for thus it became possible to incorporate here those illustrations, with appropriate text materials. For me, personally, to have met Dr. Pack and enjoyed his friendliness and simple, direct approach was rewarding, and to have collaborated with him and his associate, Dr. Abdol Islami, was an added gratification. Finally, I must say that Dr. Walton's assistance in organizing these materials was of immeasurable help.

FRANK H. NETTER, M.D.

During the seven years that have elapsed since the appearance of the original book, Volume 3, Part III, of THE CIBA COLLECTION OF MEDICAL ILLUSTRATIONS, our knowledge of liver diseases has increased considerably, and our concepts have changed as a result of the introduction of newer viewpoints and, particularly, of novel techniques. It is not possible to do justice to these almost explosive developments in a revision which, of necessity, is controlled by a straitjacket of practical considerations. Our choice of changes and additions had to be based on clinical applications. The frustration inherent in making these decisions was more than compensated for by the stimulation of working with Frank Netter, whose endeavor to present a three-dimensional visualization of biologic processes frequently leads to clarification of physiologic problems. Nevertheless, for the subjective aspect of this selection, indulgence is requested.

Among the most significant developments during this seven-year span are the expanding use of fine-structure techniques in the study of the human liver (greatly facilitated by wider application of the Menghini needle [see page 46], which seems to have reduced significantly the morbidity and mortality accompanying liver biopsy), the extension of our knowledge concerning metabolism in the liver, the introduction of additional physical methods in the diagnosis of liver disease, the revised classification of jaundice and the delineation of disease entities.

These advances called for not only a revision of some of the plates of the first edition, and the rewriting of certain texts, but also for new plates with corresponding texts. The additional materials deal with features revealed by electron microscopy, in normal and abnormal liver cells, and with their histochemistry. These are dovetailed with a schematic presentation of recent thoughts on locating metabolic pathways within these cells. All this has led to hesitant attempts to introduce organelle pathology, going beyond classic cellular pathology, with the aim of describing abnormal submicroscopic structures in viable cells, thus reflecting their altered function. The plate which suggests a two-directional disturbance in one liver cell (see page 177) represents an endeavor to use organelle pathology in the interpretation of the clinical function tests. Doubtless these initial — and, in many

ways, hypothetical — approaches will be corrected and elaborated rapidly as fine-structure analysis progresses and unites structure with function.

As to diagnostic procedures, liver function tests and the interpretation of their results have changed little in the intervening years, except for the introduction of the determination of serum activity of such enzymes as transaminases, and the increased application of the blood ammonia level to the diagnosis of hepatic precoma and, even more so, to the understanding of coma. In many institutions, however, physical techniques such as peritoneoscopy, scintillation scanning after the administration of radioisotopes, and the determination of portal pressure, as well as radiologic procedures, challenge liver function tests and liver biopsy as the most efficient laboratory procedures in the diagnosis of liver disease. Although full agreement concerning the roles of these techniques has not been reached, it was felt that their descriptions would be useful. The discovery that much of the direct-reacting bilirubin is in a conjugated form, mainly as a glucuronide, has clarified the previously mysterious van den Bergh reaction, and called for redrawing the plates devoted to bilirubin metabolism and the pathogenesis of jaundice. The recognition and explanation of the familial hyperbilirubinemias and the re-evaluation of jaundice in the neonatal period naturally followed. These, in part, also represent a description of new disease entities such as chronic idiopathic jaundice, with and without pigment (the Dubin-Johnson and the Rotor syndromes, respectively; see page 180), as well as a reclassification of jaundice in pregnancy. The delineation of chronic active hepatitis as a frequent and now better-appreciated entity, and the increasing occurrence of drug-induced hepatic injury, called for new plates, and the clarification of the pathways leading to cirrhosis stimulated redrawing for this topic also.

An account of the philosophy of this revision and supplement cannot be closed without pointing out that little has been added to the therapy of liver disease, even though the diagnosis and understanding of its pathogenesis are rapidly advancing. Future revisions will, hopefully, correct this inadequacy.

HANS POPPER, M.D., PH.D.
Pathologist-in-Chief, The Mount Sinai Hospital

Professor of Pathology, Columbia University
College of Physicians and Surgeons
New York City

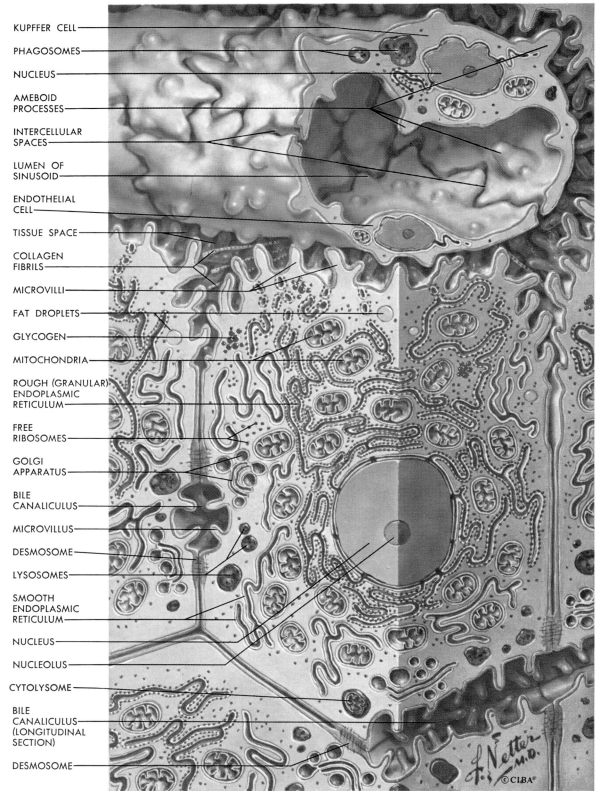

KUPFFER CELL

PHAGOSOMES

NUCLEUS

AMEBOID PROCESSES

INTERCELLULAR SPACES

LUMEN OF SINUSOID

ENDOTHELIAL CELL

TISSUE SPACE

COLLAGEN FIBRILS

MICROVILLI

FAT DROPLETS

GLYCOGEN

MITOCHONDRIA

ROUGH (GRANULAR) ENDOPLASMIC RETICULUM

FREE RIBOSOMES

GOLGI APPARATUS

BILE CANALICULUS

MICROVILLUS

DESMOSOME

LYSOSOMES

SMOOTH ENDOPLASMIC RETICULUM

NUCLEUS

NUCLEOLUS

CYTOLYSOME

BILE CANALICULUS (LONGITUDINAL SECTION)

DESMOSOME

ULTRAMICROSCOPIC STRUCTURE OF NORMAL LIVER CELLS

Electron microscopy raises the maximal magnification from 1000 times to 150,000 or more, making it possible not only to see cells but also to observe their components, called organelles. Some organelles have not yet been delineated, and the relationships, significance and functions of those now recognized will probably be interpreted differently in the future.

The border of the hepatocyte is of three types: 1. It is almost straight (except for occasional invaginations) where two neighboring cells are in close contact, with a narrow *intercellular space,* 100 angstroms (A) in width, extending between cell membranes. 2. The surface of the liver cell directed toward the perisinusoidal tissue space has many irregular extensions, designated as *microvilli.* These increase the cell's surface and indicate active resorption or secretion of fluid. This *sinusoidal* surface is further increased by extension of the *tissue spaces* between neighboring liver cells. 3. The *bile canaliculus* contains regular fingerlike microvilli projecting into its lumen. It is separated from the narrow space between neighboring cells by fusion and condensation of the cell membranes (*desmosome*). The surface directed against the perisinusoidal space is much larger than that toward the bile canaliculus, reflecting the greater function of the hepatocyte directed toward the blood stream, in contrast to that involved in bile formation.

The *nuclear* membrane consists of two layers with many pores. The outer membrane is continuous, in places, with the profiles of the *endoplasmic reticula.* The latter, probably the most specific organelles, are long, narrow, wavy channels. Most of these are lined with fine Palade *granules,* or ribosomes, which are considered to be the sites of protein formation. Some *ribosomes* are *free* in the hyaloplasm. Other profiles of the *endoplasmic reticulum* are free of ribosomes, even under normal circumstances but particularly after starvation, and they are then designated as *smooth.* Between the profiles of the endoplasmic reticulum, and frequently very close to them, are the

mitochondria, which have a double membrane, the inner one invaginating into a central matrix as cristae. Another organelle is the *Golgi apparatus,* which consists of groups of short smooth lamellae surrounded by fine vacuoles. Also, in the vicinity of the bile canaliculi are bodies designated as *lysosomes,* to indicate their identity with a cell fraction containing hydrolytic enzymes. These bodies have varied shapes and appearances and contain ferritin or other pigments, *e.g.,* lipofuscin pigment. Altered endoplasmic reticula or mitochondria are surrounded by membranes to form *cytolysomes.* The functions of these various bodies and their relation to hydrolytic enzymes, including acid phosphatase, are still problematic, and it is, therefore, preferable to designate them as pericanalicular dense bodies.

The hyaloplasm, or intracytoplasmic substance, exhibits many variations, depending greatly on nutri-

tion. It contains *glycogen,* which appears clear under the electron microscope, but which is recognized as particulate matter after lead staining. *Fat droplets* and clear vacuoles vary in size and number. The perisinusoidal space is normally narrow and is filled with a maze of hepatocellular microvilli which are in contact with the sinusoidal-lining cells; between these cells there are a few *collagen fibrils.* The continuous basement membrane, which is characteristic of all other capillaries, is missing. This enhances the exchange between liver cells and blood and justifies the distinguishing term, "sinusoids". This exchange is further facilitated by spaces between the *endothelial cells.* The *Kupffer cells,* which line the sinusoids, are either flat or bulky. The endothelial-lining cells have few organelles. The Kupffer cells have more, among them bodies designated as *phagosomes,* which resemble the lysosomes and contain acid phosphatase.

ULTRAMICROSCOPIC STRUCTURE OF ABNORMAL LIVER CELLS

In liver cell injury the organelles undergo changes which vary according to the offender and the duration of the insult. Moreover, because of continuing advances in microscopy, and as in all fine-structure studies, any explanation of these changes is bound to appear naïve in a very short time.

According to our present knowledge, the organelle responsible for the most specific function of the liver cell, the *endoplasmic reticulum,* undergoes various changes. The profiles dilate and *shatter* and are transformed into vesicles which are scattered throughout the liver cell. The *ribosomes* lose contact with the membranes, so that smooth profiles predominate. Small fragments of normal, rough endoplasmic reticulum persist only around *mitochondria.* In later stages, closely packed narrow lamellae of smooth endoplasmic reticulum appear, possibly as a regenerative change. On light microscopy, these *whorls* are seen as eosinophilic hyaline inclusions. Diffuse reduction of cytoplasmic basophilia is due to the loss of ribosomes containing ribonucleic acid (RNA), whereas an increase of ribosomes in later stages, at least in some cells, causes basophilia of regenerating cells. Injury to the endoplasmic reticulum appears to be the first alteration following administration of many poisons and drugs; it also occurs in human viral hepatitis and is the most sensitive electron-microscopic indication of liver cell injury. The energy-providing *mitochondria can swell,* and their matrices become less dense, as a result of altered permeability of their double membranes. Milder degrees of swelling possibly reflect physiologic regulation of cell respiratory function under the influence of thyroxin or other factors. Excessive swelling is produced by poisons, such as cyanide, which arrest cellular respiration and thus exhaust the supply of adenosine triphosphate (ATP) by the uncoupling of oxidative phosphorylation. This accompanies many types of cell death from various causes. Another mitochondrial alteration entails a change of their shape and *cristae,* with normal or increased density of their matrices. Giant forms occur in alcoholic hepatitis and have been experimentally produced in choline and unsaturated fatty acid deficiencies. Various *alterations of cristae* include swelling, curling, elongation and multiplication to produce "myelin" degeneration.

Most types of hepatocellular injury are associated with an increase of pericanalicular dense bodies (*lysosomes*) and their spread throughout the cells. They vary

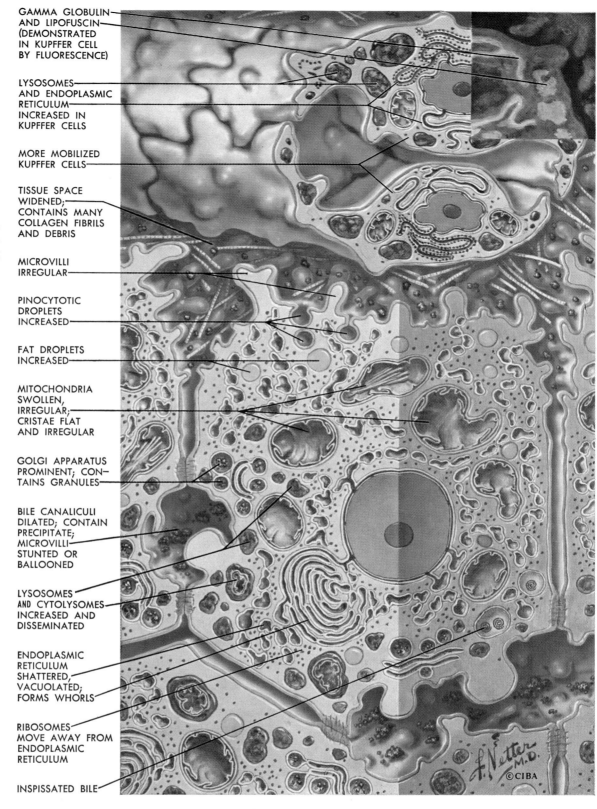

GAMMA GLOBULIN AND LIPOFUSCIN (DEMONSTRATED IN KUPFFER CELL BY FLUORESCENCE)

LYSOSOMES AND ENDOPLASMIC RETICULUM INCREASED IN KUPFFER CELLS

MORE MOBILIZED KUPFFER CELLS

TISSUE SPACE WIDENED; CONTAINS MANY COLLAGEN FIBRILS AND DEBRIS

MICROVILLI IRREGULAR

PINOCYTOTIC DROPLETS INCREASED

FAT DROPLETS INCREASED

MITOCHONDRIA SWOLLEN, IRREGULAR; CRISTAE FLAT AND IRREGULAR

GOLGI APPARATUS PROMINENT; CONTAINS GRANULES

BILE CANALICULI DILATED; CONTAIN PRECIPITATE; MICROVILLI STUNTED OR BALLOONED

LYSOSOMES AND CYTOLYSOMES INCREASED AND DISSEMINATED

ENDOPLASMIC RETICULUM SHATTERED, VACUOLATED; FORMS WHORLS

RIBOSOMES MOVE AWAY FROM ENDOPLASMIC RETICULUM

INSPISSATED BILE

f. Netter M.D. ©CIBA

in size, shape and density. Some contain degenerated organelles (a fact which reflects, for example, an increased turnover of mitochondria), whereas others include groups of organelles. This type of *cytolysome* has been considered a device to segregate focal areas of cytoplasmic degeneration. Other such bodies reflect increased, and possibly abnormal, pinocytosis. A third source of the bodies is retention of substances which are normally secreted in bile, particularly near *bile canaliculi.* The *Golgi apparatus is prominent* under these circumstances, and its vesicles contain electron-opaque material. The relation between Golgi vesicles, the endoplasmic reticulum and lysosomes is not clear. These dense bodies are also the site of deposition of pigments such as *lipofuscin.* The accumulation of fluid in the endoplasmic reticulum, in mitochondria and in *pinocytotic vacuoles* accounts for hydropic swelling.

Changes also occur on cell borders. *Bile canaliculi* can *dilate,* with swelling, *distortion* or loss of *microvilli.* The perisinusoidal *tissue space* may also dilate, and sinusoidal microvilli may swell or disappear. Alteration of bile canaliculi is typically associated with cholestatic jaundice, but changes of the sinusoidal border are not specific. If the latter are severe enough, cytoplasmic material is released into the tissue space, and, clinically, the serum activity of the serum transaminases rises (see page 175). After a long-lasting injury, the enlarged sinusoidal space also contains *collagen fibrils.*

The sinusoidal cells increase in number and enlarge, so that the *Kupffer* cells contain large numbers of phagosomes and an increase in the endoplasmic reticulum as well as lipofuscin; the latter is recognized by spontaneous *fluorescence,* and γ-globulin can be demonstrated by immunofluorescence.

METABOLIC PROCESSES IN LIVER CELLS

The advancement of fine-structure techniques and the present knowledge of organelles have shifted the emphasis, concerning metabolic activities of the liver, from the liver as a whole (relative to the "metabolic pool", see page 36), to processes within the hepatocyte or within the hepatic mesenchymal cells. Protein formation takes place on *ribosomes* that are free in the cytoplasm and also on those attached to the *endoplasmic reticulum*. They consist of ribonucleoprotein (*RNP*) particles with a molecular weight of approximately 2,000,000. In the RNP particle a genetic code is incorporated which depends on the relative position of four main bases: the purines, adenine and guanine; and the pyrimidines, uracil and cytosine. The sequence of the bases influences the position of the *amino acid* constituents in the protein molecule. This genetic code originates from the nuclear chromosomal desoxyribonucleic acid (*DNA*) which is arranged in a double helix with similar bases, except that thymine replaces uracil. Each DNA helix is assumed to act as a template for the formation of the shorter-chain messenger, RNA, the individual components of which come from the *nucleolus*. *Messenger RNA*, released from the *nucleus*, brings genetic information for the formation of *protein* to the ribosomes. The amino acid building blocks of protein in the hyaloplasm are derived either from the blood stream, as a result of intestinal absorption, or from cellular metabolism of carbohydrates or fatty acids. They obtain their amino groups by *transaminase* activity. All of the *amino acids* are *activated by enzymes* which transfer adenosine monophosphate to their carboxyl groups, with liberation of pyrophosphate. The resulting "activated" amino acid (adenylate) combines with *soluble RNA*, which has a relatively small molecular weight of 30,000. This RNA is the carrier which brings amino acids to the ribosomes, and returns to the hyaloplasm. Whether all protein formation is completed on one ribosome, or whether a chain is necessary in the form of helical polysomes, is not known. *Ribosomes attached to the endoplasmic reticulum* appear to be responsible for the proteins secreted by the liver cell into the blood. Secretion occurs with considerable speed, as indicated by observations following the administration of radioactive amino acids. These *blood proteins* include *serum albumin*, α-*globulin*, several *proteins important in blood coagulation* (prothrombin; factors V, VII and IX; and fibrinogen) and also some serum *enzymes*. The *smooth endoplasmic reticulum* is the site of *glucose-6-phosphatase* (see page 174), and thus it is the site of blood sugar formation. Also localized here are the enzymes responsible for *detoxification* and *neutralization*. These inactivate *various drugs* by oxidation, acetylation, methylation and *conjugation*. The contribution of the lamellae of the *Golgi apparatus* is not established, especially since they are not clearly differentiated morphologically from the endoplasmic reticulum. They may *conjugate bilirubin* with glucuronide. Probably *bile acids* form from *cholesterol* in the smooth endoplasmic reticulum. These are transferred to the bile by the secretory apparatus, which includes the Golgi apparatus, the pericanalicular dense bodies and the *canaliculi*. Canalicular microvilli are probably responsible for the secretion of *electrolytes* and *water*.

The metabolic processes thus far described depend on energy supplied by the *mitochondria*. The enzymes of the *Krebs citric acid cycle* are located in their matrix (see page 36). Pyruvate is converted to acetate as *acetyl Co-A* as it is fed into the cycle. It is oxidized to *carbon dioxide*, while the dehydrogenases remove *hydrogen* from the intermediates. This hydrogen, or its equivalent in *electrons*, passes to the membranes of the *mitochondria* where the enzymes of the so-called respiratory chain are localized. These electron carriers consist of *cytochromes*, *flavoproteins* and pyridine nucleotides. As hydrogen combines with oxygen to form water, *energy* is provided in specific locations. This, in turn, restores *ATP* from adenosine diphosphate (*ADP*) and inorganic phosphate. ATP is used as the immediate source of *energy* in the metabolism of the cells. The energy becomes available as high-energy phosphate bonds are split from ATP. The resulting ADP is recharged by the respiratory-chain enzymes in the mitochondrial membrane. This membrane is said to consist of two layers of protein molecules separated by lipid. Respiratory assemblies, consisting of several specific enzyme molecules, apparently representing recurring units of complete sets, are aligned on the membrane. These membrane enzymes probably regulate the shape and permeability of the mitochondrial membranes. The state of the membranes is influenced by physiological substances, such as thyroxin or ATP, and by pharmacologic agents. Alteration of their permeability results in swelling, during which oxidative phosphorylation is uncoupled, or oxidation occurs without recharge of ADP to ATP. Di- and triphosphopyridine nucleotides (*DPN*, *TPN*) are key cofactors in the *cycle* of hydrogen release and acceptance. Since they participate in many metabolic processes, their state of oxidation or reduction, which depends on mitochondrial function, determines the direction of intracellular metabolic processes, *e.g.*, *fatty acid* synthesis or oxidation. Mitochondria, therefore, not only provide energy but also influence the pathways of metabolism. Specific liver cell functions are localized in the endoplasmic reticulum, whereas mitochondria are responsible for the nonspecific provision of the necessary energy. In contrast, the supernatant fluid is the route of supply and the site of *storage* of glycogen, fat and, possibly, proteins and vitamins.

Fat is brought to the liver either as a protein complex (*chylomicrons*) or as nonesterified fatty acids (*NEFA*). *Fatty acids* in the liver come from *lipoproteins*, NEFA and other metabolic pathways via *acetyl Co-A* and *phospholipids*. Lipoproteins consist of protein complexed with *triglycerides, phospholipids* and *cholesterol*. They are considered to be the most significant vehicle for the release of lipids from the liver, whereas NEFA are the most important media for bringing fatty acids from depots to the liver cells. Interference with lipoprotein formation, from insufficient protein synthesis in general or from the lack of ATP, is important in the development of hepatic steatosis. The synthesis of triglycerides and phospholipids initially follows a common pathway which begins with glycerol being activated by ATP and by an enzyme, glycerol kinase. The resulting glycerol phosphate combines with fatty acids bound to Co-A to form phosphatidic acid. This unstable compound loses its phosphate with the assistance of a *phosphatase* to form a diglyceride, a key intermediate, the further fate of which depends on available cofactors. Activated choline, in the form of cytidine diphosphate choline, shifts the synthesis toward lecithin with the help of a transferase, and cytidine diphosphate ethanolamine favors the formation of another phospholipid. In contrast, fatty acids, activated by Co-A, favor the formation of triglycerides which accumulate in steatosis. The availability of cofactors and their reduction or increase, resulting from injurious agents or specific deficiencies, are examples of the dependence of pathologic hepatic alterations on the prevalence of normal pathways. The biosynthesis of fatty acids follows three pathways, two of which are in mitochondria. One is a reversal of fatty acid oxidation and requires such cofactors as ATP, Co-A, reduced triphosphopyridine nucleotide (*TPNH*) and reduced diphosphopyridine nucleotide (*DPNH*), and this results in relatively short-chain acids. A second one, possibly responsible for longer-chain fatty acids, requires similar cofactors and a heat-stable factor probably related to pyridoxal phosphate. The third pathway, apparently in the soluble fraction, produces de novo nonmitochondrial long-chain fatty acids and requires other cofactors plus TPNH. The availability of TPNH is a key factor in directing intracellular pathways. The fatty acids also are the source of the *ketone* bodies which can be released to the blood.

The energy provided by the mitochondria and the availability of Co-A are important in the anabolic and catabolic processes of carbohydrate metabolism, which have been clarified in recent years. *Pyruvic acid* is formed from *glucose* by two pathways, and the initial step of both is the formation of *glucose-6-phosphate* by *hexokinase* and ATP. One path is the classical Embden-Meyerhof scheme via fructose and triose, whereas the other involves *pentose*. It thus supplies an ingredient for nucleic acids and, moreover, restores TPNH from TPN. Glucose-6-phosphate also is the initial step of glycogen synthesis via glucose-1-phosphate, which is formed with the help of phosphoglucomutase. This substance combines with uridine phosphate to form uridine diphosphate glucose (*UDPG*) with the help of *pyrophosphatase*. UDPG is converted to *glycogen* by *UDPG transglucosylase* and *branching enzymes*. In this process *phosphorylases* are not involved, as they are in the process of glycogenolysis in which *debranching enzymes* and probably amylase are also necessary.

Part of the energy provided by the mitochondria is also used to convert the amino group released by oxidases from amino acids to form *urea*. This process involves a complex cycle of the amino acids ornithine, citrulline and arginine, originally described by Krebs and Henseleit. *Ammonia*, in effect, is linked with carbon dioxide (see page 178).

Normally, the metabolic functions of the *Kupffer cells* are relatively few. Organelles of these cells are small, and a few profiles of the endoplasmic reticulum are visible. Most of their functions involve *phagocytosis*, with the uptake of *iron pigment, debris* and *bacteria*. Their ability to transform *hemoglobin* to nonconjugated or *free bilirubin* is referred to under Bile Pigment Metabolism, Normal and Abnormal (see page 47).

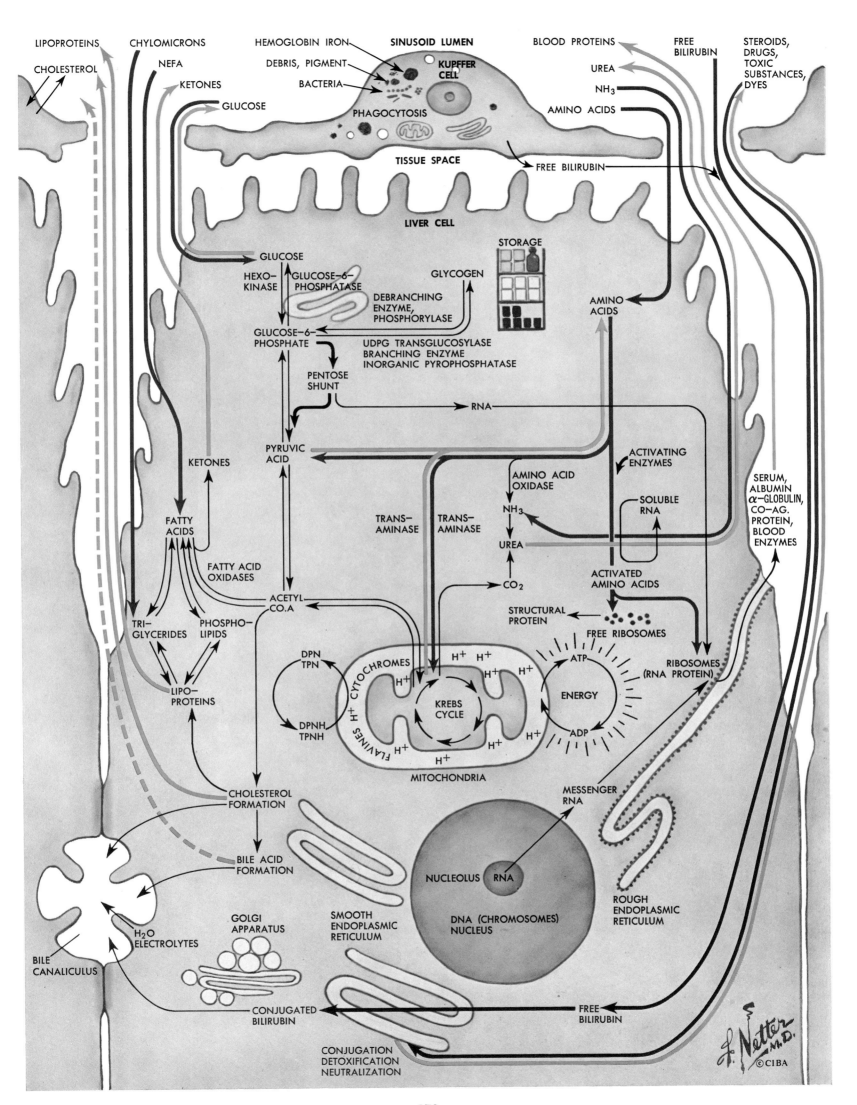

LIPOPROTEINS

CHOLESTEROL

CHYLOMICRONS

NEFA

KETONES

GLUCOSE

HEMOGLOBIN IRON

DEBRIS, PIGMENT

BACTERIA

SINUSOID LUMEN

KUPFFER CELL

PHAGOCYTOSIS

BLOOD PROTEINS

UREA

NH₃

AMINO ACIDS

FREE BILIRUBIN

STEROIDS, DRUGS, TOXIC SUBSTANCES, DYES

TISSUE SPACE

FREE BILIRUBIN

LIVER CELL

GLUCOSE

HEXO-KINASE

GLUCOSE-6-PHOSPHATASE

GLYCOGEN

STORAGE

DEBRANCHING ENZYME, PHOSPHORYLASE

GLUCOSE-6-PHOSPHATE

UDPG TRANSGLUCOSYLASE BRANCHING ENZYME INORGANIC PYROPHOSPHATASE

AMINO ACIDS

PENTOSE SHUNT

RNA

KETONES

PYRUVIC ACID

TRANS-AMINASE

TRANS-AMINASE

AMINO ACID OXIDASE

NH₃

UREA

ACTIVATING ENZYMES

SOLUBLE RNA

SERUM, ALBUMIN α-GLOBULIN, CO-AG. PROTEIN, BLOOD ENZYMES

FATTY ACIDS

FATTY ACID OXIDASES

ACETYL CO.A

CO₂

ACTIVATED AMINO ACIDS

STRUCTURAL PROTEIN

FREE RIBOSOMES

TRI-GLYCERIDES

PHOSPHO-LIPIDS

DPN TPN

CYTOCHROMES

H⁺ H⁺

H⁺

ATP

ENERGY

RIBOSOMES (RNA PROTEIN)

LIPO-PROTEINS

FLAVINES H⁺

KREBS CYCLE

DPNH TPNH

ADP

H⁺

MITOCHONDRIA

CHOLESTEROL FORMATION

MESSENGER RNA

BILE ACID FORMATION

BILE CANALICULUS

H₂O ELECTROLYTES

GOLGI APPARATUS

SMOOTH ENDOPLASMIC RETICULUM

NUCLEOLUS RNA

DNA (CHROMOSOMES) NUCLEUS

ROUGH ENDOPLASMIC RETICULUM

CONJUGATED BILIRUBIN

FREE BILIRUBIN

CONJUGATION DETOXIFICATION NEUTRALIZATION

F. Netter M.D.
©CIBA

HISTOCHEMISTRY OF LIVER CELLS

Attempts to demonstrate the function of organelles include the separation of cellular fractions by *ultracentrifugation* and histochemical or immunocytochemical localization of the chemical compounds. Serial centrifugation of tissue homogenized in sucrose solution separates various cell fractions. The *nuclear fraction* with the largest particles sediments first, and then the *mitochondrial* portion. From the latter fraction a slightly smaller one is separated; this is called the *lysosome* layer, because it contains many hydrolytic enzymes. The *microsomes* correspond to the *endoplasmic reticulum*. The supernatant or *cell sap* layer is the hyaloplasm, and the lightest fraction is lipid (*fat*).

Histochemistry indicates distribution rather than concentration. Diffusely distributed material may be less well visualized than that which is concentrated in one site.

Nuclear chromatin is indicated by the *Feulgen* reaction, which is considered specific for desoxypentose nucleic acid. Synthesis of *DNA* can be demonstrated by autoradiography after the administration of *tritiated thymidine*. Thymidine is specifically incorporated into DNA and is not reutilized. Grains or tracks in the silver emulsion over the nuclei are indications of newly formed cells. The cytoplasm of liver cells is basophilic, owing to the phosphoric acid valences of RNP in the ribosomes, both those associated with the endoplasmic reticulum and those free in the cytoplasm. Other acid valences, such as the free *RNA* in the supernatant, are dissolved during fixation, but basophilia which is recognizable by light microscopy does not differentiate *free ribosomes* (which presumably form the structural proteins of the cells) from ribosomes associated with the endoplasmic reticulum which produce the protein to be secreted. The latter protein can be visualized by yellow-green fluorescence after staining with fluoresceinated antihuman *albumin* produced in rabbits. The smooth endoplasmic reticulum can be visualized by demonstration of *glucose-6-phosphatase*. The mitochondria are the site of the *succinoxidases*, *diaphorases* and *dehydrogenases* demon-

strated by tetrazolium methods. In the mitochondria, adenosine triphosphatase (*ATP-ase*) can also be shown. The *Golgi apparatus* contains *pyrophosphatases* which are possibly related to conjugation. The pericanalicular dense bodies and the phagosomes give a variety of histochemical reactions pointing to their lack of homogeneity, also apparent on electron microscopy. Many of these entities react positively with Schiff's reagent even after *glycogen* removal, suggesting that they contain *polysaccharides*. Some have a golden to brown spontaneous fluorescence indicative of lipofuscin; others contain *ferritin granules* and give a positive iron reaction. Most, but not all, exhibit *acid phosphatase* activity. Many contain *5-nucleotidase*, which is also found in cell membranes. They may contain *β-glucuronidase* and *esterases*. The pericanalicular dense bodies are probably best considered as devices to segregate, within the cell, the material

to be absorbed or to be excreted, stored or digested. In the hyaloplasm, besides glycogen and *fat droplets*, some *esterases*, *phosphorylases* and *glycogen-branching enzymes* can be demonstrated, pointing to the *cell sap* as the site of glycogen formation and breakdown. Sinusoidal and, particularly, bile *canalicular* membranes give an ATP-ase reaction. This, however, is probably not the ubiquitous ATP-ase found in mitochondria and chemically in the cell sap, because it differs in its response to specific inhibitors and activators. Nevertheless, the histochemical ATP-ase reaction, whatever its metabolic meaning, is probably the most effective method of visualizing bile canaliculi which also give an *aminopeptidase* reaction. *Pinocytotic vacuoles*, aggregating around the sinusoidal border, account for increased *acid phosphatase* activity in cell damage, particularly in anoxia. On the sinusoidal border also, *alkaline phosphatase* can be visualized.

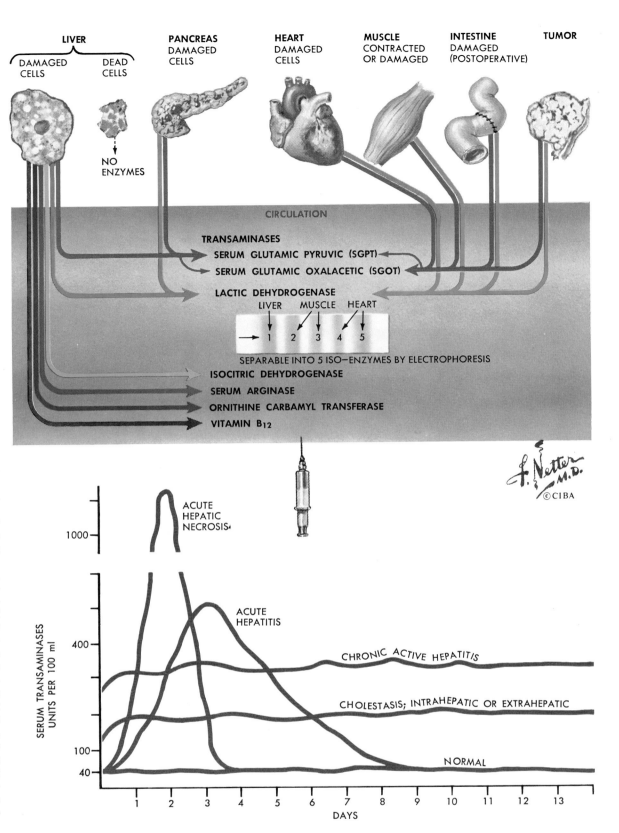

SERUM TRANSAMINASES

The diagnosis of liver diseases can be facilitated by determining the activity of certain serum enzymes, especially those formed by the liver. A reduction of the activity of choline esterase or coagulation factors (see page 40) and an elevation of alkaline phosphatase (see page 43) have long been known to indicate cholestasis. Only recently has an elevation of the serum activity of various enzymes, derived from damaged tissues, assumed practical, differential diagnostic importance. The main examples of such enzymes are the glutamic pyruvic and the glutamic oxalacetic transaminases. These transfer amino groups from amino acids, such as glutamic acid, to α-keto acids, namely, oxalacetic or pyruvic acid. This reaction would result in the conversion of glutamic acid to α-ketoglutaric acid, and the formation of aspartic acid from oxalacetic, or alanine from pyruvic acid. They require pyridoxine for their action, and most determinations measure changes of this cofactor. These enzymes are found in almost all organs.

Originally, necrosis of parenchymal cells was assumed to release enzyme protein into the circulation, and the elevation was considered to be the result of cytolysis. Actually, *dead tissues fail to release enzymes*, but *damaged cells* permit *leakage* of cytoplasmic material into the *circulation*. Thus, an elevation of the *transaminases* reflects an increased permeability of the cell membrane. This occurs after *damage to the liver*, for instance by *hepatitis*, or to the heart immediately after a *myocardial infarct*. Similar elevations result from *damage to the pancreas*, *injury to the intestine* (*postoperative*, in particular), *necrosis of tumor tissue*, or violent exercise. The latter can result in sufficient leakage from *skeletal muscles* to produce enzyme elevations in the abnormal range.

The activity of a given enzyme in the tissue far exceeds its plasma concentration. Elevation following injury of different organs reflects, to some extent, the specific organ's activity. However, the situation is complex, since the speed of removal of the enzymes also determines the degree and duration of any elevation, and therefore the differential diagnostic utilization of enzyme activity is determined more by empiric observations than by a biochemical rationale. In general, the elevation of *serum glutamic pyruvic transaminase* (*SGPT*) is relatively greater after injury to the liver and pancreas, whereas the elevation of *serum glutamic oxalacetic transaminase* (*SGOT*) is higher in myocardial infarct, muscle injury, intestinal alterations, tumors and

nonspecific damage. The ratio between SGPT and SGOT has been ascribed significance in the separation of various liver diseases. Both transaminases are usually determined, and most authorities agree that an elevation of serum activity of SGPT is more sensitive, as well as more specific, for liver injury.

Attempts are under way to increase the diagnostic usefulness of enzyme tests by various devices, such as studying groups of serum enzymes, or separating enzymes with apparently identical function into different electrophoretic serum protein fractions, called *iso-enzymes*. *Lactic dehydrogenase*, for example, is found in many organs and has recently been widely used in cancer diagnosis. It has been *separated by immunologic* or *electrophoretic methods into five fractions*. The one derived from the *liver* moves more slowly electrophoretically; that from the *heart*, faster. Of those enzymes coming specifically from the liver,

only *serum arginase* and *ornithine carbamyl transferase* (both of the urea cycle) have not yet been sufficiently sensitive to be of value. Whether *isocitric dehydrogenase* comes only from the liver is still not established. *Vitamin B_{12}* deserves mention here, because its serum level also rises in liver damage.

Regardless of any theoretical basis, at present the *transaminase* levels are the most widely used in clinical practice. They show a moderate elevation in *intrahepatic* and *extrahepatic cholestasis*, but in *hepatitis* a transient peak is noted. The peak is extremely steep and even more short-lived in *hepatic necrosis*, apparently because of the lack of release from necrotic cells. Although an overlap exists between cholestasis and hepatitis, serial determinations are frequently helpful; they are particularly useful in persisting hepatitis, since moderate elevation bespeaks continued activity.

LIVER SCANNING AND TRANSHEPATIC CHOLANGIOGRAPHY

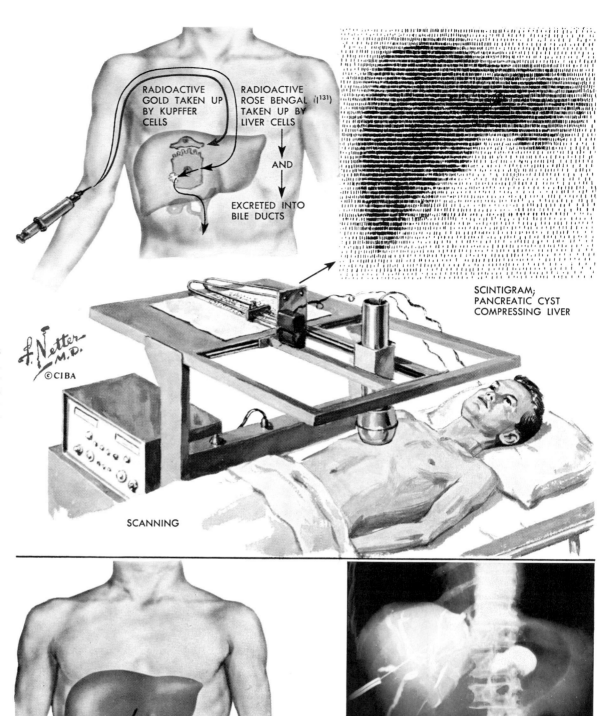

SCINTIGRAM; PANCREATIC CYST COMPRESSING LIVER

SCANNING

PERCUTANEOUS TRANSHEPATIC CHOLANGIOGRAPHY

CHOLANGIOGRAM; CARCINOMA OF PANCREAS

Originally, biochemical techniques were most widely used in the differential diagnosis of liver disease, especially jaundice. Subsequently, liver biopsy was added. Currently, physical methods are becoming more popular, since they provide a more direct answer and offer a visual record of alteration.

Scintillation *scanning* is an application of dye excretion tests (see page 45) with the demonstration of the distribution of radioactive material in the liver. This is done with a radiation detector, which is shielded to record radioactivity emanating from one direction, and which has an automatic scanning device. The detector is moved back and forth, in parallel lines, until the entire surface area of the liver has been covered. The radiation is recorded on paper by an electromagnetic or photographic dot printer, which makes a mark whenever a sufficient impulse is received. The resulting *scintigram* gives an image of the shape and contour of the liver. Two general types of radioisotopes, in doses of 50 to 200 μc, are injected. One group, taken up by the reticulo-endothelial cells, including the *Kupffer cells*, consists of colloidal *gold* or I^{131}-tagged, heat denatured albumin. The spleen usually is also visualized. The other group is represented by I^{131}-*tagged rose bengal,* which is *taken up by liver cells* and *excreted into the bile.*

Since radioactivity of the liver is recorded, by all techniques, only to a depth of several centimeters, the position of the patient may be changed to obtain various views of the scintigram. The anterior posterior position, in which the liver normally has a triangular shape with the apex toward the left hypochondrium, is most widely used. Its lower border is almost straight if *radioactive gold* is used, but, after the injection of rose bengal, the gallbladder may appear (particularly in repeat scintigrams), and even excretion of the dye into the intestine may be seen. Photoscanning demonstrates, primarily, space-occupying lesions in the liver; this, sometimes, is even more efficient than surgery. Primary and metastatic carcinoma may be seen and confirmed by subsequent biopsy of the area of the "filling defect". Similarly, intra-

hepatic abscesses or hydatid cysts produce a gap in the scintigram. Also, *pressure* from extrahepatic masses, such as *pancreatic cysts,* may be recognized. A negative scintigram is said to be more reliable than a negative laparoscopy; moreover, repetition of the procedure imposes little hardship on the patient. Whether the technique is useful in biliary disease remains to be proved; in the diagnosis of jaundice, it has been of little use.

In the differential diagnosis of biliary obstruction from intrahepatic cholestasis, which is notoriously difficult by biochemical tests and even by liver biopsy, percutaneous filling of the intrahepatic biliary tract, by blind injection of radiopaque material through a needle inserted into the parenchyma of the liver, has been applied. A needle or catheter is directed upward through the epigastrium into the middle portion of the right lobe. In biliary obstruction with consequent

dilation of bile ducts (hydrohepatosis), bile is readily aspirated, and then a contrast medium is injected to visualize the biliary tree. It is filled down to the area of the obstruction, which may be at the bifurcation of the hepatic duct, or at the lower part of the common duct, in *carcinoma of the pancreas* or the papilla of Vater. With undilated bile ducts in intrahepatic cholestasis, no bile, or little of it, is obtained on needling, and no *cholangiogram,* or an undilated one, is seen. In addition, biliary calculi and injuries or sclerosing diseases of the bile ducts, as well as anomalies, may be visualized. In view of the danger of biliary peritonitis in the presence of hydrohepatosis, *percutaneous transhepatic cholangiography* usually is followed by surgical intervention, if positive findings are obtained. With this precaution, the procedure seems safe and useful, if other diagnostic attempts have failed.

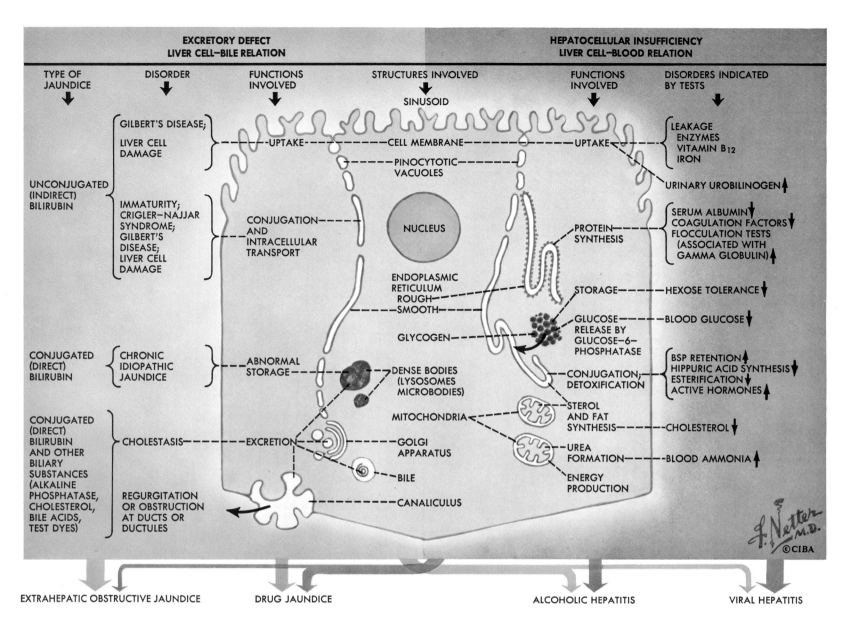

EXCRETORY DEFECT LIVER CELL–BILE RELATION				HEPATOCELLULAR INSUFFICIENCY LIVER CELL–BLOOD RELATION	
TYPE OF JAUNDICE	DISORDER	FUNCTIONS INVOLVED	STRUCTURES INVOLVED	FUNCTIONS INVOLVED	DISORDERS INDICATED BY TESTS

SINUSOID

GILBERT'S DISEASE;
LIVER CELL DAMAGE
— UPTAKE — CELL MEMBRANE — UPTAKE —
LEAKAGE
ENZYMES
VITAMIN B₁₂
IRON

PINOCYTOTIC VACUOLES

URINARY UROBILINOGEN ↑

UNCONJUGATED
(INDIRECT)
BILIRUBIN

IMMATURITY;
CRIGLER–NAJJAR
SYNDROME;
GILBERT'S
DISEASE;
LIVER CELL
DAMAGE

CONJUGATION
AND
INTRACELLULAR
TRANSPORT

NUCLEUS

PROTEIN
SYNTHESIS

SERUM ALBUMIN ↓
COAGULATION FACTORS ↓
FLOCCULATION TESTS
(ASSOCIATED WITH
GAMMA GLOBULIN) ↑

ENDOPLASMIC
RETICULUM
ROUGH
SMOOTH

STORAGE — HEXOSE TOLERANCE ↓

GLYCOGEN

GLUCOSE
RELEASE BY
GLUCOSE–6–
PHOSPHATASE
— BLOOD GLUCOSE ↓

CONJUGATED
(DIRECT)
BILIRUBIN

CHRONIC
IDIOPATHIC
JAUNDICE

ABNORMAL
STORAGE

DENSE BODIES
(LYSOSOMES
MICROBODIES)

CONJUGATION;
DETOXIFICATION

BSP RETENTION ↑
HIPPURIC ACID SYNTHESIS ↓
ESTERIFICATION ↓
ACTIVE HORMONES ↑

CONJUGATED
(DIRECT)
BILIRUBIN
AND OTHER
BILIARY
SUBSTANCES
(ALKALINE
PHOSPHATASE,
CHOLESTEROL,
BILE ACIDS,
TEST DYES)

CHOLESTASIS — EXCRETION

MITOCHONDRIA

STEROL
AND FAT
SYNTHESIS
— CHOLESTEROL ↓

GOLGI
APPARATUS

UREA
FORMATION
— BLOOD AMMONIA ↑

BILE

REGURGITATION
OR OBSTRUCTION
AT DUCTS OR
DUCTULES

CANALICULUS

ENERGY
PRODUCTION

f. Netter M.D.
©CIBA

EXTRAHEPATIC OBSTRUCTIVE JAUNDICE   DRUG JAUNDICE   ALCOHOLIC HEPATITIS   VIRAL HEPATITIS

SUPPLEMENT—PLATE 7

Two-directional Disturbances of Hepatocytes in Interpretation of Liver Function Tests

The correlation between fine-structure alterations and functional changes and the application of this knowledge to clinical differential diagnosis are challenging but fraught with uncertainty. The *structure* and *function* of the hepatocytes can be separated into those concerning the *relation between liver cells and blood* and between *liver cells and bile.* In this sense, disturbance of the *endoplasmic reticulum* is reflected in reduced *serum albumin,* impaired blood *coagulation* and abnormal results of *flocculation* tests, although the latter are also determined by an elevation of *γ-globulin.* Damage to the endoplasmic reticulum also results in an increased Bromsulphalein® (*BSP*) *retention,* a reduced *hippuric acid synthesis* and an impaired *esterification* of various substances. Faulty inactivation of *hormones,* metabolized in the liver, increases their *activity.* Only exceptionally does reduced *glucose-6-phosphatase* activity produce clinical *hypoglycemia. Cholesterol* reduction and an elevated *blood ammonia* level indicate a defective *mitochondrial activity.* Faulty *urobilinogen* uptake leads to

increased *urinary* excretion. The alterations described are laboratory evidences of hepatocellular insufficiency.

This is in contrast to those which implicate an excretory defect, particularly recognized by elevated serum *bilirubin* levels in various *types of jaundice.* Faulty uptake of *unconjugated bilirubin,* probably from altered *sinusoidal membranes,* occurs, hypothetically, in *liver cell injury* and in some instances of *Gilbert's disease.* The *conjugation* and *intracellular transport* of *unconjugated bilirubin,* presumably in the profiles of the endoplasmic reticulum as well as in the *Golgi apparatus,* is permanently impaired in the *Crigler-Najjar syndrome,* temporarily damaged in *immaturity* and diminished in some cases of Gilbert's disease.

Jaundice with normal bilirubin conjugation but with retention of the *conjugated bilirubin,* in the absence of significant fine-structure changes, is *chronic idiopathic jaundice.*

Centrolobular *cholestasis,* with its characteristic light-microscopy picture, is associated with changes in several organelles which are considered, together, as the *"bile secretory"* apparatus". These organelles include the altered *bile canaliculi,* the Golgi apparatus, and the more numerous *dense bodies.* These changes vary from cell to cell, indicating that the function of the bile secretory apparatus is interfered with to different degrees and at different sites, even in adjacent cells. These lesions are associated not only with elevation of conjugated bilirubin in serum but

also with increases in *alkaline phosphatase* activity, in *cholesterol* and in *bile acids,* and with retention of *dyes* used in function *tests.* The same biochemical alterations accompany *obstruction* of, or *regurgitation* from, *bile ducts or ductules.*

These considerations imply that damage to the hepatocyte may impair its function in two directions, each independent of the other. Formerly, cholestasis was considered by many to be the result of alterations of the bile passages and an impairment of bile flow. However, centrolobular cholestasis, at least, appears to result from damage to a specific group of hepatocellular organelles. This condition differs from that which has been called "liver cell impairment", representing damage to those organelles engaged in synthesis and energy provision. The time-honored use of hepatic tests (see page 51), therefore, still has value, except that "bile flow interference" usually also reflects an injury to the liver cell, although the latter may result from regurgitation from ducts or ductules.

This tentative summary of the present knowledge of structure and function still retains the concept of two basic alterations — namely, an *excretory* defect and a hepatocellular insufficiency — which occur in various combinations in liver diseases. The first alteration is more common in *extrahepatic obstructive jaundice,* but the latter is found more often in *viral hepatitis. Drug jaundice,* as a rule, has more of the excretory defect, whereas in *alcoholic hepatitis,* somewhat more hepatocellular insufficiency occurs.

AMMONIA METABOLISM

Some of the *amino groups* of ingested proteins are transformed within the colon, by intestinal *bacteria*, into *ammonia* or *amines*. These substances are absorbed into the portal venous system. Ammonia, with the help of glutamine synthetase, combines with glutamic acid in various tissues to form *glutamine*. In the *liver cell*, ammonia is transformed to *urea* via the urea *cycle of Krebs and Henseleit*. The ammonia combines with CO_2, and the resulting carbamyl phosphate is added to ornithine by ornithine carbamyl transferase, to form citrulline. The addition of a second ammonia results in arginine, which is transformed into urea and ornithine in the presence of arginase, to complete the cycle.

A *fourth of the urea formed* is *excreted into the intestine*, and *three fourths* are *excreted by the kidney*, which also forms ammonia from glutamine. Renal ammonia is excreted into the *urine* and, normally, only a small part enters the circulation. However, *diuretics* and renal failure increase its release into the blood. Peripheral tissues, including the brain and lung, remove ammonia. Therefore, the arterial ammonia level more closely reflects altered ammonia metabolism than does the venous level; normally, the former is less than 1.0 mg per cent. In extracellular alkalosis, as occurs in liver diseases, ammonia more readily passes into cells, making high blood ammonia levels more injurious. Abnormally high blood ammonia may result from an excess supply when ammonium salts are used as diuretics. It can also occur because of abnormal *congenital anastomoses between the portal and the systemic* parts of the circulation through *umbilical* veins. The most important cause is liver disease, which makes itself felt by two mechanisms — the *failure of the liver to form urea* via the Krebs-Henseleit cycle, as a result of injury to hepatocytes, and the *shunting* of blood past the liver, in *cirrhosis*. This bypass may be effected by *extrahepatic portasystemic collaterals* through the veins of the *esophagus* and in the anterior abdominal wall, as well as by *intrahepatic* anastomoses between branches of the *portal and the hepatic veins. Surgically* constructed shunts may produce the same effect.

Ammonia intoxication results from the influence of excess ammonia upon the Krebs tricarboxylic acid cycle, with depletion of α-ketoglutarate, which is utilized in the formation of glutamic acid and glutamine. This has been considered to be the cause of *coma,* since the brain depends, for most of its energy, on aerobic glycolysis derived from the Krebs cycle. Ammonia intoxication is corre-

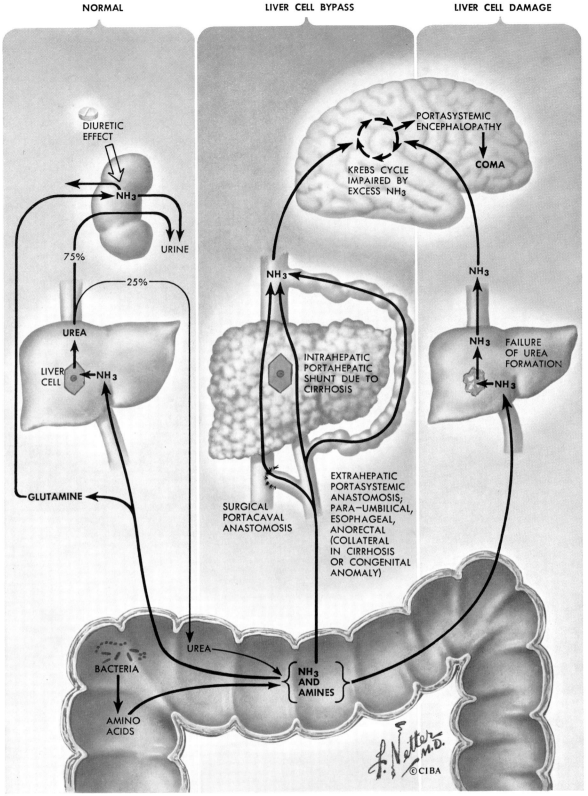

lated with the central nervous system manifestations of confusion, somnolence and flapping tremor, occurring in liver disease, designated as *portasystemic encephalopathy* or precoma. There is a good correlation between central nervous system manifestations and blood ammonia levels above 2 mg per cent. However, in the individual patients, this elevation frequently is missing. Therefore, some authorities recommend determination of the glutamine level of the serum or the spinal fluid as a better guide. Moreover, other enterogenic amines may be important in hepatic coma, as is the associated electrolyte imbalance.

Hepatic coma (see page 75) follows accidental or therapeutic increases of the ammonia supply in the form of high protein intake, excessive use of diuretics, particularly acetazolamide or thiazides, ammonia administration, gastrointestinal hemorrhage, azotemia and amino acid infusion. Thus, the most effective

therapeutic procedures in hepatic coma, or in the attempt to avoid neuropsychiatric complications, are reduction of the intake of nitrogenous substances, particularly proteins; removal, by enemas, of ammonia precursors from the intestine; and the suppression, by oral broad-spectrum antibiotics, of bacterial ammonia formation in the intestine. Other procedures are still in the experimental stage: *e.g.,* removal of the colon; production of urease antibodies, to prevent ammonia formation by intestinal bacteria; and hemodialysis, as used in renal disease. The administration of glutamic acid to take up ammonia, thus forming glutamine, and the administration of arginine to enhance urea formation, have more theoretical than practical efficiency. In general, the therapeutic procedures are more effective in hepatic coma resulting from shunts, as seen in cirrhosis, than in the hepatocellular defect of hepatitis.

CLINICAL DETERMINATION OF PORTAL HYPERTENSION

To understand the causes of *portal hypertension* (see page 72) and to assess the possibility of surgical management (see page 73), exact information about the degree of pressure elevation and the site of *obstruction*, if any, to the flow of blood is important, as is also a knowledge of the surgical anatomy of the portal venous system. *Pressure* is estimated either by *wedging* a catheter into the *hepatic vein* or by percutaneous measurement of *intrasplenic pressure*.

In the first method a radiopaque catheter is inserted into the antecubital vein, under fluoroscopic control, as in catheterization of the right side of the heart. However, the catheter is advanced into the *inferior vena cava* until it meets resistance in one of the tributaries of the hepatic veins. The proximal end is then connected via a *transducer* to a pressure-recording device. With an adequately wedged catheter, the blood flow through the catheterized hepatic vein tributary is blocked, and the pressure thus recorded is that in the surrounding hepatic sinusoids. This is *normally 50 to 180 mm water pressure* or the corresponding amount (*3.5 to 13.5 mm*) *of mercury*. During this procedure, pressures in the inferior vena cava, above and below the diaphragm, are also recorded.

Pressure in the spleen is determined by inserting a fine needle which is connected, by a flexible polyethylene tube, to a manometer. The normal splenic pulp pressure is in the same range as the wedged hepatic vein pressure.

In *cirrhosis*, in which *regenerative nodules* compress hepatic vein branches, the wedged pressure represents the pressure in the sinusoids which are drained by the noncatheterized neighboring tributaries of the hepatic veins. It is as high as the splenic pressure and thus reflects *postsinusoidal* hypertension, indicating that the liver cells are being exposed to increased pressure. In *portal fibrosis*, in which the hepatic parenchyma, as such, is not involved (*e.g.*, in *schistosomiasis* or *sarcoidosis*), the splenic pressure is raised. Since the drainage from the hepatic veins is not altered, however, the wedged pressure is normal. This represents *presinusoidal* portal hypertension, with stasis in the splanchnic system but without significant functional effect on the liver itself. Such *intrahepatic* presinusoidal portal hypertension may occur

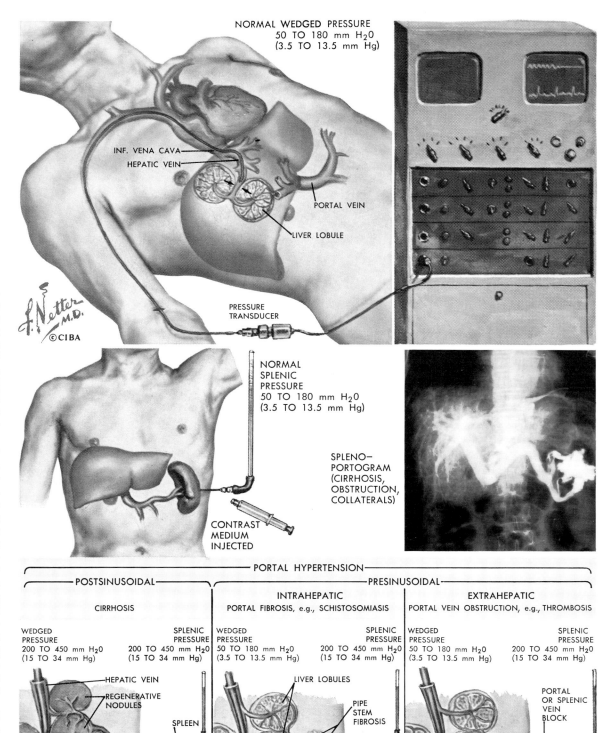

in some types of cirrhosis in which the pressure from regenerative nodules is functionally less significant than from either scarring in the portal tract or compression of the portal vein branches by nodules. The relation, therefore, between splenic and hepatic wedged pressure may be quite variable in cirrhosis. Other causes of presinusoidal intrahepatic portal hypertension are congenital hepatic *fibrosis*, developmental defects, and hepatic infiltrations, as, for instance, in hematologic disorders. In hepatitis (alcoholic or viral) transient elevations of splenic and, frequently, of the wedged pressure are reported.

Extrahepatic presinusoidal portal hypertension results mainly from *obstruction* of the *portal vein* (see page 72), but a block of the splenic vein alone also raises the splenic pulp pressure.

The portal venous system can be visualized by percutaneous *injection of radiopaque material* into the spleen, with rapid multiple film exposures immediately thereafter. The initial filling of the veins produces a "vasculogram", followed by a "hepatogram", which represents a diffuse opacification of the entire liver by the contrast medium in the sinusoids. In cirrhosis, venous filling may be normal, but *collaterals* are also visualized, in which the width and tortuosity of the coronary vein are important observations. Moreover, a characteristic picture is given in a patient with esophageal varices; with a partial or complete obstruction of the portal vein by a thrombus; or with a patent portacaval shunt.

The application of this technique for the detection of intrahepatic or epigastric masses or neoplasms has not yet been fully evaluated. Splenic puncture for pressure measurement or for splenoportography is contraindicated in patients with a bleeding tendency, and it is seldom done on icteric patients.

CONGENITAL AND FAMILIAL HYPERBILIRUBINEMIAS

Most benign hyperbilirubinemias are congenital and frequently familial. Formerly, they were designated as retention jaundice (see page 48), but they are now better understood, owing to the improved knowledge of bilirubin transport through the liver cell. Rare extremes of these diseases may have major clinical — even fatal — consequences, but most cases are important only because of differentiating them from hepatic disorders with a graver prognosis. *Unconjugated bilirubin* passes through the liver cell membrane facing the sinusoid, probably without the participation of the Kupffer cell, and is conjugated by the enzyme, *glucuronyl transferase,* with glucuronic acid. This acid is derived from glucose, linked to uridine phosphate, and oxidized to uridine diphosphate glucuronic acid (*UDPGA*). The prompt-reacting *bilirubin glucuronide* is excreted into the bile.

Bilirubin transport through the liver cell may be partially or completely *blocked* at any of four sites. *Uptake* of unconjugated bilirubin by the liver cell may be blocked, but this is difficult to prove. It has been associated with a frequently familial disorder, *Gilbert's disease* (chronic intermittent juvenile jaundice), familial nonhemolytic jaundice and nonhemolytic acholuric jaundice. However, this has not been universally accepted, and inhibitory effects from progestinlike substances have been postulated.

The inhibition of conjugation is better established, since *deficient* glucuronyl transferase activity can be measured in liver homogenates. However, it is not certain whether glucuronide conjugation, with test substances other than bilirubin, mirrors the clinical disease. Not all conjugating and other drug-handling mechanisms are fully developed at birth, and this fact largely accounts for the physiologic hyperbilirubinemia of the newborn, with retention of the unconjugated bilirubin in the blood. This is more severe in prematurity. Moreover, progestational *steroids* from the mother *inhibit transferase* activity and may contribute to the hyperbilirubinemia. Drugs, particularly antibiotics and vitamin K preparations, favor hyperbilirubinemia by competitive inhibition with conjugation. *Permanent incomplete* conjugation defects, on an apparently congenital basis, explain most cases of Gilbert's disease, particularly those with bilirubin levels above 5 mg per cent. The pathogenesis of this disorder with lower bilirubin levels is questionable, and differentiation from mild hemolytic jaundice or low-grade hepatitis is important. Some patients with typical viral hepatitis have persistent elevation of unconjugated bilirubin without other functional alterations. Glucuronyl transferase is *completely* absent in the

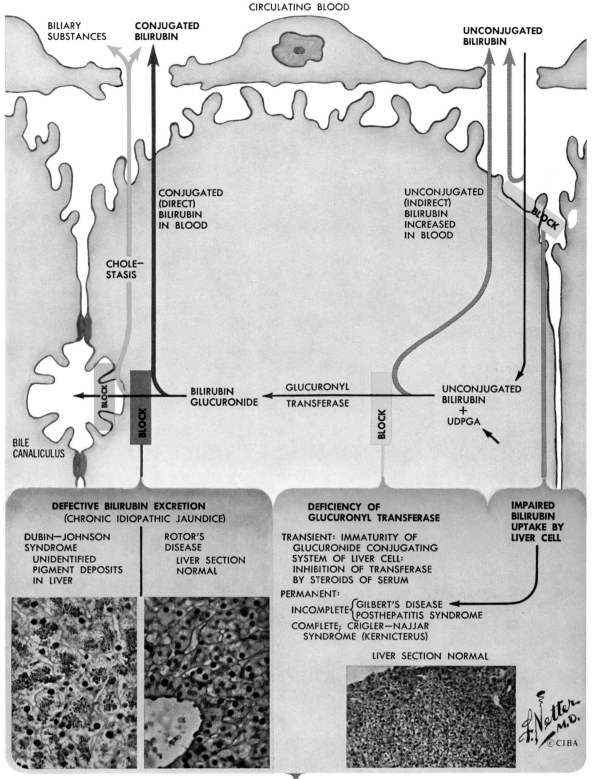

ALSO OCCUR TO VARIABLE DEGREE IN ACQUIRED LIVER CELL INJURIES

Gunn strain of rats and in the *Crigler-Najjar syndrome,* and few afflicted individuals reach adulthood. In all these conditions the *liver* is morphologically *normal,* and no alteration of hepatic tests is noted except for elevated unconjugated bilirubin in the serum. The prognosis in Gilbert's disease and in the posthepatitis syndrome is good, even if minor constitutional complaints are present. With bilirubin levels above 20 mg per cent in immaturity and in the Crigler-Najjar syndrome, *kernicterus* develops.

Another block involves the biliary *excretion* of *conjugated bilirubin,* with an increase of serum conjugated and unconjugated bilirubin but not of other *biliary substances.* In the absence of *cholestasis,* this is usually a familial disorder, designated as *chronic idiopathic jaundice.* One form, the *Dubin-Johnson syndrome,* is associated with accumulation of a golden-brown *pigment* in the liver cells, predominantly in the

lobular center and around undilated *bile canaliculi.* The Kupffer cells are free of pigment. This abnormality may be detected at any age and is associated with vague constitutional symptoms, faulty excretion of test dyes and a lack of visualization of the gallbladder on cholecystography. The intensity of the disease varies in different persons and, particularly, in siblings of known cases; jaundice is seldom severe. The prognosis is excellent. In the other form, designated as *Rotor's disease,* which also is often familial, hardly any pigment deposition is noted, but the prognosis is similar. Cholecystography yields normal results.

The fourth block occurs in cholestasis. It is associated with characteristic morphologic changes, including dilatation of the bile canaliculi, and is accompanied by elevation of other biliary substances in the serum (see page 171). All four types of block occur in liver cell injury.

Drug-induced Hepatic Injuries

The incidence of liver injuries following the administration of *drugs* is rapidly increasing, in view of the greater use and variety of chemically complex drugs. Since reactions occur sporadically, and the types of hepatic responses to injury are limited, it is frequently difficult to decide whether disordered hepatic function after medication is caused by the drug, is a manifestation of the underlying ailment or is an independent liver disease, such as viral hepatitis or *extrahepatic* biliary *obstruction*.

Drug-induced hepatic injuries can be divided conveniently into four groups. The first group results from therapeutic administration of substances which, because of their established hepatotoxic activity, are *poisons*. They are represented by *carbon tetrachloride* used as an anthelmintic, by *chloroform* as an anesthetic or by *phosphorus*. However, most intoxications come from occupational or accidental exposure. Areas of *necrosis* are distributed regularly throughout the *liver,* usually with *zonal* predominance, *with or without* steatosis (*fatty metamorphosis,* see pages 62 and 91). The *lesion depends* on the *dose* taken, and it is *universally* found with sufficiently *high doses.* Alcoholic patients and pregnant women are usually more susceptible. The *mortality depends on the dose* of the responsible substance. There is little mystery about this type of injury, the problem being mainly the detection of the exposure.

The second type of drug-induced injury is associated with *jaundice,* having all the clinical and laboratory manifestations of *extrahepatic biliary obstruction* (see page 83). Histologically, *centrolobular cholestasis* is seen, but the *portal* tracts usually exhibit an *inflammatory* reaction which may be severe enough to be designated as allergic cholangiolitis (see page 97). This portal reaction is transient, or even missing, following the administration of some drugs. It is, therefore, not responsible for the intrahepatic cholestasis (see page 51). Many drugs, particularly *sulfonylurea derivatives,* have been incriminated in producing cholestasis. Of these, the *phenothiazines,* especially chlorpromazine, are frequently held responsible, as well as *oral antidiabetic agents* and also *diuretics.* Also included in this general category are the 17-α-*alkyl-substituted androgenic steroids* and organic *arsenicals.* Following the administration of any of these, the *incidence* of *cholestatic jaundice* rarely exceeds 1 *to* 2 *per cent* of the patients exposed, and it is much lower with some drugs. There is *no clear relation to the*

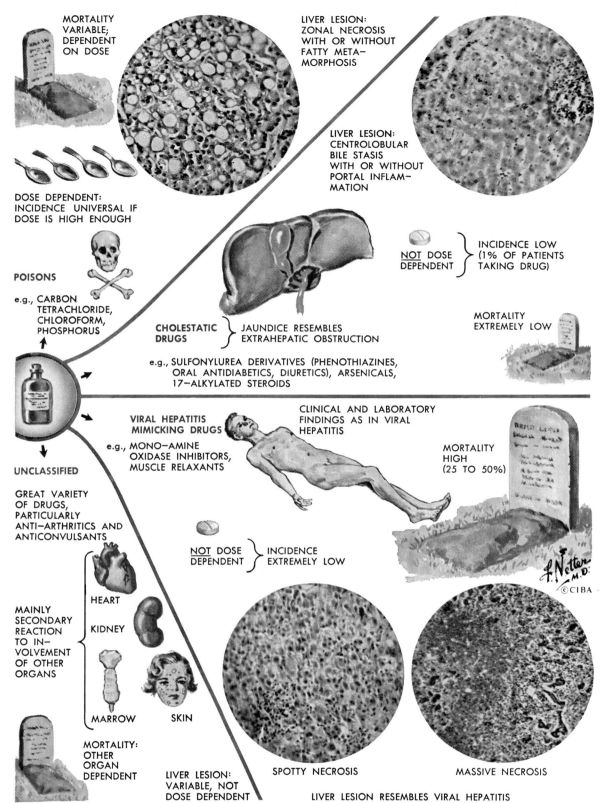

MORTALITY VARIABLE; DEPENDENT ON DOSE

LIVER LESION: ZONAL NECROSIS WITH OR WITHOUT FATTY METAMORPHOSIS

LIVER LESION: CENTROLOBULAR BILE STASIS WITH OR WITHOUT PORTAL INFLAMMATION

DOSE DEPENDENT: INCIDENCE UNIVERSAL IF DOSE IS HIGH ENOUGH

POISONS

e.g., CARBON TETRACHLORIDE, CHLOROFORM, PHOSPHORUS

NOT DOSE DEPENDENT } INCIDENCE LOW (1% OF PATIENTS TAKING DRUG)

MORTALITY EXTREMELY LOW

CHOLESTATIC DRUGS } JAUNDICE RESEMBLES EXTRAHEPATIC OBSTRUCTION

e.g., SULFONYLUREA DERIVATIVES (PHENOTHIAZINES, ORAL ANTIDIABETICS, DIURETICS), ARSENICALS, 17-ALKYLATED STEROIDS

VIRAL HEPATITIS MIMICKING DRUGS

CLINICAL AND LABORATORY FINDINGS AS IN VIRAL HEPATITIS

e.g., MONO-AMINE OXIDASE INHIBITORS, MUSCLE RELAXANTS

MORTALITY HIGH (25 TO 50%)

UNCLASSIFIED

GREAT VARIETY OF DRUGS, PARTICULARLY ANTI-ARTHRITICS AND ANTICONVULSANTS

NOT DOSE DEPENDENT } INCIDENCE EXTREMELY LOW

MAINLY SECONDARY REACTION TO INVOLVEMENT OF OTHER ORGANS

HEART

KIDNEY

MARROW   SKIN

MORTALITY: OTHER ORGAN DEPENDENT

LIVER LESION: VARIABLE, NOT DOSE DEPENDENT

SPOTTY NECROSIS

MASSIVE NECROSIS

LIVER LESION RESEMBLES VIRAL HEPATITIS

dose given; sometimes jaundice follows the administration of only a few tablets. The disease is usually short-lived and disappears soon after discontinuation of the therapy. Since protracted jaundice is rare, a *fatal outcome is extremely uncommon.*

By contrast, the administration of some drugs (the third group) is followed by *clinical and laboratory manifestations of viral hepatitis.* Morphologically also, the whole spectrum from acute *spotty necrotic* hepatitis (see page 93) to acute *massive* or submassive *necrosis* (see pages 94 and 95) is seen, and, as a rule, the structural changes are even more severe than would be expected from the clinical picture. The *resemblance to viral hepatitis* has made it difficult to establish a causal connection, and usually a number of cases must be observed before suspicion is aroused and a relation between drug intake and hepatitis is confirmed. Among the drugs thus implicated are cin-

chophen, *mono-amine oxidase inhibitors* and *muscle relaxants.* Again, dose dependency is not clear, and, although the *incidence* of hepatitic manifestations is *extremely low,* the *mortality* rate is relatively *high.* If, therefore, a drug is associated with hepatitic reactions, most probably on a hypersensitivity basis, its further use should not be attempted.

A fourth drug reaction, designated as *"unclassified",* is produced by a great variety of drugs, particularly *antiarthritics* and *anticonvulsants.* They cause many different hepatic alterations, again not dependent on the dose given. However, the *changes in the liver* are probably not primary but, rather, *secondary* to lesions in other organs, such as *heart, kidney,* bone *marrow* and *skin,* and they thus correspond to a nonspecific reactive hepatitis (see page 91). The myocarditis, dermatitis, nephritis and hematologic changes *determine* the clinical picture and *mortality* rate.

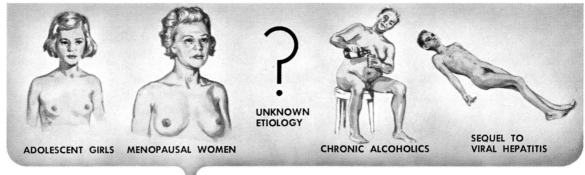

ADOLESCENT GIRLS   MENOPAUSAL WOMEN   UNKNOWN ETIOLOGY   CHRONIC ALCOHOLICS   SEQUEL TO VIRAL HEPATITIS

CHRONIC ACTIVE HEPATITIS

The incidence, diagnosis and prognosis of chronic hepatitis are still not well established. This malady occurs with persistent symptoms and signs after acute liver disease; it may be recognized, initially, with manifestations of chronic disease; or it may be detected during a routine physical examination. In the first two instances, the clinical manifestations may be mild or conspicuous, and associated with jaundice of variable degrees. If the disease follows acute hepatitis, the etiology is considered more or less well established. It seems to be viral hepatitis in most cases, as recognized by the epidemiologic background or by a fairly characteristic histologic picture (see page 93). It may pass through either a transient or a prolonged chronic state (see page 96). Alcoholic hepatitis (see page 78) and, occasionally, drug-induced hepatic injury (see page 181) can also become chronic. Etiologically, however, the least-understood entity is *chronic active hepatitis*. It has no established etiology but presents characteristic clinical and laboratory manifestations; these cases are found more frequently in *women*, particularly during *adolescence* or near the *menopause*, suggesting endocrinologic involvement. In some instances this disease is considered to be a *sequel to* anicteric *viral hepatitis*, although the incidence of this illness, in relation to icteric viral hepatitis, is unknown. The importance of *alcoholism*, in view of its widespread incidence, often cannot be assessed.

Even when an offending agent, such as a virus disease or a metabolic disorder, is present initially, it may disappear despite the continuous progression of the liver disease. This persistence of activity has led to the concept of self-perpetuation, applied both to hepatitis and to the cirrhotic state. Self-perpetuation in cirrhosis was originally considered to be the result of ischemic necrosis, induced by circulatory disturbances (see pages 68 and 116). Since ischemic necrosis is seen only at autopsy and is not found in biopsy specimens, it probably represents a cause of death rather than of self-perpetuation. A study of biopsy specimens indicates that there is a rather indistinct border between the parenchyma and the connective tissue septa, with *necrosis* of single *liver cells* (mainly on the parenchymal periphery) and an *accumulation* of *lymphoid* and *plasma cells*. These

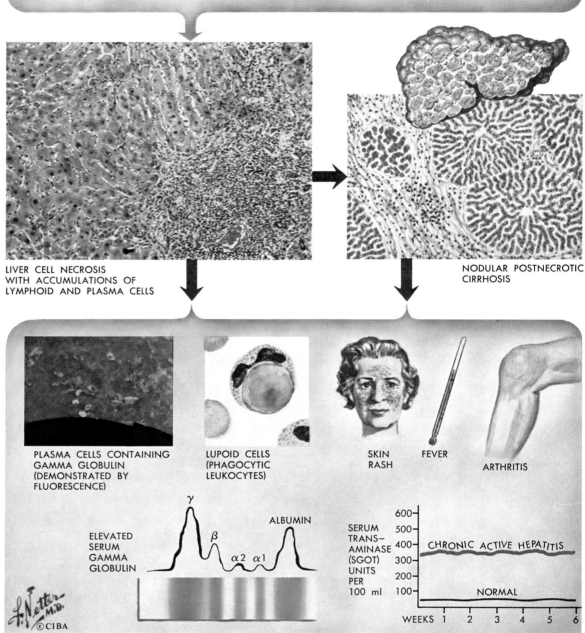

LIVER CELL NECROSIS WITH ACCUMULATIONS OF LYMPHOID AND PLASMA CELLS

NODULAR POSTNECROTIC CIRRHOSIS

PLASMA CELLS CONTAINING GAMMA GLOBULIN (DEMONSTRATED BY FLUORESCENCE)

LUPOID CELLS (PHAGOCYTIC LEUKOCYTES)

SKIN RASH   FEVER   ARTHRITIS

ELEVATED SERUM GAMMA GLOBULIN — γ, β, $\alpha2$, $\alpha1$, ALBUMIN

SERUM TRANSAMINASE (SGOT) UNITS PER 100 ml — 600, 500, 400, 300, 200, 100 — CHRONIC ACTIVE HEPATITIS — NORMAL — WEEKS 1 2 3 4 5 6

correlate best with a progression of the disease and thus reflect self-perpetuation.

The final stage of this disorder is *postnecrotic cirrhosis* (see page 81), presumably resulting from relentless progression of piecemeal *liver cell necrosis*. Some authorities have assumed that destruction of the hepatic parenchyma by auto-immune processes causes the persistent progression. They have offered, in support of this concept, the conspicuous *elevation of the serum γ-globulin* level, and the presence of γ-globulin-producing *cells* in the liver which are demonstrated by immunocytochemical techniques (based on staining with *fluoresceinated* antihuman γ-globulin produced in rabbits).

A positive reaction for lupus erythematosus has been found, in a few cases, giving rise to the term, "*lupoid* hepatitis". This reaction occurs most often in women with chronic active hepatitis, who have other serologic reactions, such as positive Wassermann tests, and certain systemic manifestations, particularly *arthralgias, skin rashes* and *fever*. Despite these findings, most observers believe that this positive reaction represents not lupus erythematosus but, rather, a peculiar chronic hepatitis with transitions to those forms without systemic manifestations. The role of immune processes in this disorder is questionable, although some immune disturbance is probable in the group in which systemic manifestations are prominent, and for which the term "lupoid hepatitis" is used.

The clinical manifestations of hepatic insufficiency and cirrhosis vary, depending on the stage, as do the laboratory findings. Persistent but moderate elevation of *SGOT* activity is the most indicative. The long-term prognosis is generally poor, but it is somewhat better in young girls. The response to steroid therapy is unpredictable and frequently transient.

REFERENCES

General References

POPPER, H., AND SCHAFFNER: *Progress in Liver Disease,* Grune & Stratton, Inc., New York, 1961.

SHERLOCK, S.: *Diseases of the Liver and Biliary System,* Blackwell Scientific Publications, Oxford, 1963.

Specific References

PLATE
NUMBER

ARIAS, I. M.: *Chronic unconjugated hyperbilirubinemia without overt signs of hemolysis in adolescents and adults,* J. clin. Invest., 41:2233, 1962. — 10

BARTHOLOMEW, L. G., HAGEDORN, CAIN AND BAGGENSTOSS: *Hepatitis and cirrhosis in women with positive clot tests for lupus erythematosus,* New Engl. J. Med., 259: 947, 1958. — 12

BILLING, B. H., COLE AND LATHE: *The excretion of bilirubin as a diglucuronide giving the direct van den Bergh reaction,* Biochem. J., 65:774, 1957. — 3, 10

DEDUVE, C.: *Lysosomes, a new group of cytoplasmic particles;* page 128 in *Subcellular Particles,* Hayashi, T., ed., The Ronald Press Company, New York, 1959. — 1, 2

ESSNER, E., AND NOVIKOFF: *Localization of acid phosphatase activity in hepatic lysosomes by means of electron microscopy,* J. biophys. biochem. Cytol., 9:773, 1961. — 4

PLATE NUMBER

GOLDFISCHER, S., ARIAS, ESSNER AND NOVIKOFF: *Cytochemical and electron microscopic studies of rat liver with reduced capacity to transport conjugated bilirubin,* J. Exp. Med., 115:467, 1962. — 10

ISSELBACHER, K. J., AND MCCARTHY: *Studies on bilirubin sulfate and other nonglucuronide conjugates of bilirubin,* J. clin. Invest., 38:645, 1959. — 10

LEEVY, C. M., ZINKE, BABER AND CHEY: *Observations on the influence of medical therapy on portal hypertension in hepatic cirrhosis,* Ann. intern. Med., 49:837, 1958. — 9

MACKAY, I. R.: *The problem of persisting destructive disease of the liver,* Gastroenterology, 40:617, 1961. — 12

MARTINI, G. A., DÖLLE AND STROHMEYER: *Liver Disease,* Gastroenterology, 44:866, 1963. — 8

NAGLER, W., BENDER AND BLAU: *Radioisotope photoscanning of the liver,* Gastroenterology, 44:36, 1963. — 6

NOVIKOFF, A. B., AND ESSNER: *The liver cell: Some new approaches to its study,* Amer. J. Med., 29:102, 1960. — 1, 2, 4

PANKE, W. F., BRADLEY, MORENO, RUZICKA, JR. AND ROUSSELOT: *Technique, hazards, and usefulness of percutaneous splenic portography,* J. Amer. med. Ass., 169: 1032, 1959. — 6

PLATE NUMBER

POPPER, H., AND SCHAFFNER: *The liver and its diseases,* Gastroenterology, 40:536, 1961. — 3

SCHMID, R.: *Hyperbilirubinemia;* page 226 in *The Metabolic Basis of Inherited Disease,* Stanbury, J. B., Wyngaarden, and Fredrickson, eds., The Blakiston Division, McGraw-Hill Book Co., Inc., New York, 1960. — 10

SHALDON, S., BARBER AND YOUNG: *Percutaneous transhepatic cholangiography. A modified technique,* Gastroenterology, 42: 371, 1962. — 6

SHERLOCK, S.: *Primary biliary cirrhosis (chronic intrahepatic obstructive jaundice),* Gastroenterology, 37:574, 1959. — 12

—— AND TURNER: *Liver Disease,* Gastroenterology, 42:612, 1962. — 9

STEINER, J. W., AND CARRUTHERS: *Studies on the fine structure of the terminal branches of the biliary tree. II. Observations of pathologically altered bile canaliculi,* Amer. J. Path., 39:41, 1961. — 2

WACHSTEIN, M.: *Enzymatic histochemistry of the liver,* Gastroenterology, 37:525, 1959. — 4

WRÓBLEWSKI, F.: *The clinical significance of transaminase activities of serum,* Amer. J. Med., 27:911, 1959. — 5

SUBJECT INDEX

(For Plates 1 Through 12 of Supplement)

(Numerals refer to pages, *not* plates)

CONTENTS

INTRODUCTION

Although infrequent attempts to remove cancerous portions of the liver were made in the latter part of the last century, it was only quite recently (1952) that Lortat-Jacob reported a successful resection of the right lobe of the liver. This organ, or any part of it, had generally been considered inviolate to surgery, because its location, blood supply and extremely friable nature presented serious problems. The excessive leakage of blood and bile attending surgical section of such a highly vascular, bile-forming tissue militated against ready acceptance of surgical treatment.

Today, the situation is entirely different. Certain tumefactions of the liver are treated, like those of most other organs, in clinics especially equipped to handle this type of surgery. Some tumors now lend themselves to surgical removal because of improvements in techniques and pre- and postoperative treatment. Contributing to these improvements are the patient's nutritional buildup and maintenance, expert anesthetic manipulation and the control of infections, as well as skillful surgical intervention based on thorough knowledge of the anatomical structure of the liver, with special reference to possible abnormal locations of its arteries (see pages 16 and 17), veins (see page 19) and bile ducts (see page 23). Also, there is the very reassuring fact that even a small segment of liver (one fifth of the normal volume) has an enormous capacity to regenerate and function normally within the relatively short period of 4 or 5 months after subtotal hepatectomy.

The following plates and corresponding texts are intended to present only the significant highlights of certain surgical approaches to the treatment of liver tumors. Detailed information concerning signs, symptoms, diagnosis, treatment and prognosis is available elsewhere (see References, page 198).

GEORGE T. PACK, M.D.
Attending Surgeon Emeritus
Memorial Cancer Center
New York, N. Y.

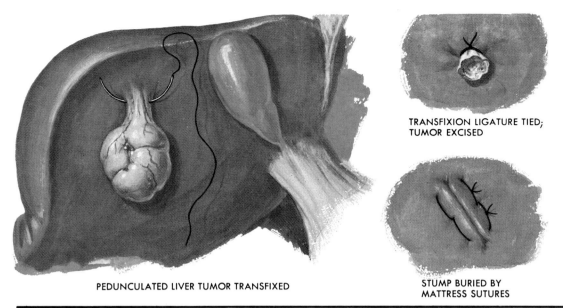

PEDUNCULATED LIVER TUMOR TRANSFIXED

TRANSFIXION LIGATURE TIED; TUMOR EXCISED

STUMP BURIED BY MATTRESS SUTURES

Operative Procedures

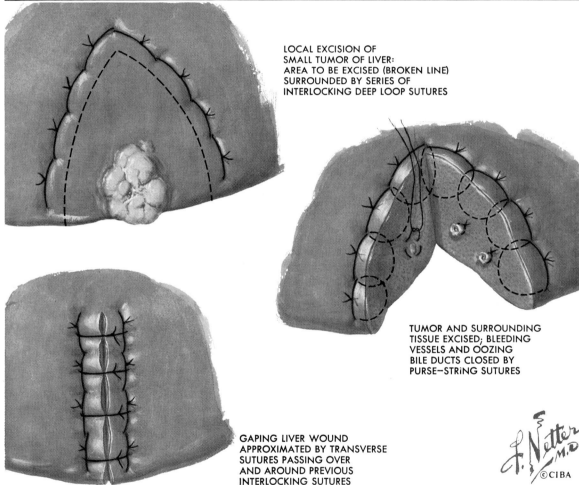

LOCAL EXCISION OF SMALL TUMOR OF LIVER: AREA TO BE EXCISED (BROKEN LINE) SURROUNDED BY SERIES OF INTERLOCKING DEEP LOOP SUTURES

TUMOR AND SURROUNDING TISSUE EXCISED; BLEEDING VESSELS AND OOZING BILE DUCTS CLOSED BY PURSE—STRING SUTURES

GAPING LIVER WOUND APPROXIMATED BY TRANSVERSE SUTURES PASSING OVER AND AROUND PREVIOUS INTERLOCKING SUTURES

Excision of Pedunculated Tumors

Certain slowly growing tumors, such as the cavernous hemangioma, the hamartoma and even the rare benign hepatomas, may become extruded from the liver, to which, however, they remain attached by a pedicle. Patients with tumors of this sort may have, on changing posture, the sensation of a ball rolling in the upper abdomen. These tumors may be simply *excised,* with immediate closure of the pedicle by *transfixion* and *mattress sutures.*

Hemostatic Excision

When a tumor is accessible and located near the periphery, it may be removed by *local excision.* Often, an encapsulated tumor, such as a hemangioma, may be removed with the capsule intact. Even multiple *small* metastases may be excised in this way, albeit with the knowledge that the procedure will, very probably, prove to have been entirely futile as far as arrest of the cancer is concerned.

Liver tissue is extremely friable. Even the capsule of Glisson is a rather delicate structure. Therefore, in order to reduce the tendency of sutures to cut through, as well as to diminish bleeding and, perhaps, to decrease the possibility of air embolism through an open hepatic vein, sutures are placed distal to the proposed excision before any incision is made. Parallel to and beyond the planned lines of incision, a *series of interlocking,*

deeply looped sutures is passed until the tumor-bearing region is surrounded. These ligatures are firmly tied. The bulk of the *tissue* to be sacrificed is then quickly *excised,* and hot laparotomy pads are placed against the cut surfaces. Individual *bleeding vessels* and leaking *bile ducts* are meticulously *closed by purse-string sutures.* Once bleeding has been controlled, apposition *sutures* are placed *transversely,* using long, full-curved needles so as *to pass over and around* the longitudinal loops *previously* placed. Other methods of providing temporary hemostasis include gentle manual compression of the cut surfaces, between the thumbs and fingers of a skillful assistant, or digital compression of the hepatoduodenal ligament. One should never resort to the clumsy, traumatizing and undependable liver clamps.

Segmental Excision

Occasionally, in the case of an apparently isolated metastasis or a small benign tumor not amenable to simple excision, segmental excision may be preferred to lobectomy. The segmental arrangement of the liver has already been described (see page 13). Unfortunately, the hepatic venous system follows an independent course, unrelated to other vessels. Because of this interdigitation of efferent and afferent venous systems, the entire right half of the liver should be considered a surgical unit to be excised in toto. However, the superior left (lateral superior), inferior left (lateral inferior) and inferior quadrate (medial inferior) areas can be excised with impunity, as individual units.

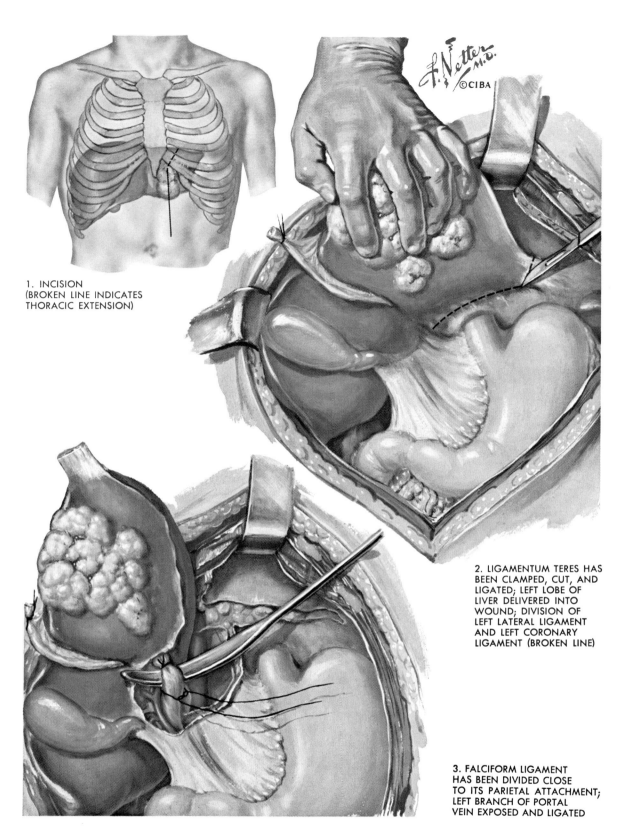

1. INCISION
(BROKEN LINE INDICATES
THORACIC EXTENSION)

LOBECTOMY

2. LIGAMENTUM TERES HAS
BEEN CLAMPED, CUT, AND
LIGATED; LEFT LOBE OF
LIVER DELIVERED INTO
WOUND; DIVISION OF
LEFT LATERAL LIGAMENT
AND LEFT CORONARY
LIGAMENT (BROKEN LINE)

3. FALCIFORM LIGAMENT
HAS BEEN DIVIDED CLOSE
TO ITS PARIETAL ATTACHMENT;
LEFT BRANCH OF PORTAL
VEIN EXPOSED AND LIGATED

Removal of an entire lobe is infinitely better than any less extensive operation, except for those procedures already mentioned. There are several reasons for this point of view:

1. Blood loss is greatly reduced, because vessels and ducts can be identified and ligated before excision rather than afterward.

2. When dealing with metastases, local excision has a very low cure rate. The reasons are obvious: the likelihood of a single palpable lesion being the sole metastatic involvement is certainly remote, considering the ease with which cancer cells from intra-abdominal viscera reach the liver via the portal vein. Moreover, the speed with which cancer cells grow in such a nutritious environment, and the manner in which they are spread throughout the liver must be considered.

3. Less than 20 per cent of normal liver tissue is necessary to maintain life, and liver tissue regenerates very rapidly. Therefore, the entire right lobe may be removed with the assurance that sufficient liver function will be preserved for even a stressful life.

LEFT LOBECTOMY

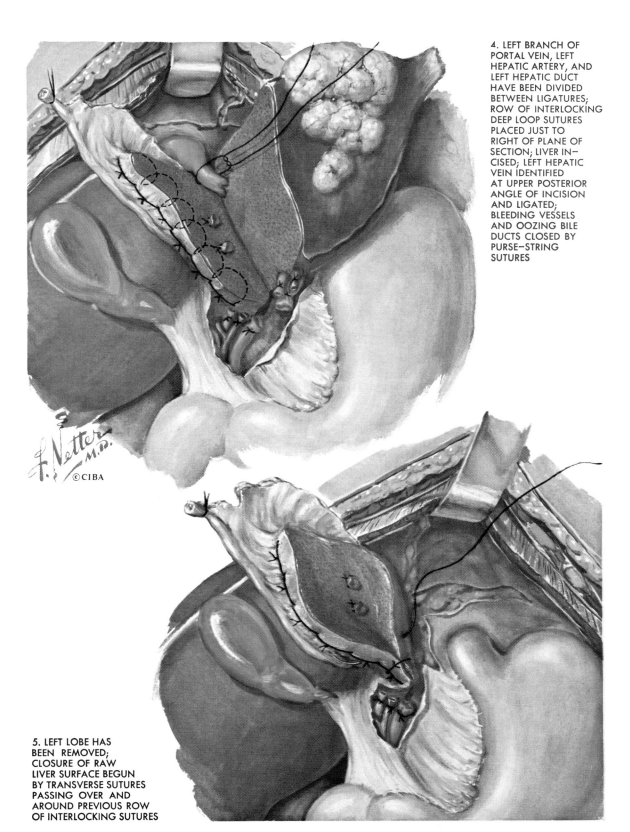

4. LEFT BRANCH OF PORTAL VEIN, LEFT HEPATIC ARTERY, AND LEFT HEPATIC DUCT HAVE BEEN DIVIDED BETWEEN LIGATURES; ROW OF INTERLOCKING DEEP LOOP SUTURES PLACED JUST TO RIGHT OF PLANE OF SECTION; LIVER INCISED; LEFT HEPATIC VEIN IDENTIFIED AT UPPER POSTERIOR ANGLE OF INCISION AND LIGATED; BLEEDING VESSELS AND OOZING BILE DUCTS CLOSED BY PURSE-STRING SUTURES

5. LEFT LOBE HAS BEEN REMOVED; CLOSURE OF RAW LIVER SURFACE BEGUN BY TRANSVERSE SUTURES PASSING OVER AND AROUND PREVIOUS ROW OF INTERLOCKING SUTURES

Left lobectomies, as carried out in the past, usually were subtotal in nature, accomplished by a guillotine excision and dependent on previously placed mattress sutures for hemostasis. Although this procedure may be adequate for nonneoplastic diseases and benign tumors, it should not be employed for malignant tumors, and, in any case, it is inferior to total ablation of the left lobe. The latter procedure is carried out in the following manner:

In opening the abdomen, an *incision* is made in such a way that it can be *extended* to open the *thorax*, if the diagnosis is verified and the criteria for lobectomy are established. As opposed to laparotomy, laparothoracotomy has a number of advantages. Better exposure is obtained, the operation may be shortened, and a better opportunity is afforded to secure and maintain the hemostasis so important to the safety of the patient. In preparation for this, a vertical incision, which may be extended obliquely through the rib cartilages, is made in the epigastrium.

The *ligamentum teres hepatis* is *clamped, cut and ligated*; the hepatic end is used for gentle traction downward, and then upward, *to deliver* the *left* lateral *lobe into the wound*. The long *left lateral ligament* and then the *left coronary ligament* are *severed*.

The *falciform ligament* is *cut* as far away from the liver as possible, so that its fan-shaped base along the superior aspect of the interlobar fissure is kept intact, later to cover the denuded liver segment. This concludes the procedures of mobilization.

The left lobe is now withdrawn outward and rotated toward the right, in order to expose the undersurface of the liver and the portal fissure. This brings the posterolateral aspect of the pedicle into view, so that the *left branch of the portal vein* is the first structure encountered. This vein is *ligated*. The *left hepatic duct* is next ligated and *divided*, after which the *left* branch of the *hepatic artery* is ligated and divided between ligatures.

(Continued on page 192)

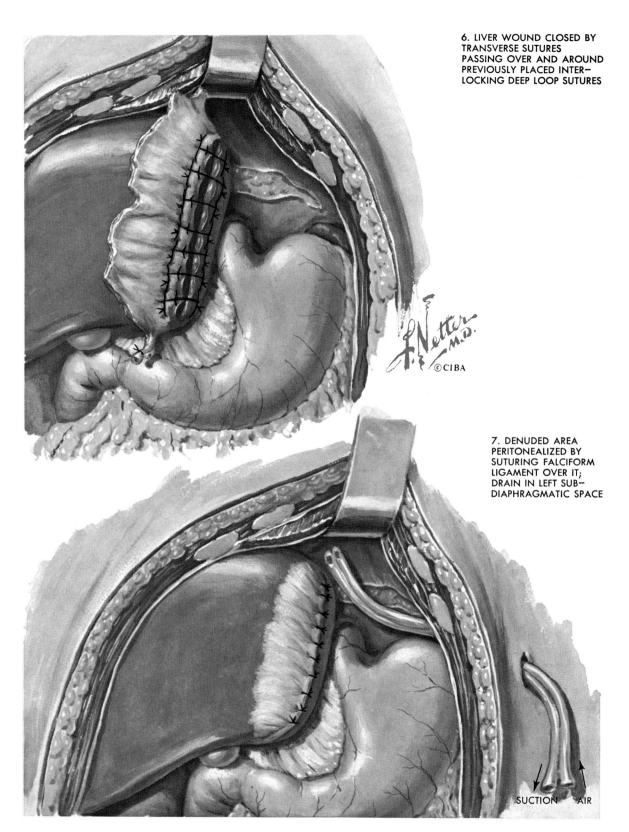

6. LIVER WOUND CLOSED BY
TRANSVERSE SUTURES
PASSING OVER AND AROUND
PREVIOUSLY PLACED INTER-
LOCKING DEEP LOOP SUTURES

LEFT LOBECTOMY

(Continued from page 191)

7. DENUDED AREA
PERITONEALIZED BY
SUTURING FALCIFORM
LIGAMENT OVER IT;
DRAIN IN LEFT SUB-
DIAPHRAGMATIC SPACE

SUCTION   AIR

About 25 per cent of these patients have an anomalous arterial supply to the left lobe. Therefore, the surgeon must make a careful search for the presence of accessory, or even replaced, left hepatic arteries originating from the left gastric artery or the celiac trunk (see page 16).

All vessels (with the exception of the

hepatic vein) now having been ligated, the excision follows the less vascular and relatively fibrous plane of cleavage between the lobes. The incision starts at the sagittal fissure and continues along the septum, backward and downward, until the *left hepatic vein* is encountered and isolated at the *superoposterior angle* (see page 191). *Ligation* and severance of this vessel are the final steps in removal of the lobe.

Mattress sutures are placed along the wound edge of the liver. Because of the fibrous tissue in the septum, these may be tied with sufficient firmness to provide hemostasis. The *denuded area* is then further reinforced by suturing the peritoneal sheet of the *falciform ligament* in place so as to *peritonealize* the wound. The *left subdiaphragmatic space* is *drained*, in case there should be some slight leakage of bile.

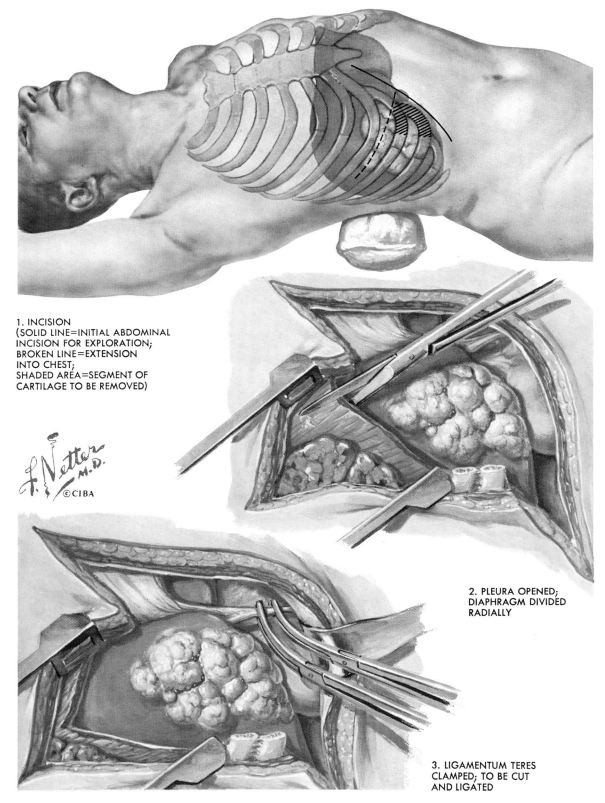

1. INCISION
(SOLID LINE=INITIAL ABDOMINAL
INCISION FOR EXPLORATION;
BROKEN LINE=EXTENSION
INTO CHEST;
SHADED AREA=SEGMENT OF
CARTILAGE TO BE REMOVED)

2. PLEURA OPENED;
DIAPHRAGM DIVIDED
RADIALLY

3. LIGAMENTUM TERES
CLAMPED; TO BE CUT
AND LIGATED

EXTENDED RIGHT LOBECTOMY

In this operation the entire right lobe is removed, along with the medial segment of the left lobe. Thus, all liver tissue to the right of the left segmental fissure is sacrificed.

From animal experiments and clinical experience, it has been found that this operation still leaves a sufficient amount of liver tissue to support metabolic needs. Moreover, it offers better control of blood loss and gives greater hope of cure than is possible with less extensive operations, the inadequacies of which have been responsible for the general pessimism as to the possibility of cure in the presence of hepatic metastasis.

Indications: Neoplasms involving only the right lobe of the liver, without evidence of regional or distal spread, should be excised in this way. These include (1) primary malignant tumors of the right lobe, regardless of size; (2) primary benign tumors, if large enough to involve the entire lobe; (3) cancers of the gallbladder; (4) metastatic cancer limited to the right lobe, if the primary cancer has previously been removed with a reasonable expectation of freedom from local recurrence.

Contraindications: These include (1) involvement of the lateral segment of the left lobe by intrahepatic spread or generalized metastasis; (2) obliterating endophlebitis of the hepatic veins; (3) involvement of vessels or biliary ducts at the porta hepatis, rendering resection technically impossible; (4) advanced cirrhosis affecting the left lobe.

Although hepatic insufficiency is often mentioned as a contraindication, an immediate improvement in liver function, which often follows ligation with shunting of blood to the intact left lobe, sometimes renders this contraindication questionable.

Technique: The patient is placed in a supine position and raised on a kidney rest, with the trunk rotated about 15 degrees to the left. A right paracostal (Marwedel) *incision* is made 2 fingerbreadths below the costal margin and extending from the left costal arch to the right midaxillary line. The various muscular layers of the *abdominal* wall are individually divided in routine fashion, exposing the peritoneum. The peritoneum is opened, allowing examination of the liver in order to determine the extent of the cancer and whether total ablation of the right lobe is both desirable and technically possible.

If it is decided that the cancerous portion of the liver is resectable, a satisfactory exposure for the operation is accomplished by opening the right *chest* through the seventh interspace, thus forming a T-shaped incision. A small wedge of the right costal arch is removed to prevent postoperative intercostal pain.

The *pleura* is *opened*, exposing the *diaphragm* from above. This, in turn, is then incised *radially* toward the inferior vena cava. A medium-sized Finochietto retractor is inserted. The *ligamentum teres* is *clamped, cut* and tied with oo silk. The visceral extremity of the ligament is used for traction to aid in the manipulation of the liver.

(Continued on page 194)

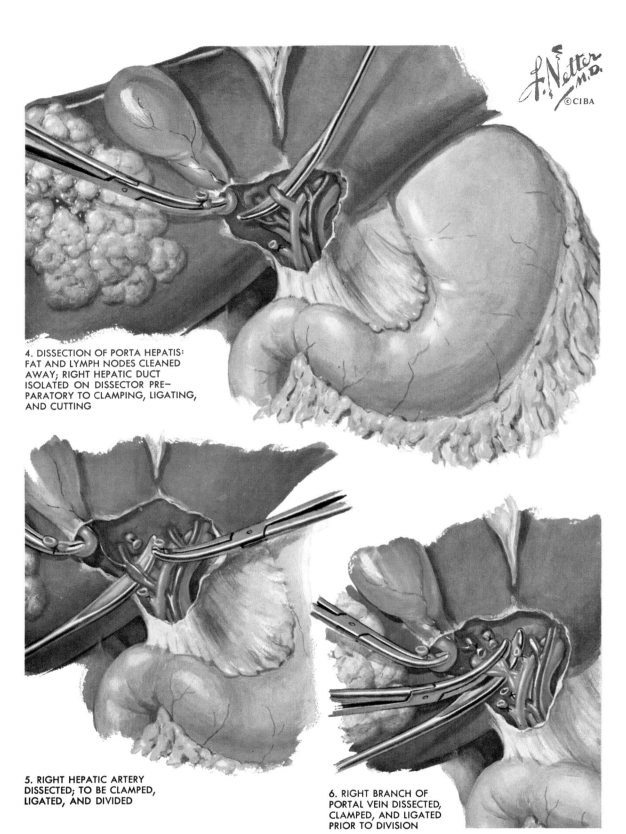

4. DISSECTION OF PORTA HEPATIS:
FAT AND LYMPH NODES CLEANED
AWAY; RIGHT HEPATIC DUCT
ISOLATED ON DISSECTOR PRE-
PARATORY TO CLAMPING, LIGATING,
AND CUTTING

5. RIGHT HEPATIC ARTERY
DISSECTED; TO BE CLAMPED,
LIGATED, AND DIVIDED

6. RIGHT BRANCH OF
PORTAL VEIN DISSECTED,
CLAMPED, AND LIGATED
PRIOR TO DIVISION

EXTENDED RIGHT LOBECTOMY

(*Continued from page 193*)

Dissection is begun at the hilus (porta hepatis) of the liver by incising the peritoneum overlying the common duct. The proper hepatic artery is identified and followed to its bifurcation into the right and left branches (rami). The cystic duct is doubly clamped and cut between the clamps, then tied with oo black silk. By using traction on the stump of the cystic duct, the portal vein is exposed. A Kocher *dissector* is inserted posterior to the *right hepatic duct,* and two Adson *clamps* are applied. The duct is then ligated and cut.

The *right hepatic artery* is exposed and handled in a similar manner. Exposure is facilitated by leaving the hemostats on the cystic duct, the right hepatic duct and the right hepatic artery.

Since anomalies may occur in the blood supply of the liver, a search should be made for any accessory right hepatic arteries (see page 16), which should be ligated if found.

The retrohepatic space is entered, exposing the inferior vena cava, which will be found in close proximity to the portal vein. The *right branch of the portal vein* is then isolated. With the aid of a Kocher dissector, a *ligature* is placed around the vessel and tied. A *clamp* is placed proximally, and the right branch of the portal vein is severed.

(*Continued on page 195*)

EXTENDED RIGHT LOBECTOMY

(Continued from page 194)

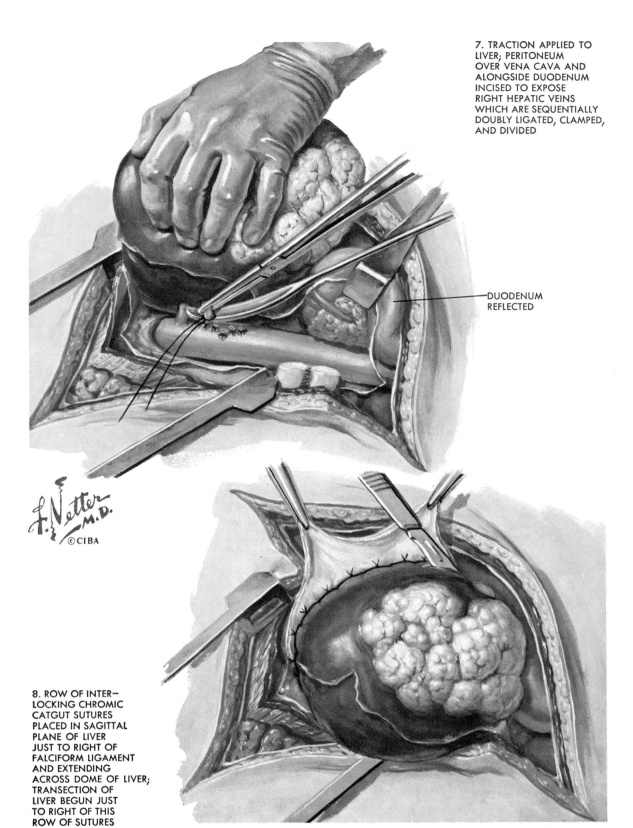

7. TRACTION APPLIED TO LIVER; PERITONEUM OVER VENA CAVA AND ALONGSIDE DUODENUM INCISED TO EXPOSE RIGHT HEPATIC VEINS WHICH ARE SEQUENTIALLY DOUBLY LIGATED, CLAMPED, AND DIVIDED

DUODENUM REFLECTED

8. ROW OF INTERLOCKING CHROMIC CATGUT SUTURES PLACED IN SAGITTAL PLANE OF LIVER JUST TO RIGHT OF FALCIFORM LIGAMENT AND EXTENDING ACROSS DOME OF LIVER; TRANSECTION OF LIVER BEGUN JUST TO RIGHT OF THIS ROW OF SUTURES

The assistant now rotates the right lobe of the liver to the patient's left, assisted by traction on the round ligament. The *peritoneum overlying* the *vena cava is incised to expose the right hepatic veins.* The liver is now retracted caudad and detached from the surface of the diaphragm for additional exposure. The first right hepatic vein encountered is mobilized with a Kocher dissector. It is *doubly* tied in continuity, on the vena caval side,

with oo black silk. An Adson *clamp* is placed on the hepatic side of the vein, which is then carefully *cut* between the *clamp* and the *ligature.* Three or more other right hepatic veins are treated in the same manner.

At this stage of the procedure, one must use extreme care to preserve the hepatic vein of the left lobe.

After ligation of all right hepatic veins, the right lobe of the liver will be completely deprived of its extrahepatic blood supply. Any additional bleeding will come from the left lobe.

A double *row* of *interlocking* No. 1 *chromic catgut*

sutures, on atraumatic liver needles, is *placed* in the *sagittal plane just to the right of the falciform ligament.* These interlocking sutures are tied with surgeon's knots. This row of sutures is continued *across the dome* of the *liver.* Separation of the two lobes, with a scalpel, is now begun. As the dissection is carried deeper into the liver substance, additional sutures are placed across the larger vessels and bile ducts. This technique allows only minimal blood loss during the dissection of the liver parenchyma.

(Continued on page 196)

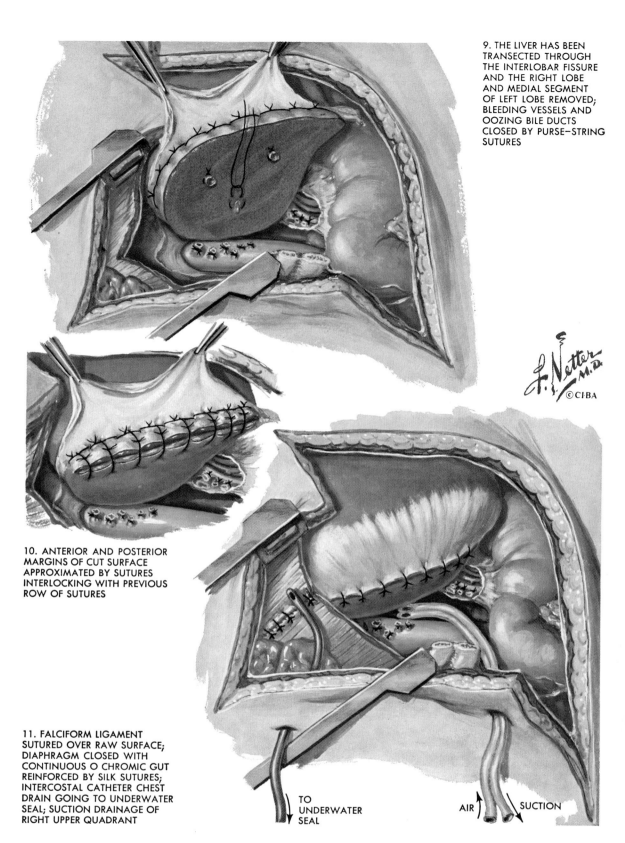

9. THE LIVER HAS BEEN TRANSECTED THROUGH THE INTERLOBAR FISSURE AND THE RIGHT LOBE AND MEDIAL SEGMENT OF LEFT LOBE REMOVED; BLEEDING VESSELS AND OOZING BILE DUCTS CLOSED BY PURSE-STRING SUTURES

EXTENDED RIGHT LOBECTOMY

(*Continued from page 195*)

10. ANTERIOR AND POSTERIOR MARGINS OF CUT SURFACE APPROXIMATED BY SUTURES INTERLOCKING WITH PREVIOUS ROW OF SUTURES

11. FALCIFORM LIGAMENT SUTURED OVER RAW SURFACE; DIAPHRAGM CLOSED WITH CONTINUOUS O CHROMIC GUT REINFORCED BY SILK SUTURES; INTERCOSTAL CATHETER CHEST DRAIN GOING TO UNDERWATER SEAL; SUCTION DRAINAGE OF RIGHT UPPER QUADRANT

TO UNDERWATER SEAL

AIR   SUCTION

At this point the right lobe is completely mobilized and removed. *Sutures are now placed so as to interlock with the previous layer,* thus *approximating the anterior and posterior surfaces* of the left lobe. These sutures are cut. The left lobe will be found to be engorged, with rounded edges, because this remaining 20 per cent of the liver is now receiving the entire portal venous and hepatic arterial blood supply.

The *falciform ligament* is now *sutured over the raw surface,* to decrease the possibility of biliary fistula. The *diaphragm* is *closed with continuous* o *chromic catgut* sutures and reinforced with oo black silk. These reinforcing sutures are then cut closely.

A stab wound is made, and an *intercostal catheter* is inserted in the eighth interspace in the midaxillary line. This is connected to an *underwater seal.* The chest wall is approximated with a Bailey rib approxi-

mator, and the intercostal muscles are closed with interrupted sutures of oo black silk. The right pleural cavity is sealed by joining the cut edge of the diaphragm to the intercostal muscles. The *right upper quadrant* is *drained* through a separate stab wound, and the peritoneum is closed. The abdominal wall is closed, in layers, with oo black silk; the skin is closed with interrupted sutures. The junction of the abdominal and thoracic incision is reinforced with stay sutures.

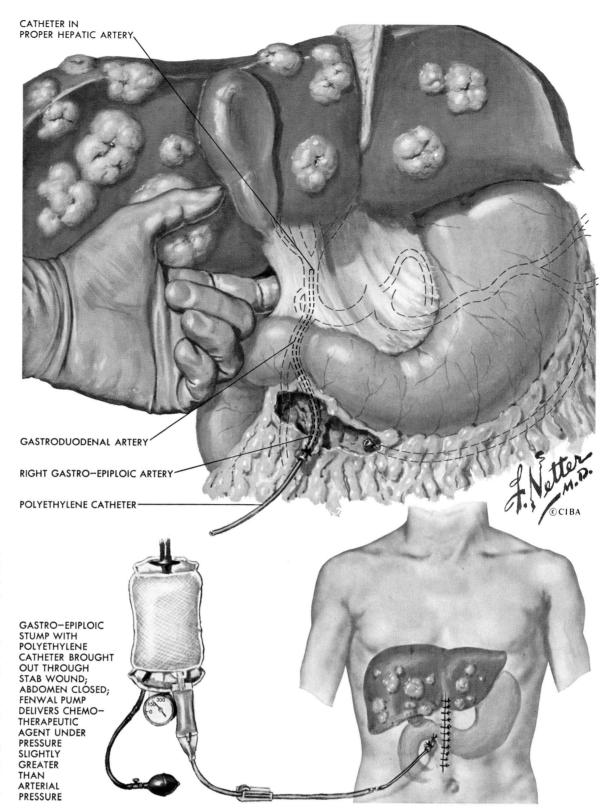

CATHETER IN
PROPER HEPATIC ARTERY

GASTRODUODENAL ARTERY

RIGHT GASTRO-EPIPLOIC ARTERY

POLYETHYLENE CATHETER

GASTRO-EPIPLOIC
STUMP WITH
POLYETHYLENE
CATHETER BROUGHT
OUT THROUGH
STAB WOUND;
ABDOMEN CLOSED;
FENWAL PUMP
DELIVERS CHEMO-
THERAPEUTIC
AGENT UNDER
PRESSURE
SLIGHTLY
GREATER
THAN
ARTERIAL
PRESSURE

Palliative Therapy in Inoperable Cases

Infusion of Chemotherapeutic Agents

Because cancers of the liver, both primary and metastatic, receive their blood supply through the arterial system, palliative chemotherapy has been given by way of the hepatic artery. At laparotomy, the *right gastro-epiploic artery* is isolated from the stomach and severed; the proximal end is intubated with a tiny *polyethylene catheter* which is guided upward into the proper hepatic artery. This vascular pedicle is withdrawn from the abdomen through a *stab wound* so that, at the completion of the infusion, the tube is withdrawn and the artery is ligated at the skin level, thus avoiding internal hemorrhage as well as the necessity of a secondary laparotomy. The heparinized polyethylene catheter is connected either with a *Fenwall* pressure infusion apparatus or with a Sigma finger pump, whereby the fluid is forced, drop by drop, into the artery by a *pressure greater than* the patient's own *arterial pressure*. Methotrexate® is the drug commonly employed, 50 mg in 1 liter of 5 per cent glucose in distilled water being infused slowly and continuously the first day. Then 10 to 20 mg are given daily. A total dose of 150 mg can be given in this way with comparative safety. At the same time, the patient receives the citrovorum factor* intramuscularly, every 6 hours, in order to

*A dietary element found necessary for the growth of Leuconostoc citrovorum.

diminish the toxic effect of Methotrexate® on the bone marrow. In inoperable cases some palliation has thus been achieved.

Infusion of Radioactive Ceramic Microspheres

Radioactive yttrium[90] has been incorporated, in aliquot parts, in tiny ceramic microspheres measuring 60 microns in diameter. These ceramic particles, being too large to pass through the capillary bed of the liver, become incarcerated there and emit radiation throughout the duration of their activity. For the treatment of metastases diffusely disseminated throughout the liver, a dose of 50 to 100 millicuries can be given safely through the hepatic artery. Some

patients have experienced appreciable palliation, whereas others have had no relief.

Infusion of Radioactive (I[131]) Rose Bengal

The concentration and excretion of radioactive (I[131]) rose bengal for photoscanning of the liver has already been described (pages 45 and 176). Most patients with bile duct cancer manifest evidence of biliary obstruction and increased retention of administered radioactive rose bengal, sometimes for 7 to 30 days compared with less than 24 hours in the normal individual. An intravenous injection of 10 to 20 millicuries, repeated as signs and symptoms warrant, over a period of 3 to 12 weeks, has resulted in some degree of palliation in 64 per cent of the patients treated.

REFERENCES

PACK, G. T., AND ISLAMI: *Surgical Treatment of Tumors of the Liver;* page 380 in *Treatment of Cancer and Allied Diseases, Volume V,* Pack, G. T., and Ariel, eds., Hoeber Medical Division, Harper and Row, Publishers, New York, 1962.

PACK, G. T., AND ISLAMI: *Operative Treatment of Hepatic Tumors,* Clinical Symposia, 16:38, 1964.

SUBJECT INDEX

(For Plates 13 Through 21 of Supplement)

(Numerals refer to pages, *not* plates)

GLOSSARY

In the preface to this revised edition, it was stated that most anatomical terms were made to conform to the *Nomina Anatomica* of 1961. To have made changes in every instance would have involved very expensive modifications of certain plates and some text materials, especially when the latter required the insertion or deletion of one or more words. In such instances, as a rule, in the text preceding or following the change, a resetting of all type for the sentence, paragraph, column or entire page, as the case demanded, would have been necessary. Therefore, editorial judgment was exercised with reference to frugality as well as to accuracy and clarity. In addition, this inconsistency permits a more gradual transition from the old to the new terminology, *e.g., celiac trunk* for *celiac artery, left gastric vein* for *coronary vein, suprarenal* for *adrenal,* etc. The reader's attention is directed particularly to the following:

New Term	Old Term
Anterior vagal trunk[1]	Left vagus nerve[1]
Area nuda (bare area)	— —
Atrium	Auricle — old clinical term
Celiac nodes (in part)	Right suprapancreatic nodes
Celiac trunk	Celiac artery
Fissure for ligamentum teres	Fossa for umbilical vein = fetal ligamentum teres = adult
Fissure for ligamentum venosum	Fossa for ductus venosus = fetal ligamentum venosum = adult
Gallbladder fossa	Gallbladder bed
Hepatogastric ligament	Gastrohepatic ligament
Hepatorenal recess	Right inferior infrahepatic space
Inferior margin (of liver)	Anterior margin (of liver)
Inferior rectal veins	Inferior hemorrhoidal veins
Internal iliac artery	Hypogastric artery
Left gastric nodes	Superior gastric nodes
Left gastric vein	Coronary vein
Left inferior anterior subhepatic recess	Left inferior anterior infrahepatic space
Left inferior posterior subhepatic recess (omental bursa)	Left inferior posterior infrahepatic space
Left ramus of hepatic artery proper	Left hepatic artery
Left superior subphrenic recess	Left superior suprahepatic space
Major papilla (of Vater)	Papilla (of Vater)
Mesenteric nodes	Transverse mesocolic nodes
	Superior mesenteric nodes
Middle rectal veins	Middle hemorrhoidal veins
Muscular layer (of gallbladder)	Fibromuscular layer (of gallbladder)
— —	Neck of pancreas[2]
Pancreaticolienal nodes	Left suprapancreatic nodes
Pars anterior of diaphragmatic surface of liver	Anterior surface of liver
Pars dextra of diaphragmatic surface of liver	Right lateral surface of liver
Pars posterior of diaphragmatic surface of liver	Posterior surface of liver
Pars superior of diaphragmatic surface of liver	Superior surface of liver
Perivascular fibrous capsule	Glisson's capsule
Posterior vagal trunk[1]	Right vagus nerve[1]
Pyloric nodes	Superior pancreatic nodes
Rami pancreatici	Splenic artery branches
Right gastric vein	Pyloric vein
Right ramus of hepatic artery proper	Right hepatic artery
Right superior anterior subphrenic recess	Right superior anterior suprahepatic space
Right superior posterior subphrenic recess	Right superior posterior suprahepatic space
Spiral fold (of Heister)	Spiral valve (of Heister)
Sulcus for interior vena cava	Fossa for inferior vena cava
Superior rectal veins	Superior hemorrhoidal veins
Suprarenal gland	Adrenal gland
Suprarenal impression	Adrenal impression
Uncinate process (of pancreas)	Pancreatic lingula
Visceral surface (of liver)	Inferior surface

1. Vagus nerves become vagal trunks at the esophageal plexus.
2. Neck (of pancreas) is no longer an official N.A. term.

INFORMATION ON CIBA COLLECTION VOLUMES

Since publication of its first volume, THE CIBA COLLECTION OF MEDICAL ILLUSTRATIONS has enjoyed an almost "unheard-of" reception from members of the medical community. The remarkable illustrations by Frank H. Netter, M.D. and text discussions by select specialists make these books unprecedented in their educational, clinical, and scientific value.

In the United States, copies of all CIBA COLLECTION books may be purchased from the Medical Education Division, CIBA Pharmaceutical Company, Division of CIBA-GEIGY Corporation, Summit, New Jersey 07901. In other countries, please direct inquiries to the nearest CIBA-GEIGY office.